History of Nursing Source Book

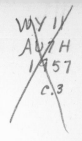

History of Nursing
Source Book

By ANNE L. AUSTIN, R.N., B.S., A.M.

FORMERLY PROFESSOR OF NURSING
WESTERN RESERVE UNIVERSITY
CLEVELAND, OHIO

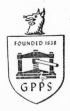

G. P. Putnam's Sons   New York

To

my teacher, Isabel Maitland Stewart

and to

my students everywhere

Preface

THIS book is an outgrowth of a conviction that the study of nursing history can most effectively be undertaken when the student has access to the writings of those who made the history, or were very close to them in point of time. It is an attempt to bring together for the student and the teacher, without the intrusion of too much interpretation of the contents on the part of the compiler, some of the literature in English which comprises or illustrates the history of nursing, and which serves to correlate general history with nursing history to the end that the relation of the latter to the former may be better understood.

A large proportion of the literature of nursing history, particularly of the early periods, may be consulted only in the most extensive libraries, and in many cases is not even then available to the nursing student. This may be because it is rare or because it exists in bulky volumes on other subjects, of which it forms only a small part. Later secondhand sources are, of course, valuable, but they do not take the place of the words of those who witnessed or participated in the events, or lived at a period close to that in which the events were happening.

The values to be obtained from consultation of early sources for the study of history may be briefly stated. Sigerist, the eminent historian, says of medical history, "By analyzing developments and trends it permits us to understand a situation more clearly and to act more intelligently. We all know that success or failure of our medical work depends not only on the scientific knowledge we possess but also on a great variety of other nonmedical factors, on economic, social, religious, philosophical, political factors that are the result of historical developments. Unless we are aware of them and understand them many of our efforts will be wasted." *

Direct contact with the actual words of those who took part in the

* Henry E. Sigerist, "The Need for an Institute of the History of Medicine in India," *Bulletin of the History of Medicine,* February, 1945, pp. 113–116.

events being studied has the power to evoke a strong sense of reality, as well as to make a deep and lasting impression not always created by a secondhand account. Those who were eyewitnesses or participants have much to teach us, if we listen to them judiciously. We read them to gain not only a feeling of the times but also the facts recorded at the time, albeit with human bias but without the intrusion of the interpretation of others which may throw shadows on them or detract from their charm. The language of the old records, according to today's standards, is often simple and monotonous but, for this reason, has the ability to recreate for us an illusion of the times in which the events took place, and thus to recreate reality. The extent to which it is possible for the reader to enter into the spirit of the times of which the narrator writes will somewhat determine his degree of understanding of the present. Such an approach to historical study coupled with modern research (which, although viewing the events from a greater distance utilizes more exact methods) holds promise of a greater understanding of present-day nursing conditions.

In this book use has been made of primary and secondary sources, both early and more recent, in prose and in poetry. An attempt has been made to include excerpts from the most significant writings comprising the history of nursing from the era before the birth of Christ up to the founding of the first professional school of nursing in America in 1873. Chronology forms a convenient and necessary framework for historical events, and the arrangement is mainly chronological, although an attempt has also been made to follow the development of movements and trends. Since it is intended that the book shall be used in conjunction with one or more of the existing textbooks on the subject, this is not a narrative history. The actual items selected represent some of the sources which are adjudged enlightening, although not of equal value, for a study of this nature. The selection has been influenced by many factors, among which were the plenitude of sources on some subjects and the paucity of them on others, and the accessibility of the sources to the compiler, together with the feasibility of their use. It is hoped that this effort, which is regarded as a beginning only, will lead to other and similar ones.

In presenting the sources themselves, an attempt has been made to preserve the writer's meaning, insofar as it was understood and to the extent to which it was thought possible. The materials presented are direct quotations as they were found in the literature. Since some of the quotations were, of practical necessity, secured from secondary sources, the writers of which had in turn quoted, translated, or paraphrased them, changes may have occurred in the wording or spelling before the present compiler obtained them. In utilizing these, however, the exact wording of the source consulted has been preserved. Attention is called in this connection to the preservation of the punctuation (or lack of it), and the ancient spelling. Examples of the latter are: "hear" for "here"; "yt" for "that"; "then" for "than"; "of" for "off"; and "pat" for "that."

A further word of explanation needs to be said concerning the limitations of the book. It is realized that, traditionally, the books on history of nursing have dealt not only with nursing itself but also with related fields, such as the fields of medicine and social work. This is particularly true of the earliest periods before the emergence of nursing as a distinct vocation in human society. It has been thought that this book would be more useful to the student and the teacher if it utilized chiefly the more distinctly nursing elements of the history. With reference to the period covered, it has been deemed advisable to carry it only to the time of the founding of the first schools of nursing in America. The reasons for this include such considerations as the fact that after that time, the literature is large, making selection difficult and impracticable; that literature concerning nursing from that time on to the present is available in the majority of nursing or general libraries, or if not now available may be made so with a minimum of effort and expense; and that many of the early documents of American nursing history have recently been made accessible by the National League of Nursing Education and by interested publishers of nursing books.

The plan of organization has been designed to give wide representation to the various phases of nursing history. The chapter headings reflect the literary approach to the history rather than the narration of historical events and, in general, follow the chronological pattern often found in books on history. The latter framework is associated with the developments in nursing history as they are usually conceived. It is hoped that this plan will aid teachers and students in utilizing the source book in conjunction with the textbooks in use in nursing schools.

The plan followed in the separate chapters is as follows: first, an introduction consisting of a short outline of the historical period covered, together with a brief statement of the sources to be used; second, a presentation of the sources themselves; and third, a brief concluding statement which highlights the significance of the readings and forms a bridge between chapters. The readings are preceded by short historical notes giving a few biographical details concerning the writer, comments on the book or article, and notes on the quotation from the writings.

The appendix is comprised of two documents expressive of the growing concern of the medical profession and the public concerning the preparation of qualified persons for the care of the sick.

The notes referred to by superior figures in the text are placed, by

9

chapters, in the section following the appendix. It is hoped that this will be more helpful to the reader than placing them at the bottoms of the text pages. The notes are, in the main, documentation of sources, and are given in abbreviated form. The complete citations of the references are given in the bibliography. A complete bibliography on the subject of the source book would be very extensive; therefore the one included here consists only of the works used.

The index has been compiled to conform to the requirements of the large number of topics touched on in the book, and to act as a list of the readings included.

The source book has been designed to be used in the programs in nursing leading to a diploma, where a short course in history of nursing may be given in the first year, as well as in those leading to baccalaureate or higher degrees, in which the trend is toward giving this course in the last year. The materials in the book may also be utilized by senior students or graduate nurses who are investigating some aspect of nursing as a research project. It is intended that the book should be used in conjunction with other histories of nursing and with the publications of the National League for Nursing and its predecessors which bear on the evolution of the profession of nursing.

In the diploma programs the study may proceed in chronological order, selections from the source book being made to highlight the main topics and to add interest to the textbook being used. The teacher will find it possible to select from the readings for this purpose. Three examples follow: for a study of "Nursing in India," Reading No. 4, *Charaka-Samhita,* and Reading No. 5, *Sushruta Samhita;* for the "Reform of Nursing in England in the First Half of the Nineteenth Century," Readings Nos. 176, Lionel S. Beale, "Nursing the Sick in Hospitals, Private Families, and Among the Poor," *Medical Times and Gazette,* December 6, 1875, pp. 630-632, and 180, *Memoirs of the Life of Elizabeth Fry;* for "Early Nursing in Canada," No. 421, *The Jesuit Relations and Allied Documents,* and No. 247, John Knox, *An Historical Journal of the Campaigns in North America.*

For the more mature student the study may proceed in the usual way, or more unconventionally, and perhaps more realistically, by beginning with the present. Chronological continuity may be provided by lectures by the teacher and by group discussions placed at strategic intervals, as the course progresses and as the interest and knowledge of the student warrant it. Interests, both large and small, may be pursued in this way, utilizing the readings. The development of such major aspects of nursing history as the following, may be studied: "Evolution of Organized Nursing in the Home," Readings Nos. 21, 72 (latter part), 84, 97, 132, 133,

145, 165, 183, 227, 228 (last part), 235, 236, 237, 258; "Chief Characteristics of the Nightingale System of Nursing and Nursing Education," as described by Miss Nightingale herself, Readings Nos. 218, 219, 228; as described by two Nightingale probationers, Readings Nos. 216, 217.

It is hoped also that senior students and graduate nurses in degree programs will find the readings, biographical and literary notes and the bibliography helpful in research in history of nursing, not only in themselves, but also as a means of leading them to investigate other important and valuable materials not found in the source book itself. The following interests might be pursued, using the readings: "Hospital Administration," "Qualifications of the Nurse," "Economic Status of Nurses," et cetera.

It is the hope of the compiler that the source book may stimulate readers to further exploration of the richness of the subject, and may amplify and extend the horizons of nursing history of the student and the teacher.

Anne L. Austin.

North Hollywood, California.

Acknowledgments

MANY people have contributed to the production of this book. The indebtedness of the writer to books and periodicals is obvious from the contents, and acknowledgment is made in the proper places. That to people is more intangible in many instances, but none the less real and substantial. The thanks of the writer are rendered with grateful appreciation to all of them, whether or not it has been possible to mention them by name.

Anyone attempting the production of a book on the history of nursing is forever indebted to Mary Adelaide Nutting and Lavinia Lloyd Dock. Not only did they themselves utilize source materials extensively, but their research and its scholarly result came at a time when nursing was but beginning to emerge as a profession. Their work therefore, at an early date, set a high standard in historical writing in nursing.

Not the least among those to whom the present writer owes a word of sincere thanks are those to whom the book is dedicated, "To my teacher, Isabel Maitland Stewart, and to my students everywhere." To the former, the writer owes thanks for her first insight into history of nursing as an important part of the education of the nurse, and for continued encouragement in various ways; and to the latter, appreciation of the inspiration coming from the interest of both basic and advanced professional nursing students in enriching their backgrounds through a knowledge of the history of their vocation.

It is a privilege to record here a special word of grateful recognition to two who have contributed outstandingly, though in different ways, to the writing of the book:

To Edell F. Little, Executive Director of the Visiting Nurse Association of Los Angeles, for encouragement and understanding, for helpful suggestions, and for assistance at all stages of the work; and to Dr. Genevieve K. Bixler, Head, Nursing Education Project, Southern Regional Education Board, and Chairman, Editorial Board of The

13

Acknowledgments

Modern Nursing Series of G. P. Putnam's Sons, for a critical reading of the manuscript, for valuable suggestions, and for conspicuous assistance in the preparation and publication of the manuscript.

It is a pleasure to say a special word of thanks to Mrs. Geraldine Mink, Librarian of the School of Nursing, Western Reserve University, who contributed much by her consistently prompt, accurate, complete, and cheerful responses to many requests. The library itself, with its rich resources in history of nursing, was at all times at the disposal of the writer.

Thanks are also given to Associate Professor Margaret S. Taylor, of the School of Nursing, University of California at Los Angeles, for assistance in obtaining certain reference materials.

Sister Rosarita, Secretary General and Archivist, Sisters of Charity, Mount St. Joseph, Ohio, was of the greatest help in the research on the Sisters of Charity.

Dorothy Schullian, Curator of Rare Books, History of Medicine Division of the Armed Forces Medical Library, Cleveland, Ohio, kindly assisted in the transcription of the bill rendered by David Field for nursing soldiers in the French and Indian Wars.

Irwin Stein of the History Division of the Los Angeles Public Library, and Henriette Callot, were helpful in translating important passages in the sources. Specific annotations of these will be found in the notes.

Librarians of several libraries contributed more than could reasonably be expected of them. Of particular assistance were the staffs of the Library of Western Reserve University; the Cleveland Public Library, especially the John G. White Collection; the Los Angeles Public Library, in particular the History Division; the Library of the University of California at Los Angeles, including the William Andrews Clark Library; the Library of the University of Southern California; the History of Medicine Division of the U.S. Armed Forces Medical Library; the Cleveland Medical Library Association; and the Henry E. Huntington Library.

In addition, thanks are given to the following libraries which assisted in many ways: Library of Congress, Library of Dr. Elmer Belt; Buffalo Public Library; University of California at Berkeley; Chicago Public Library; University of Chicago; John Crerar Library; College of Mount Saint Mary, Los Angeles; Grosvernor Library; Los Angeles County Medical Association; San Francisco College for Women; and the Western Reserve Historical Society.

Other libraries which loaned materials are: Brown University; Duke University; University of Illinois; Loyola University, Los Angeles; Oberlin College; Yale University; Xavier University, Cincinnati; Ameri-

14

can Antiquarian Society; Library Company of Philadelphia; Newberry Library; and U.S. National War College.

Grateful acknowledgment is made to the following individuals and organizations for the use of manuscripts in their possession, specific details of which are given in the bibliography: Armed Forces Medical Library, History of Medicine Division; Virginia M. Dunbar, Dean, Cornell University–New York Hospital School of Nursing; Ladies Benevolent Society; Library of Congress; School of Nursing, Western Reserve University; and Sisters of Charity of Mount St. Joseph, Ohio.

It is a pleasure also to thank the following publishers for granting permission to quote from their publications, specific information concerning which is given in the bibliography: Academia Nacional de Medicina de México; Alumnae Association of the St. Luke's Hospital School of Nursing, New York; *Annals of Medical History;* Edward Arnold (Publishers) Ltd.; J. W. Arrowsmith, Ltd.; Beaver Printing Company; *Bulletin of the History of Medicine;* Burns, Oates & Washburne, Ltd.; Cambridge University Press; Catholic University of America; Champlain Society; Chatto & Windus; Columbia University Press; J. M. Dent & Sons, Ltd.; The Dolphin Press; Doubleday & Company, Inc.; E. P. Dutton & Co., Inc.; Harvard University Press; William Heinemann, Ltd.; Hodder & Stoughton, Ltd.; Paul B. Hoeber, Inc.; Houghton Mifflin Company; Henry E. Huntington Library; International Council of Nurses; *Journal of the American Medical Association;* P. J. Kenedy & Sons; Alfred A. Knopf, Inc.; John Lane, The Bodley Head, Ltd.; Longmans, Green & Co., Inc.; Longmans, Green & Co., Ltd.; *Louisiana Historical Quarterly;* The Macmillan Company, New York; Methuen & Co., Ltd.; Minnesota Historical Society; John Murray (Publishers) Ltd.; North Carolina State Department of Archives and History; Pennsylvania Historical and Museum Commission; Princeton University Press; Remington Putnam Book Company; Routledge and Kegan Paul, Ltd.; Ryerson Press; St. Martin's Press, Inc.; Charles Scribner's Sons; Society for Promoting Christian Knowledge; University of Chicago Press; University of Pennsylvania Press; and *The Yale Review.*

Anne L. Austin.

North Hollywood, California.

Editorial Introduction

IN keeping with its policy of providing through the *Modern Nursing Series* books having broad scope and the present day approach to nursing, the latest of the series is here being introduced to the reading public. The book entitled *History of Nursing Source Book* by Anne L. Austin represents to an unusual degree the application of modern systematic study to the accumulations of the remote and near past as these affect modern nursing.

As nursing makes progress toward professional stature it is concerned about the ways in which the past has contributed to the present, not alone for the understanding of the present in nursing but also for the appreciation of the elements of man's slow advance in the conservation of human resources, the Christian ethic of the value of the individual. Nursing history lives in the excerpts and fragments of earlier times which reveal practices of nursing and healing in the broad setting of the early and mediaeval Christian Church, and in the colonial period of American history, and the history of its wars, to mention some of the outstanding periods covered.

The compiler has made an essentially literary approach to her task, for she has, first, selected much new material, including many primary sources which give the reader direct contact with the accounts of eye witnesses; second, she has organized and interpreted the materials in such a way as to relate all to the on-going stream of history; and, third, she has availed herself of the methods of documentation and indexing most accepted in sound modern historical research. These methods will prove invaluable to the research worker in the history of nursing for they will facilitate the tracking down of clues from one source to others, so essential in historical research.

The book provides in its Preface and elsewhere several practical suggestions for use which are beyond and beside the traditional uses of historical materials in nursing. As indicated, its use can be extended into

17

Editorial Introduction

graduate study and research in the history of nursing, for it identifies issues, and raises questions for which no answers are provided. To deal with some of these it will be helpful to plan for seminars and to assist in the organization of systematic study, both of which constitute education on a high intellectual level. If this presupposes in the teacher marked competence in educational method as well as knowledge and appreciation of history (including nursing history), this is no more than is being expected of today's teachers of history in secondary and higher education, and is only another challenge to nursing to measure up to the demands and the standards of the times.

To speak of the value of this compilation for students of nursing on advanced levels is not to say it has limited possibilities for others. From the compiler's considerable experience in teaching history of nursing to students in both basic and advanced programs it can be stated that the Source Book has great potentiality for the young basic nursing student with limited library facilities. In fact, it seems much more likely to awaken interest than does the traditional approach to history of nursing. A third extension of use seems likely to be the scrutiny of persons who are not concerned primarily with nursing education. Such persons will use the book as an example of good organization in a professional field with which they are relatively unfamiliar, and its acquaintance will enable them to understand better the contribution nursing has made to the well being of mankind.

The Editorial Board of the *Modern Nursing Series* takes great pleasure in introducing this scholarly work to educators everywhere.

Genevieve K. Bixler
Chairman

Contents

Contents

PART III

*Some Sources for the Study of Nursing
in the Western Hemisphere Before 1873*

APPENDIX

PART I

Some Sources for the Study of Nursing in the Old World Before 1860

Chapter 1

The Nurse in the Literature
of Early Civilizations

INTRODUCTION

THE beginnings of nursing are unknown to us. They lie in a time of which no written records exist. For a true understanding of the evolution of nursing, it would be desirable to search not only the written history of the past but also the obscurity of prehistory. The folkways and mores of preliterate peoples without doubt included certain customary ways of nursing the sick. In order to reconstruct them it would be necessary to find means of learning of the life of primitive man, but since by definition he is "preliterate," this has been difficult to accomplish except by deductions from studies of contemporary groups.

In spite of the importance of preliterate nursing, for the purposes of this book the study will begin with early civilizations, since some of these left a literature. For information concerning their care of the sick, it is necessary to turn to religious and medical manuscripts, secular prose and poetry, letters, legal codes, official archives, inscriptions on temples, tombs, and monuments, votive tablets, and remains of buildings and public works. While an examination of these is rewarding with reference to the healing art and sanitation, showing that these peoples felt a greater or lesser degree of concern for the maintenance of health and the care of the sick, it yields little concerning the art of nursing as it is understood today. This may be because the nursing of the sick took place in the home, as part of the everyday life of the women of the family, and was therefore not noteworthy. Nurses are mentioned in some literatures, but with one possible exception, that of India, they are obviously not the ancestors of the modern professional nurse. They are, rather, children's nurses or nursemaids, or wet nurses. However, if nursing is interpreted in its broadest sense as health conservation as well as therapeutic care of the sick, these women may be regarded as nurses.

The quotations which follow illustrate the relative scarcity of definite

23

information concerning nurses and nursing in these groups. They do, however, give inklings of the existence of children's nurses and wet nurses.

In this chapter, selections have been made from among a larger number, where reference to nurses is to be found. The Babylonian literature yields the account of the creation, in which there is mention of a child's nurse (1).* The Hebrew literature includes the query of Pharaoh's sister from the Old Testament concerning the nursing of the infant Moses by a wet nurse (2); and passages from the *Talmud,* from which one is chosen which gives the remedy for a scorpion's sting, as told by a nurse (3).

From the medical writings of India comes the only reference to attendants of the sick in the modern sense. The treatises of Charaka (4) and of Sushruta (5) mention the nurse and describe his relation to the physician. These also specify the qualifications of the nurse, who, in these instances, was a man.

Greek literature contains many allusions to nurses; these, however, are children's nurses, and not primarily attendants of the sick. Selections are made from these for presentation in this chapter. *The Iliad* and *The Odyssey* mention nurses (6). Other Greek nurses are alluded to in *The Idylls of Theocritus* (7) and in *Plutarch's Lives* (8). That children's nurses were a definite part of Greek society is also attested to by Plato, who speaks of them in his treatise on *Laws* (9). Xenophon, in *Oeconomicus,* indicates that wives of Greek estate owners assumed the care of their servants when ill (10). Certain nursing procedures, such as bandaging and baths, are described in detail in the writings of Hippocrates, while in the same source the medical student is represented as carrying out some of the functions of the present-day nurse (11).

Among the Roman writers, three which refer to nurses or nursing are quoted here. In Vitruvius' *On Architecture,* in the legend of the origin of the Corinthian capital, a nurse figures in a small way (12); Pliny, in his *Letters,* asks a friend to care for the farm which Pliny had given his nurse (13); and Celsus, in *De Medicina,* describes the use of cupping (a procedure remembered by older present-day nurses) in the treatment of a patient (14).

References to nursing in English from the literature of northern Europe are relatively rare. Included here is one from *The Ancient Laws of Ireland,* alluding indirectly to a nurse, in detailing the allowances of food and other payments which were prescribed by law (15).

* Figures in parentheses refer to the numbers of the readings.

THE SOURCES

1. *The Babylonian Genesis*

[This epic, the Babylonian story of the Creation, was recorded on seven clay tablets. Parts of it were discovered by Layard between 1848 and 1876, among the ruins of King Ashurbanipal's library; others were found at later dates. It was probably composed about 1000 B.C., or even earlier.[1]]

> Ea (and Damkina, his wife, dwelt therein) in splendor.
> In the chamber of fates, the abode of destinies,
> The most skilful, the wisest of gods [was begotten (?)].
> Within the Apsu Marduk was born,
> Within the holy Apsu [Marduk] was born.
> He who begot him was [Ea], his father;
> Damkina, his mother, was she who bore him;
> He sucked the breast of goddesses;
> The nurse who cared for him filled (him) with
>   awe-inspiring majesty![2] *

2. The Old Testament. Exodus, 2:7–9 (King James Version)

[This passage is taken from the story of Moses' childhood. It is assumed that a wet nurse is meant here.]

Then said his sister to Pharaoh's daughter, Shall I go and call to thee a nurse of the Hebrew women, that she may nurse the child for thee?

And Pharaoh's daughter said to her, Go. And the maid went and called the child's mother.

And Pharaoh's daughter said unto her, Take this child away, and nurse it for me, and I will give thee thy wages. And the woman took the child, and nursed it.

3. *The Talmud.* Kethuboth, 50a

[According to the *Encyclopaedia Britannica,*[3] the *Talmud* is the Hebrew codification of the law, which grew up during the first four centuries of the Christian Era. It is a systematic compilation of already-existing law, and contains innumerable references to health and disease.]

Abaye stated, Nurse [from whom he learned many proverbs and maxims, legends and folklore] told me: A child of the age of six whom a scorpion has bitten on the day on which he has completed his sixth year does not

---

* Reprinted from *The Babylonian Genesis* by Alexander Heidel, by permission of The University of Chicago Press. Copyright, 1942, by the University of Chicago.

survive [as a rule]. What is his remedy?—The gall of a white stork in beer. This should be rubbed into the wound [and the patient] be made to drink it. A child of the age of one year whom a bee has stung on the day he has completed his first year does not survive [as a rule]. What is his remedy?— The creepers of a palm-tree in water. This should be rubbed in and [the patient] be made to drink it.[4]

4. *Charaka-Samhita*

[The *Charaka-Samhita* is a treatise on medicine by Charaka, an Indian physician. The date is uncertain, some authorities placing it as early as between 800 and 600 B.C.,[5] while others assign Charaka to the first century of our era.[6] In all likelihood the latter date is more accurate. The meaning of the word *Samhita* is "collection."]

Part IV. Lesson IX.

And now we shall explain the Lesson called the Brief Aggregate of Four. Thus said the illustrious son of Atri.

The Physician, Drugs, Nurse, and Patient, constitute an aggregate of four. Of what virtues each of these should be possessed so as to become causes for the cure of disease should be known.

The absence of harmony in respect to the ingredient humours (of the body) is Disease; while their harmony constitutes our normal condition. Health, again, is otherwise called Happiness; while Disease is Sorrow or Misery. In Disease, the well-known tale of four commencing with Physician has active agency. The course that is adopted for restoring the harmony of the ingredient humours is called Treatment.

A thorough mastery of the Scriptures (bearing on the science of life), large experience (of actual results), cleverness, and purity (of both mind and body), are regarded as the four (principal) qualifications of the Physician.

Abundance of virtue, adaptability to the disease under treatment, capacity of being used in diverse ways, and undeterioration numbering the fourth, are the attributes of Drugs.

Knowledge of the manner in which drugs should be prepared or compounded for administration, cleverness, devotedness to the patient waited upon, and purity (of both mind and body) are the four qualifications of the attending Nurse.

Memory, obedience to directions (given by the Physician), fearlessness, and communicativeness (with respect to all that is experienced internally and all that is done by him during the intervals of the Physician's visit), are the qualifications of the Patient.

If this tale of four be possessed of these sixteen qualifications then does it constitute the cause for the achievement of success (in Treatment). The Physician, in this aggregate of four, is the chief cause (for the achievement of success) since he is the ascertainer (of the character of the disease), the director (with respect to what the patient and the nurse should do), and the minister (who applies the remedies that bring about the cure).

As in the task of cooking, a vessel, fuel, and fire are means in the hands of the cook; as a field, an army, and weapons are means in the victor's hands for achieving a victory in battle; even so the patient, the nurse, and drugs are objects that are regarded as the physician's means in the matter of achieving a cure. In the act of treatment, the physician is regarded as the chief cause.

Section XV.

In this Lesson, however, we shall lay down in brief those diverse articles that require to be kept ready in view of the dangers [sickness] to which we allude. They are as follows:

In the first place a mansion should be constructed under the supervision of an engineer well-conversant with the service of building mansions and houses. It should be spacious and roomy. The element of strength should not be wanting in it. Every part of it should not be exposed to strong winds or breezes. One portion of it should be open to the currents of the wind. It should be such that one may move or walk through it with ease. It should not be exposed to smoke, or the Sun, or dust, or injurious sound and touch and taste and form and scent. It should be furnished with staircases, with pestles and mortars, privies, accomodation for belting, and cook-rooms.

After this should be secured a body of attendants of good behavior, distinguished for purity or cleanliness of habits, attached to the person for whose service they are engaged, possessed of cleverness and skill, endued with kindness, skilled in every kind of service that a patient may require, endued with general cleverness, competent to cook food and curries, clever in bathing and washing a patient, well-conversant in rubbing or pressing the limbs; or raising the patient, or assisting him in walking or moving about, well-skilled in making or cleaning beds, competent to pound drugs, or ready, patient and skillful in waiting upon one that is ailing, and never unwilling to do any act that they may be commanded (by the physician or the patient) to do. A number of men should also be secured that are skilled in vocal and instrumental music, in hymning enconiums and eulogies, conversant with and skilled in reciting verses and pleasant discourses and narratives and stories of legendary histories, clever in reading the face and understanding what is wanted by the patient, approved and liked by him upon whom they are to wait, fully conversant with all the requirements of time and place, and possessed of such politeness as to become agreeable companions . . .[7]

5. *Sushruta Samhita*

[Most writers place Sushruta, the ancient Indian surgeon, after Charaka, or in the second century A.D. The dates of both Charaka and Sushruta are uncertain. This translation is based on the original Sanskrit text.]

27

Now we shall discuss the Chapter which treats of the management or nursing of a patient with an ulcer etc.

First of all a suitable chamber must be sought and selected for a patient, suffering from an ulcer. It should be roomy and spacious and situated in a commendable site.

Diseases, which are physical, mental or traumatic in their origin, can never attack a person who dwells in a clean and spacious chamber, protected from excessive heat, and strong gusts of wind.

The bed should be spread clean, ample and comfortable, with the head of the beadstead [sic] turned towards the east, and provided with some kind of a weapon.

In a spacious and well-spread bed, an ulcer patient can toss about and move his limbs with the greatest comfort. The reason for the head being turned towards the east is that the patient may easily make obeisance to the (demons and) celestial spirits, who inhabit that quarter of the sky. Thus the patient shall lie in comfortable posture, attended upon by his sweet-talking friends and relations.

The friends and relations of a patient shall alleviate the pain of his ulcer with pleasant and interesting topics, and by solacing him with the prospect of a speedy recovery.... An ulcer patient should always be clad in clean and white garments, having his hair and nails closely clipped and pared off ...

. . . .

The physician, the patient, the medicine, and the attendants (nurses) are the four essential factors of a course of medical treatment. Even a dangerous disease is readily cured, or it may be expected to run a speedy course in the event of the preceding four factors being respectively found to be (qualified, self-controlled, genuine and intelligently watchful).

In the absence of a qualified physician the three remaining factors of treatment will prove abortive.... A qualified physician is alone capable of relieving the pain of many a suffering patient, just as only a helmsman is capable of taking his boat across a river even without the help and co-operation of a single oarsman.

Qualities of physician:—A physician who is well versed in the science of medicine and has attended to the demonstrations of surgery and medicine, and who himself practises the healing art: and is clean, courageous, light-handed, fully equipped with supplies of medicine, surgical instruments and appliances, and who is intelligent, well read, and is a man of ready resources, and one commands a decent practice, and is further endowed with all moral virtues, is alone fit to be called a physician.

Patient:—The patient, who believes in a kind and all-merciful Providence, and possesses an unshakable fortitude and strong vital energy, and who is laid up with a curable form of disease, and is not greedy, and who further commands all the necessary articles at his disposal, and firmly adheres to the advice of his physician, is a patient of the proper or commendable type.

28

Medicine:—The (proper) medicine is that which consists of drugs grown in countries most congenial to their growth, collected under the auspices of proper lunar phases and asterisms, and compounded in proper measures and proportions, and which is pleasing (exhilirating to the mind) and has the property of subduing the deranged bodily humours without creating any discomfort to the patient, and which is harmless even in an overdose, and is judiciously administered at the opportune moment.

Nurse:—That person alone is fit to nurse or to attend the bedside of a patient, who is cool-headed and pleasant in his demeanour, does not speak ill of any body, is strong and attentive to the requirements of the sick, and strictly and indefatigably follows the instructions of the physician.[8]

6. The Works of Homer

[Little is known about the life of Homer, the Greek writer of *The Iliad* and *The Odyssey,* except from his writings. It is thought, however, that he lived about 700 B.C., probably in Asia Minor. Legends about him were numerous in ancient times, one of them being that he was blind.[9]]

The Iliad

Then a busy housedame spake in answer to him: "Hector, seeing thou straitly chargest us tell thee true, neither hath she [Andromache] gone out to any of thy sisters or thy brothers' fair-robed wives, neither to Athene's temple, where all the fair-tressed Trojan women are propitiating the awful goddess; but she went to the great tower of Ilios, because she heard the Trojans were hard pressed, and great victory was for the Achaians. So hath she come in haste to the wall, like unto one frenzied; and the nurse with her beareth the child . . ."

.   .   .   .

So spake glorious Hector, and stretched out his arm to his boy. But the child shrunk crying to the bosom of his fair-girdled nurse, dismayed at his dear father's aspect, and in dread at the bronze and horsehair crest that he beheld nodding fiercely from the helmet's top.[10]

The Odyssey

But Telemachus, where his chamber was builded high up in the fair court, in a place with a wide prospect, thither betook himself to his bed, pondering many thoughts in his mind; and with him went trusty Eurycleia, and bare for him torches burning. She was the daughter of Ops, son of Peisenor, and Laertes bought her on a time with his wealth; while as yet she was in her first youth, and gave for her the worth of twenty oxen. And he honoured her even as he honoured his dear wife in the halls, but he never lay with her, for he shunned the wrath of his lady. She went with Telemachus, and bare for him the burning torches: and of all the women of the household she loved him most, and she had nursed him when a little one. Then he opened the door of the well-builded chamber and sat down on the bed and took off his soft doublet, and put it in the wise old woman's hands. So she folded the doublet and smoothed it, and hung it on a pin by the jointed bedstead, and went forth on her way from the room, and pulled to the door with the silver handle, and drew home the bar with the thong. There, all night through, wrapt in a fleece of wool, he meditated in his heart upon the journey that Athene had showed him.

Then wise Penelope answered him: "Dear stranger, for never yet has there come to my house, of strangers from afar, a dearer man or so discreet as thou, uttering so heedfully the words of wisdom. I have an ancient woman of an understanding heart, that diligently nursed and tended that hapless man my lord, she took him in her arms in the hour when his mother bore him. She will wash thy feet, albeit her strength is frail. Up now, wise Eurycleia, and wash this man, whose years are the same as thy master's. Yea and perchance such even now are the feet of Odysseus, and such too his hands, for quickly men age in misery." [11]

7. *The Idylls of Theocritus*

[Theocritus, the Greek poet, sometimes called "the creator of pastoral poetry," lived in the third century B.C. The authorship of some of the *Idylls* has been questioned, but many are commonly attributed to him. He has had numerous imitators.[12]]

> Alcmena once had washed and given the breast
> To Heracles, a babe of ten months old,
> And Iphicles his junior by a night;
> And cradled both within a brazen shield,
> A gorgeous trophy, which Amphitryon erst
> Had stript from Pterelaus fall'n in fight.
> She stroked their baby brows, and thus she said:
> "Sleep, children mine, a light luxurious sleep,
> Brother with brother: sleep, my boys, my life:
> Blest in your slumber, in your waking blest!" [13]

8. *Plutarch's Lives*

[The greatest work of Plutarch (c. A.D. 45–120), Greek biographer, is usually said to be *The Parallel Lives*. Forty-six of these survive, arranged in pairs—a Greek life and a Roman one. While the biographies show a pride in the Greeks, there is evidence of an effort to be fair to all. These works have been described by many as without peer in the literature.[14]]

Plutarch's Lives: Alcibiades

Certain it is that Nicias, Demosthenes, Lamachus, Phormio, Thrasybulus, and Thermamenes were prominent men, and his [Alcibiades'] contemporaries and yet we cannot so much as name the mother of any one of them; whereas, in the case of Alcibiades, we even know that his nurse, who was a Spartan woman, was called Amycla, and his tutor Zopyrus. The one fact is mentioned by Antisthenes, and the other by Plato.[15]

Plutarch's Lives: Lycurgus

There was much care and art, too, used by the nurses; they had no swaddling bands; the children grew up free and unconstrained in limb and form, and not dainty and fanciful about their food; not afraid in the dark, or of being left alone; without peevishness or ill humor or crying. Upon this account, Spartan nurses were often bought up, or hired by people of other countries; and it is recorded that she who suckled Alcibiades was a Spartan; who, however, if fortunate in his nurse, was not so in his preceptor; his guardian, Pericles, as Plato tells us, chose a servant for that office called Zopyrus, no better than any common slave.[16]

9. The Works of Plato

[This great Athenian philosopher (427?–347? B.C.) was the son of noble parents. He was a friend and pupil of Socrates and established the first great philosophical school. All of Plato's known writings have survived. The *Laws* are written in the form of dialogues, as are Plato's other works. Plato was also of a poetic turn of mind.[17]]

... Shall we risk ridicule, and lay down a law that the pregnant woman shall walk, and that the child, while still soft, shall be moulded like wax, and be kept in swaddling clothes till it is two years old? And shall we also compel the nurses by legal penalties to keep carrying the children somehow, either to the fields or to the temples or to their relatives, all the time until they are able to stand upright; and after that, still to persevere in carrying them until they are three years old, as a precaution against the danger of distorting their legs by overpressure while they are still young? And that the nurses shall be as strong as possible? and shall we impose a written penalty for every failure to carry out these injunctions?[18]

10. Xenophon's Oeconomicus

[Xenophon, the Greek historian, was born in Athens about 430 B.C. The *Oeconomicus* is, in a sense, a continuation of the *Memorabilia*, which was written to defend Socrates against the charges brought against him. The *Oeconomicus* deals with the management of the house and farm, and the home duties of the Greek wife. It is written in the form of a dialogue.[19]]

31

"Then shall I too have to do these things?" said my wife.

"Indeed you will," said I. "Your duty will be to remain indoors and send out those servants whose work is outside, and superintend those who are to work indoors, and to receive the incomings and distribute so much of them as must be spent, and watch over so much as is to be kept in store; and take care that the sum laid by for a year be not spent in a month. And when wool is brought to you, you must see that cloaks are made for those that want them. You must see too that the dry corn is in good condition for making food. One of the duties that fall to you, however, will perhaps seem rather thankless: You will have to see that any servant who is ill is cared for."

"Oh no," cried my wife, "it will be delightful, assuming that those who are well cared for are going to feel grateful and be more loyal than before." [20]

11. The Writings of Hippocrates

[Hippocrates, the Greek philosopher and writer, called the "Father of Medicine," was born at Cos, in 460 B.C.[21] His works represent the rational approach to the practice of medicine, in contrast to the magical, as exemplified by the worship of Asklepios, the Greek god of medicine. In the following, Hippocrates describes in detail several nursing procedures.]

[On hot applications]

... Of hot applications the most powerful is hot water in a bottle or bladder, or in a brazen vessel, or in an earthly one; but one must first apply something soft to the side, to prevent pain. A soft large sponge, squeezed out of hot water and applied, forms a good application, but it should be covered up above, for thus the heat will remain the longer, and at the same time the vapor will be prevented from being carried up to the patient's breath, unless when this is thought of use, for sometimes it is the case.

[On baths]

The bath is useful in many diseases. . . . And if the patient be not bathed properly, he may be thereby hurt in no inconsiderable degree, for there is required a place to cover him that is free of smoke, abundance of water, materials for frequent baths, but not very large, unless this should be required. It is better that no friction should be applied, but if so, a hot soap must be used in greater abundance than is common, and an effusion of a considerable quantity of water is to be made at the same time and afterwards repeated. There must also be a short passage to the basin, and it should be of easy ingress and egress. But the person who takes the bath should be orderly and reserved in his manner, should do nothing for himself, but others should pour the water upon him and rub him, and plenty of water, of various temperatures, should be in readiness for the douche, and the affusions quickly made; and sponges should be used instead of the comb, and the body should be anointed when not quite dry. But the head should be rubbed by the sponge until it is quite dry; the extremities should be protected from cold, as also the head and the rest of the body . . .

[On bandaging]

There are two views of bandaging; that which regards it while doing, and that which regards it when done. It should be done quickly, without pain, with ease, and with elegance; quickly, by despatching the work; without pain, by being readily done; with ease, by being prepared for everything; and with elegance, so that it may be agreeable to the sight. By what mode of training these accomplishments are to be acquired has been stated. When done, it should fit well and neatly; it is neatly done when with judgment, and when it is equal and unequal. The forms of it (the bandage?) are the simple, the slightly winding (called a scia), the sloping (sima), the monoculus, the rhombus, and the semi-rhombus. The forms of the bandage should be suitable to the form and the affection of the part to which it is applied.

There are two useful purposes to be fulfilled by bandaging: first, strength, which is imparted by the compression and the number of folds. In one case the bandage effects the cure, and in another it contributes to the cure. For these purposes this is the rule—that the force of the construction be such as to prevent the adjoining parts from separating without compressing them much, and so that the parts may be adjusted but not forced together; and that the constriction be small at the extremities, and least of all in the middle. The knot and the thread that is passed through should not be in a downward but in an upward direction, regard being had to the circumstances under which the case is presented; to position, to the bandaging, and to the compression. The commencement of the ligatures is not to be placed at the wound, but where the knot is situated [meaning?]. The knot should not be placed where it will be exposed to friction, nor where it will be in the way, nor where it will be useless. The knot and the thread should be soft, and not large.

Second. One ought to be well aware that every bandage has a tendency to fall off towards the part that declines or becomes smaller; as, for example, upward, in the case of the head, and downward, in the case of the leg. The turns of the bandage should be made from right to left, and from left to right, except on the head, where it should be in a straight direction. When opposite parts are to be bandaged together, we must use a bandage with two heads; or if we make use of a bandage with one head, we must attach it in like manner at some fixed point; such, for example, as the middle of the head; and so in other cases. These parts which are much exposed to motion, such as the joints, where there is a flexion, should have few and slight bandages applied to them, as at the ham; but where there is much extension, the bandage should be single and broad, as at the kneepan; and for the maintenance of the bandage in its proper place, some turns should be carried to those parts which are not much moved, and are lank, such as the parts above and below the knee. In the case of the shoulder, a fold should be carried round by the other armpit; in that of the groin, by the flanks of the opposite side; and of the leg, to above the calf of the leg. When the bandage be secured below, and *vice versa;* and where there is no means of doing this, as in the case of the head, the turns are to be made mostly on the level part of the head, and the folds are to be done with as little obliquity as possible, so that the firmest part being last applied may secure the portions which are more movable. When we cannot secure the bandaging by means of folds of the cloth, nor by suspending them from the opposite side, we must have recourse to stitching it with ligatures, either passed circularly or in the form of a seam.

The bandages should be clean, light, soft, and thin. One should practice rolling with both hands together, and with each separately. One should also choose a suitable one, according to the breadth and thickness of the parts. The heads of the bandages should be hard, smooth, and neatly put on. That sort of bandaging is the worst which quickly falls off; but those are bad bandages which neither compress nor yet come off.[22]

[While a medical student is indicated in the following, his duties as outlined are those of a nurse.]

Let one of your pupils be left in charge, to carry out instructions without unpleasantness, and to administer the treatment: Choose out those who have been already admitted into the mysteries of the art, so as to add anything necessary, and to give treatment with safety. He is there also to prevent those things escaping notice that happen in the interval between visits . . .[23]

12. Vitruvius. *On Architecture*

[Little is known of the life of Vitruvius (1st cen.? A.D.), the first Roman writer on architecture. His one work, *De Architectura,* discusses city planning, building materials, and other pertinent subjects. It is written in ten volumes, and was much used by other architects.[24] In the following account of the origin of the Corinthian capital, a nurse plays a minor role.]

But the third order, which is called Corinthian, imitates the slight figure of a maiden; because girls are represented with slighter dimensions because of their tender age, and admit of more graceful effects in ornament. Now the first invention of that capital is related to have happened thus. A girl, a native of Corinth, already of age to be married, was attacked by disease and died. After her funeral, the goblets which delighted her when living, were put together in a basket by her nurse, carried to the monument, and placed on the top. That they might remain longer, exposed as they were to the

34

weather, she covered the basket with a tile. As it happened the basket was placed upon the root of an acanthus. Meanwhile about spring time, the root of the acanthus, being pressed down in the middle by the weight, put forth leaves and shoots. The shoots grew up the sides of the basket, and, being pressed down at the angles by the force of the weight of the tile, were compelled to form the curves of volutes at the extreme parts. Then Callimachus, who for the elegance and refinement of his marble carving was nick-named *Catatechnos* by the Athenians; was passing the monument, perceived the basket and the young leaves growing up. Pleased with the style and novelty of the grouping, he made columns for the Corinthians on this model and fixed the proportions. Thence he distributed the details of the Corinthian order throughout the work.[25]

13. *Pliny's Letters*

[Pliny the Younger (A.D. 62?–c. 113), the nephew of Pliny the Elder, was an orator and a statesman. His fame rests mainly on his letters, which were probably written for publication. In addition to these, he wrote a biography of Pliny the Elder. He held many public offices, and died in the province of Pontus-Bithynia.[26]]

To Verus.

I am much obliged to you for undertaking the care of the little farm I gave to my nurse. It was worth, when I made her a present of it, an hundred thousand sesterces, but the returns having since diminished, it has sunk in its value: however, that will rise again, I doubt not, under your management. But, remember, what I recommend to your attention is not the fruit-trees and the land (which yet I by no means except), but my little benefaction; for it is not more the good woman's concern as a recipient, than mine as the donor, that it should be as profitable as possible. Farewell.[27]

14. Celsus. *De Medicina*

[A. Cornelius Celsus (A.D. 14?), called "one of the most judicious medical authors of antiquity," [28] wrote *De Medicina* in A.D. 30. It is his only extant work.[29] The procedure of cupping, described below, is remembered by some nurses.]

Now there are two kinds of cups, one made of bronze, the other of horn. The bronze cup is open at one end, closed at the other; the horn one, likewise at one end open, has at the other end a small hole. Into the bronze cup is put burning lint, and in this state its mouth is applied and pressed to the body until it adheres. The horn cup is applied as it is to the body and when the air is withdrawn by the mouth through the small hole at the end, and after the hole has been closed by applying wax over it, the horn cup likewise adheres. Either form of cup may be made, not only of the above materials, but also of anything else suitable; when others are lacking, a small drinking cup or porridge bowl with a narrowish mouth may be adapted conveniently for the purpose . . .[30]

15. *The Ancient Laws of Ireland*

[The ancient laws of Ireland, the Brehon Laws, were probably compiled from the eighth to the thirteenth centuries, and from codified laws much more ancient.[31] They contain allusions to "lawful" and "unlawful" physicians, and fees and compensations to be paid under certain conditions. There is also an occasional reference to a nurse.]

These are the allowances for food and a physician, and for a substitute, and for a man to act as nurse-tender.[32]

From the twice seven "cumhals" [a unit of payment] which we mentioned a while ago, take now six cows for concealment from the physician [33] or for facility of division: (and it is no concealment from the physician, where he is entitled to nothing, that he should get nothing out of it). You have then twice eighteen cows: give eighteen cows of them to the substitute alone; you have then eighteen other cows remaining: divide these among the physician, the nurse-tender, and the procuring of food; so that four cows and a "samhaisc"—heifer [34] is the share of each of them, and nine cows are for food alone.[35]

CONCLUDING STATEMENT

The quotations from the literature of early civilizations presented in this chapter are inconclusive regarding nurses and nursing. Accounts of nurses resembling those of today are not found in the writings of pre-Christian groups, with the exception of those of India.

In the Babylonian, the Hebrew, and the Greek and Roman writings quoted here, the nurse is either a child's nurse or a wet nurse. Many references illustrating this are available, especially in Greek prose and poetry. From these, and from other sources, a few examples were chosen. In the literature of India, nurses were mentioned and their characteristics described. These nurses seem to have been men, and it is clear from a reading of Charaka and Sushruta that the nurses would have had no function except working under the direction of physicians in a hospital. Nurses are occasionally mentioned in Irish literature in connection with the laws governing payment of physicians in injuries involving patients.

It has been assumed that one reason for the silence of the writings on the subject of nursing is that the care of the sick was a function of the home, there being no hospitals, except in India. It was presumably done by women, since, in most groups, the care of the family in sickness and in health was their province.

When we consider the literature of the Christian Era, with its concern for the welfare of individuals, we will find more attention centered on the care of the sick by groups outside the home, chiefly under the auspices of the Christian church. The writings of the early Christian Era therefore provide instances of nurses caring for the sick. It is with this phase that the next chapter is particularly concerned.

Chapter 2

Some Sources for the Study of Nursing in the Early Christian Era

INTRODUCTION

THE beginnings of Christianity introduced a new element into human relations which had a profound influence on the care of the sick. This change was gradual, remnants of the old ideas lingering even for centuries. The gods of healing of the ancient religions, relating closely to the lives of the people, were often difficult to supplant. From the beginning of Christianity there is noted a definite concern for the welfare of the individual, and this eventually led to special emphasis on the care of the sick. The ideal of service to one's fellow man was intrinsic in Christ's teachings, Jesus himself performing many miracles of healing. In three of the four Gospels, the disciples of Christ are directed to heal the sick. The ideal of service is also implicit in the institutions established by the early Church to carry out the Christian philosophy. The results of these facts have been far-reaching in the history of nursing, even up to the present day.

The Church, in implementing Christ's teachings, very early created offices designed to carry out acts of service in behalf of the members of the Church community. The bishops and other ecclesiastical officers were charged with dispensing church funds for charitable purposes. Personal service was emphasized, and this not infrequently included ministration to the sick. This service is indicated by the Greek words *diakonia,* "service," and *diakonein,* "to serve," or "to minister," and the service was carried out by such groups as the widows, the virgins, and the deacons and deaconesses.

The literary sources for a study of this part of nursing history illustrate the activities of the Church with regard to the care of the sick, including the appointment, qualifications, and duties of officers of the Church who ministered to the sick; the work of individual men and women; the establishment of monasteries where, among other good works, the sick

38

were cared for; and the work of early Christian hospitals. In some references, mention is made of "visiting the sick," while in others, there is definite indication that the workers actually "ministered to the needs of" the sick. It is desirable to make a distinction between these two functions whenever possible; the former being a religious or social function, possibly without any actual ministration, while the latter was evidently nursing the sick.

The New Testament references include the well-known description from the Gospel of St. Matthew of the early Christian works of charity, and the parable of the good Samaritan (16, 17). They also indicate the status, appointment, qualifications, and functions of the virgins, the widows, and the deacons and deaconesses (18–20). We cannot be sure that all the men and women mentioned by St. Paul in his Epistle to the Romans were deacons and deaconesses, or that they had formal recognition by the Church. This may have been the case, however. The most certain is probably Phoebe who is called *diaconos* (18), but this may simply mean that she was in the ministry of the Church without having any official status. On this point, Bishop Lightfoot says: "As I read my New Testament, the female diaconate is as definite an institution as the male diaconate. Phoebe is as much a deacon as Stephen or Philip is a deacon." [1] Dean Howson adds: ". . . the case might with strict accuracy have been stated more strongly, for Stephen and Philip are nowhere designated by this term whereas Phoebe is expressly so designated." [2] Deaconess Cecilia Robinson states that this is the only instance in the New Testament in which a woman is specifically referred to by the word *diakonos*.[3] This is an interesting point in the light of later Church history with reference to the deaconesses. It is thought, however, that Phoebe cared for the sick.

The *Didascalia Apostolorum* and the *Apostolical Constitutions* make provision for the offices of widows, virgins, deacons, and deaconesses (21–27). The canons or decisions of certain Church councils and synods speak directly of these Church officers also (28–41).[4] They indicate that at certain periods the widows and virgins wore a distinctive dress, took the vow of chastity, and sometimes lived in their own homes, from which they went out to do good works; on other occasions they lived in monasteries. The age for consecration is also given. The canons provide for ordination of deaconesses, and later forbid it. They are confusing on this point. Reference is made in them also to the *xenodochia,* or inns for strangers, for which the Church was responsible.

The earliest monastic communities probably concerned themselves only with the sick within their own walls. The *Rule of St. Benedict,* compiled about A.D. 528, provides for the care of the sick of the monastic

39

community. An infirmary was part of the religious house. Later a hospital became a part of the monastery. The Benedictine Rule comprises seventy-two "Instruments of Good Works," the sixteenth of which is, "To visit the sick" (42). Later monastic rules, one of which is the Rule of Abelard for the nuns of the Paraclete (43), followed rather closely the Rule of St. Benedict.

In the writings of other Church Fathers, some references to the care of the sick are found. St. Gregory of Nyssa, in his *Life of St. Macrina,* written in the form of a letter, not only describes briefly the nursing done by Macrina but speaks of Lampadia, a deaconess (44). Palladius, a Syrian monk, writes of Olympias, the deaconess, and of St. Ephrem, the deacon of Edessa, in *The Paradise of the Holy Fathers* (45). St. John Chrysostom, in *Homilies on the Gospel of Matthew,* mentions the widows and virgins cared for by the Church, and refers to the sick in the inns, for which the Church assumed responsibility (46). The "Panegyric on S. Basil," in Gregory's *Orations,* dwells on the work of St. Basil's hospital in caring for the lepers (47). Another Gregory, St. Gregory the Great, in his *Dialogues,* describes an incident involving a mentally ill patient in a hospital of the period (48).

Letters constitute an important source of information concerning the times. St. Gregory of Nyssa's letter, referred to above, gives a hint of the nursing done by St. Macrina. Abelard's Rule is contained in a letter to Heloise. There is probably little doubt that the two women mentioned by Pliny the Younger, in his letter to the Emperor Trajan in 112, were deaconesses who were tortured to elicit their admission that they were Christians (49). Some of the most useful information concerning certain eminent women and men of Rome comes from the letters of St. Jerome. From among the many which describe charitable acts performed by certain of the women, two have been chosen for inclusion here—those eulogizing the good works of Fabiola and Paula (50–51). The extreme asceticism of some of the women workers and the high regard in which this was held at the time are illustrated by the contents of these communications.

The names of many deaconesses have come down to us in letters. St. John Chrysostom gives the names of five: Olympias, Sabiniana, Pentadia, Amprucla, and Procla.[5] St. Basil writes "To the Deaconesses, Daughters of Count Terentius," who were deaconesses at Samosata.[6] Theodoret, the church historian, writes letters to two deaconesses, "To the Deaconess Casiana," and "To the Deaconess Celarina." [7] Included in this chapter are quotations from four of St. Basil's letters, touching on the affairs of early hospitals (52–55).

Contemporary and later historians and travelers provide us with information concerning the social service of the Church, and the hospitals of the period. Such ecclesiastical histories as those of Eusebius, Sozomen, and Theodoret (56–58), and the writings of Procopius (59) and William of Tyre (60), tell of the charitable work of the early Christians. This included hospital building and nursing. Of the travel accounts of this era, that of Antoninus Martyr, traveling in the Holy Land, tells of the hospices and hospitals which he observed there (61).

A source of interest concerning the deaconesses is provided in the epitaphs of two deaconesses (62), one at Pavia, Italy, and the other at Hellespontus, in Asia Minor. The latter provides the name of the last early deaconess to be known by her name, Aeria.[8]

A modern novel, *Hypatia,* written by Charles Kingsley, purporting to follow closely authentic history, portrays the work of the *parabolani,* a minor religious group of the fifth century in Alexandria, in their care of the sick of that city (63).

THE SOURCES

The New Testament

16. The Gospel According to St. Matthew, 25:35–40 (King James Version)

[These words were spoken by Christ to his disciples as he sat on the Mount of Olives. In them he sets an example of love and charity which has been the ideal of Christians since that time.]

For I was an hungered, and ye gave me meat: I was thirsty and ye gave me drink: I was a stranger, and ye took me in:

Naked, and ye clothed me: I was sick, and ye visited me: I was in prison, and ye came unto me.

Then shall the righteous answer him, saying, Lord, when saw we thee an hungered, and fed thee? or thirsty, and gave thee drink?

When saw we thee a stranger, and took thee in? or naked, and clothed thee?

When saw we thee sick, or in prison, and came unto thee?

And the King shall answer and say unto them, Verily I say unto you, Inasmuch as ye have done it unto one of the least of these my brethren, ye have done it unto me.

17. The Gospel According to St. Luke, 10:30–35 (King James Version)

[The story of the good Samaritan has become a symbol of good works for Christians of all times.]

And Jesus answering said, A certain man went down from Jerusalem to Jericho, and fell among thieves, which stripped him of his raiment, and wounded him, and departed, leaving him half dead.

And by chance there came down a certain priest that way: and when he saw him, he passed by on the other side.

And likewise a Levite, when he was at the place, came and looked on him, and passed by on the other side.

But a certain Samaritan, as he journeyed, came where he was: and when he saw him, he had compassion on him,

And went to him, and bound up his wounds, pouring in oil and wine, and set him on his own beast, and brought him to an inn, and took care of him.

And on the morrow when he departed, he took out two pence, and gave them to the host, and said unto him, Take care of him; and whatsoever thou spendest more, when I come again, I will repay thee.

18. The Epistle of Paul the Apostle to the Romans, 16:1-2 (King James Version)

[Deaconess Cecilia Robinson says: "This is the only instance in the New Testament in which the word *diakonos* is explicitly used of a woman, and it is valuable as proving that women as well as men had a recognized share in the ministry of the Church." [9]]

I commend unto you Phebe our sister, which is a servant of the church which is at Cenchrea:

That ye receive her in the Lord, as becometh saints, and that ye assist her in whatsoever business she hath need of you; for she hath been a succourer of many and of myself also.

19. The First Epistle of Paul the Apostle to Timothy, 3:8-13 (King James Version)

[The qualifications of deacons, as outlined by St. Paul, are given in the following quotation.]

Likewise must the deacons be grave, not double-tongued, not given to much wine, not greedy of filthy lucre;

Holding the mystery of faith in a pure conscience.

And let them also first be proved: then let them use the office of a deacon, being found blameless.

Even so must their wives [10] be grave, not slanderers, sober, faithful in all things.

Let the deacons be the husbands of one wife, ruling their children and their own homes well.

For they that have used the office of deacon well purchase to themselves a good degree, and great boldness in the faith which is in Christ Jesus.

20. The First Epistle of St. Paul to St. Timothy, 5:9–10 (Douay Version)

[The necessary qualifications of widows are here outlined by St. Paul.]

Let a widow be chosen of no less than threescore years of age, who hath been the wife of one husband,

Having testimony for her good works; if she have brought up children, if she have received to harbour, if she have washed the saints' feet, if she have ministered to them that suffer tribulations, if she have diligently followed every good work.

The *Didascalia Apostolorum* and the *Apostolical Constitutions*

[The *Apostolical Constitutions* are a collection of ecclesiastical regulations, professedly drawn up by the Apostles and transmitted to the Church by Clement of Rome. They were probably compiled by an unknown Syrian at the end of the fourth century. In them the authors are represented as speaking sometimes jointly, and sometimes singly. The writings are believed to be based on the *Didascalia Apostolorum,* a collection of moral and ecclesiastical instructions of the middle of the third century, of which they are an amplification. The *Didascalia Apostolorum* is best known through a Syriac version and a fragmentary Latin one. Both the *Didascalia Apostolorum* and the *Apostolical Constitutions* are probably the climax of a gradual process of crystallization of unwritten custom, made at various places and at different times for the purpose of putting into writing the order of the Church for private instruction, and also for the use of the officers of the Church.[11] Selections have been made from them to illustrate the characteristics of those caring for the sick.]

21. *Didascalia Apostolorum*, II, ii

About the election of Deacons. Let the Deacon be ordained; when he has been elected according to what has been already said, if he be of good behavior; if he be pure, if he have been elected on account of his purity, and because of his exemptions from distractions.

. . . .

Let then the service be like this: first, those things that are commanded by the Bishop, so that they only may be done at the ministration, and of all the clergy he may be the Counselor and secret of the Church. He who ministers to the sick, he who ministers to the strangers, who helps the widows, and goes round all the houses of those who are in want; lest there should be any one in distress or sickness or in misery he goes round to the houses . . .

43

Let twelve Elders be known in the Church, seven Deacons, and fourteen subdeacons; and let those Widows who sit first be thirteen.

· · · · · · ·

Cephas said, Let three widows be appointed, two who shall be continually in prayer for all those who are in temptation and in regard to revelations and signs, for what is necessary, but one to be continually with the women who are tried by sickness, who is good at service, watchful to make known what is required to the Elders. [Let them] not be lovers of filthy lucre, not accustomed to much wine, so that they may be able to be watchful in the night services of the sick, and in any other good works that any one wishes to do, for these things are the first good treasures that are desirable.

22. *Didascalia Apostolorum,* III, i

Let widows then be appointed; she who is not less than fifty years of age and over, in order that by reason of her years she may be removed from the thought of having another husband. . . . Let not then young widows be appointed to the office of widows, but let them be taken care of and trained . . .

23. *Didascalia Apostolorum,* III, xvi

This service of Deaconess is necessary also to thee for many things, for in the houses of the heathen where there are believing women, a Deaconess is required, that she may go in and visit those who are sick, and serve them with whatever they need, and anoint those who are healed from sicknesses.[12]

24. *Apostolical Constitutions,* Book III, Sect. I, Parts I, III, V, VII

Concerning Widows.
Choose your "widows not under sixty years of age," that in some measure the suspicion of a second marriage may be prevented by their age . . .

· · · · · ·

But the true widows are those which have had only one husband, having a good report among the generality for good works; widows indeed, sober, chaste, faithful, pious, who have brought up their children well, and have entertained strangers unblameably, which are to be supported as devoted to God . . .

· · · · ·

Let every widow be meek, quiet, gentle, sincere, free from anger, not talkative; not clamorous, not hasty of speech, not given to evil-speaking, not captious, not doubletongued, not a busy-body. . .

· · · · · ·

The widows therefore ought to be grave, obedient to their bishops, and their presbyters, and their deacons, and besides these to the deaconesses, with piety, reverence, and fear; not usurping authority, nor desiring to do anything beyond the constitution without the consent of the deacon . . .

25. *Apostolical Constitutions*, Book III, Sect. II, Part XIX

Ordain also a deaconess who is faithful and holy, for the ministrations toward women. . . . For we stand in need of a woman, a deaconess, for many necessities; and first in the baptism of women . . .

Let the deacon be in all things unspotted, as the bishop himself is to be, only more active. . . . And let the deaconess be diligent in taking care of the women . . .

26. *Apostolical Constitutions*, Book VIII, Parts XIX, XX

Concerning a deaconess, I Bartholomew make this constitution: O bishop, thou shalt lay thy hands upon her in the presence of the presbytery, and of the deacons and deaconesses, and shalt say:

O Eternal God, the Father of our Lord Jesus Christ, the Creator of man and of woman, who didst replenish with the Spirit Miriam, and Deborah, and Anna, and Huldah; who didst not disdain that Thy only begotten Son should be born of a woman; who also in the tabernacle of the testimony, and in the temple, didst ordain women to be keepers of Thy holy gates, do Thou now look down upon this Thy servant, who is to be ordained to the office of a deaconess, and grant her Thy Holy Spirit, and cleanse her from all filthiness of flesh and spirit, that she may worthily discharge the work which is committed to her to Thy glory and the praise of Thy Christ, with whom glory and adoration be to Thee and the Holy Spirit forever. Amen.

27. *Apostolical Constitutions*, Book VIII, Parts XXIV, XXV

I, the same [James, the son of Alphaeus], make a constitution in regard to virgins: *A virgin is not ordained, for we have no such command from the Lord; for this is a state of voluntary trial, not for the reproach of marriage, but on account of leisure for piety.*

And I, Lebbaeus, surnamed Thaddaeus, make this constitution in regard to widows: *A widow is not ordained; yet if she has lost her husband a great while, and has lived soberly and unblameably, and has taken extraordinary care of her family, as Judith and Anna—these women of great reputation— let her be chosen into the order of widows. But if she has lately lost her yoke- fellow, let her not be believed, but let her youth be judged of by the time; for the affections do sometimes grow aged with men, if they be not restrained by a better bridle.*[13]

Canons of Church Councils

[In the early Christian literature, the term "canon" designates decrees of Church councils, and, beginning with the Council of Trent (1545–

1563), it was reserved to designate dogmatic pronouncements of ecumenical councils. The canons form the basis of canon or ecclesiastical law.[14] Many of the canons of Church councils through the early Christian Era specify the behavior of Church officers such as the deaconesses, the virgins, and the widows. Others refer to the *xenodochia,* maintained by the Church. The following canons are arranged according to the chronological order of the councils where the pronouncements were made. It will be noted in the first canon cited that the statement concerning deaconesses comes as somewhat of an afterthought at the end of a longer dissertation on another subject, but one related to it. The canons are contradictory with reference to the ordination of deaconesses.]

28. Council of Nicaea, A.D. 325

Canon XIX. Concerning the Paulists who have flown for refuge to the Catholic Church, it has been decreed that they must by all means be rebaptised; and if any of them who in past time have been numbered among their clergy should be found blameless and without reproach, let them be rebaptised and ordained by the Bishop of the Catholic Church; but if the examination should discover them to be unfit; they ought to be deposed. Likewise in the case of their deaconesses, and generally in the case of those who have been enrolled among their clergy, let the same form be observed. And we mean by deaconesses such as have assumed the habit, but also, since they have no imposition of hands, are to be numbered only among the laity.[15]

29. Fourth Synod of Carthage, A.D. 398

Canon XI. If a virgin is to be presented to the bishop for consecration, it must be in the same clothes which, in accordance with her sacred calling, she will henceforth wear.

Canon CIV. If a widow who has dedicated herself to God and taken a religious habit, marries again, she shall be entirely shut out from the communion of Christians.

30. Synod of Orange, A.D. 441

Canon XXVI. Deaconesses shall no longer be ordained, and (in divine service) they shall receive the benediction only in common with the laity (not among those holding clerical offices).

31. Council of Chalcedon, A.D. 451

Canon XV. No woman shall be ordained a deaconess before she is forty years old, and then after careful trial. If, however, after she has received ordination and has been for some time in the service, she marries, disparaging the grace of God, then she shall be anathemized, together with him who has united himself with her.

Canon XVI. A virgin who has dedicated herself to the Lord God, and

46

also a monk, shall not be allowed to marry. If they do so, they shall be excommunicated. But the bishop of the place shall have full power to show them kindness.

32. Synod of Agde (Agatha in Gaul), A.D. 506

Canon XIX. Nuns (Sanctimoniales), however their morals may be approved, must not receive the veil before they are forty years old.[16]

33. Synod at Epaon in Burgundy, A.D. 517

Canon XXI. The dedication of deaconesses shall be given up through the whole kingdom. Only the *benedictio poenitentiae* may be given them if they go back (i.e., lay aside the votum castitis).[17]

34. Second Synod at Orleans, A.D. 533

Canon XVII. Women who, in opposition to the canons have received the benediction as deaconesses, if they marry again, must be excommunicated. If, at the admonition of the bishop, they give up such a union, they may, after undergoing penance, be admitted to communion again.

Canon XVIII. To no woman must henceforth the *benedictio diaconalis* be given, because of the weakness of the sex.

35. Fifth Synod of Orleans, A.D. 549

Canon XIII. No one must keep back or alienate what has been given to churches, monasteries, xenodochia or the poor. If anyone does so he shall in accordance with the old canons, as a murderer of the poor, be excommunicated until he gives back what he has withdrawn.

Canon XV. In regard to the xenodochion, which King Childebert and his consort Ultrogotho founded in Lyons, the bishop of Lyons must claim none of its goods for himself or his church. And, in general, if anyone of any position attacks the rights of this xenodochion, he shall be smitten with perpetual anathema.

36. Synod at Barcelona, A.D. 599

Canon IV. A virgin who has laid aside lay attire; has put on the habit of the religious, and has vowed chastity may no longer marry. Nor one who has received the *benedictio poenitentiae*.

37. Synod at Paris, A.D. 613

Canon XV. Virgins and widows who, remaining in their abodes, have put on the religious habit, or on whom their parents have put it, may not marry.

38. Alexandrian Synod, A.D. 633

Canon LVI. There are two kinds of widows, the secular and those dedicated to God (sanctimoniales). The latter have laid aside the secular dress, and have assumed the religious habit of the church. They may no longer marry.

39. Synod at Toledo, A.D. 656

Canon LV. A widow who wishes to take the vow of chastity, must do so in writing, and then wear the dress unaltered which the bishop or minister of the Church has given her. She shall cover her head with a red or black cloth (pallium), so that she may be known, and that no one may permit himself anything against her.

40. Synod at Latona (Frankish), A.D. 670 or 671

Canon XIII. Those widows (dedicated to God) who live piously according to the judgment of the bishops, may remain in their homes. If, however, they are negligent in regard to chastity, they shall be shut up in a convent.

41. Trullan Synod, A.D. 692

Canon XIV. In accordance with the ancient laws, no one shall be ordained priest before thirty years, or deacon before twenty-five. A deaconess must be forty years old.[18]

Monastic Rules

42. The *Rule of St. Benedict*

[The *Rule of St. Benedict,* compiled about 528, set a precedent for all succeeding monastic rules. The original manuscript of the *Rule* was destroyed in a disastrous fire in the monastery of Teano, where it had been taken for safekeeping during a Saracen invasion of Italy. The oldest extant manuscript is of England of the seventh or eighth century.[19]]

Ch. XXXVI. Of the Sick Brethren.

Before all things and above all things special care must be taken of the sick so that in every deed they be looked after as if it were Christ Himself who was served. He Himself has said, *I was sick, and ye visited Me; and what ye did to one of these, My least brethren, ye did to Me.*

But let the sick themselves bear in mind that they are served for the honour of God, and should not grieve their brethren who serve them by their superfluous demands. These, nevertheless, must be borne with patience, since from such a more abundant reward is obtained. Let the abbot, therefore, take the greatest care that the sick suffer no neglect.

For them let a separate cell be set apart with an attendant who is God-fearing, diligent and painstaking: Let baths be granted to the sick as often as it shall be expedient, but to those in health, and especially to the young, they shall be seldom permitted. Also for the recovery of their strength the use of meat may be allowed to the sick and those of very weak health. As soon, however, as they shall mend they must all in the accustomed manner abstain from flesh meat. Let the abbot take special care that the sick be not neglected by the cellarer or the attendants, because he is responsible for what is done amiss by his disciples.[20]

43. Rule Given by Abelard to Heloise for the Nuns of the Paraclete

[As far as is known, eight letters passed between Abelard and Heloise. They were probably written between 1128 and 1139. The first six are often designated "the love letters of Abelard and Heloise." The seventh defines various church officers. Letter Eight, a portion of which is quoted below, contains the Rule given by Abelard to Heloise for the nuns of the Paraclete, a monastery built by Abelard near Troyes, and later given to Heloise, who was the abbess.[21] The close resemblance of Abelard's provisions for the sick of the monastic community to those of St. Benedict is apparent.]

The Infirmarian shall provide for the sick, and shall preserve them as well from sin as from want. Whatsoever their sickness shall demand, as well as of food as of baths, or aught else that may be, is to be allowed them. For there is a proverb known in such cases: "The law was not made for the sick." Let flesh meat in no way be denied them save on the sixth day of the week or on the chief vigils or the fasts of the Four Seasons, or of Lent. . . . There must always be a careful guardian present by the sick, who, should the need arise, may straightway come to them, and the house must be furnished with all things that are necessary to their infirmity. Of medicines also, if need be, provision shall be made according to the resources of the place. Which can more easily be done if she who is over the sick is not lacking in knowledge of medicine. And to her also the charge shall pertain of those that have an issue of blood. But there ought to be some one skilled in bleeding lest it be necessary for a man to enter among the women for this purpose . . .

And once every day at the least let the Deaconess with the cellaress visit the sick person, as she were Christ, that they may carefully provide for her needs as well in bodily as in spiritual things; and may deserve to hear it said by the Lord: "I was sick, and ye visited me." [22]

Other Writings Concerning the Early Christian Era

44. *Saint Gregory of Nyssa: The Life of Saint Macrina*

[The life of St. Macrina, as told by St. Gregory of Nyssa, is in the form of a letter, written about 380, and addressed to the monk Olympius. This Gregory was the brother of St. Basil and St. Macrina, and was born about 335, probably at Caesarea. He lived until about 395. St. Macrina established a monastery which was under the direction of St. Basil. The text of the letter given here is that of Migne's *Patrologia*

Graeca.[23] Not only is St. Macrina eulogized in it, but there is mention also of Lampadia, a deaconess.]

Never did she even look for help to any human being, nor did human charity give her the opportunity of a comfortable existence. Never were petitioners turned away, yet never did she appeal for help, but God secretly blessed the little seeds of her good works till they grew into a mighty fruit.

Saddest of all in their grief were those who called on her as mother and nurse. These were they whom she picked up, exposed by the roadside in the time of famine. She had nursed and reared them, and led them to the pure and stainless life.[24]

45. Palladius. *The Paradise of the Holy Fathers*

[Palladius, a Syrian monk, was born in Galatia about 364. He wrote this manuscript in 420, at the request of Lausus, a man of high rank in Constantinople. The present translation is from a Syrian manuscript probably written in the thirteenth or fourteenth century.[25]]

Ch. VIII. Of the Blessed Woman Olympias.

And she gave herself unto tears which were without measure both day and night, and she submitted herself unto all sorts and conditions of the children of men for the sake of God, and she bowed down reverently before the holy Bishops, and she paid homage to the elders, and she entreated in an honourable manner the clergy, as well as the order of monks who dwelt in the monastic houses, and she received with welcome the virgins, and she visited the widows, and she reared the orphans, and she strengthened [those who were in a state of] old age, and she had care for the sick and she mourned with the sinners, and she led the erring into the right path, and she tended everyone, and she converted many women among those who did not believe, and prepared them for life.

Ch. LVIII. Of the Blessed Man Ephraim, the Deacon of the Church of Edessa.

And he took money, and he began to fence off in the streets places which were suitable for his purpose, and he provided with great care three hundred beds, some of which were intended for those who were dying, and others were intended for those who, it was thought, would live; and in short, he brought in from the villages which were outside the city all those whom famine had stricken, and put them to bed, and every day he performed for them with the greatest solicitude the constant service of which they were in need, [paying for the same] with the money which came to him, and he rejoiced by means of those who supported him in the matter.[26]

46. St. John Chrysostom. *Homilies on the Gospel of Matthew*

[St. John Chrysostom, called by many the greatest of the Greek Fathers, became patriarch of Constantinople in 398.[27] As such he attempted to reform the life of the capital. Admired at first, and later exiled, he wrote many brilliant homilies on the gospels. His *Homilies on the Gospel of Matthew* is thought to have been delivered at Antioch between 381 and 398, when he became archbishop.[28]]

And that thou mayest learn the inhumanity of the others, when the church is possessed of a revenue of one of the lowest among the wealthy, and not of the very rich, consider how many widows it succors every day, how many virgins; for indeed the list of them hath already reached into the number of three thousand. Together with these, she succors them that dwell in the prison, the sick in the caravansera, the healthy, those that are absent from their home, those that are maimed in their bodies, those that wait upon the altar, and with respect to food and raiment, those that casually come every day, and her substance is in no respect diminished.[29]

47. St. Gregory of Nazianzen. *Orations*, XLIII, 63. The Panegyric on S. Basil

[This Gregory is known as one of the four great Fathers of the Eastern Church. He was born in 329 at Nazianum in Cappadocia. Forty-five of his orations are extant;[30] the one quoted, written soon after 381,[31] relates to the founding of St. Basil's hospital.]

What more? A noble thing is philanthropy, and the support of the poor, and the assistance of human weakness. Go forth a little way from the city, and behold the new city [a hospital for the sick], the storehouse of piety, the common treasury of the wealthy in which superfluities of their wealth, aye, and even their necessaries, freed from the power of the moth [S. Matt. vi, 19] no longer gladdening the eyes of the thief, and escaping both the emulation of envy, and the corruption of time: where disease is regarded in a religious light, and disaster is thought a blessing, and sympathy is put to the test.... There is no longer before our eyes that terrible and piteous spectacle of men who are living corpses, the greater part of whose limbs have mortified, driven away from their cities and homes and public places and fountains, aye, and from their dearest ones ... they are no longer brought before us at our gatherings and meetings, in our common intercourse and union, no longer objects of hatred, instead of pity on account of their disease.... He ... it was, who took the lead in pressing upon these who were men, that they ought not to despise their fellowmen ... by their inhuman treatment of them.... He did not therefore disdain to honour with his lips this disease, noble and of noble ancestry and brilliant reputation though he was, but saluted them as brethren. . . . Basil's care was for the sick, the relief of their wounds, and the imitation of Christ, by cleansing leprosy, not by a word, but in deed.[32]

48. *Dialogues of St. Gregory, Surnamed the Great*

[The *Dialogues* were written by St. Gregory the Great, in 593, at the request of certain monks of his household.[33] St. Gregory was the first pope of that name, of which there were sixteen, and was the fourth and last of the great Latin Fathers. His relation to the revision of the liturgy and music of the Church is a matter of dispute.[34] The following passage describes the care of a mentally ill patient in the hospital.]

Ch. 35: Of Amantius, a Priest in the Province of Tuscania.
Dial. III, 35.
At that time, there was one amongst them beside himself, being fallen into a phrensy: who one night did so cry out like a mad man, that with his noises he disquieted all the rest that were sick, so that they could not sleep or take any rest: and so it fell out very strangely that, one being ill, all the rest fared the worse. But as I had before learned of the Reverent Bishop Floridus, who was at that time there present with the said Priest, and afterwards also plainly understood of him that attended that night upon the sick persons, the foresaid venerable Priest, rising out of his bed, went softly to the place where the mad man lay, and there prayed, laying his hands upon him; whereupon the man became somewhat better. Then he carried him away into the higher part of the house, into the oratory; where more plentifully he prayed unto God for his recovery: and straight after he brought him back to his own bed safe and sound, so that he cried out no more, neither troubled any of the other sick persons.[35]

49. *Pliny's Letters*

[Pliny the Younger, the author of the *Letters*, lived from about A.D. 62 to 113. His *Letters* are said to provide a good picture of Roman life of his time. The following excerpt from his numerous communications to the Emperor Trajan, written in 112 from Bithynia, where he was governor,[36] reveals the methods used to extract confessions from prisoners. The reply of the Emperor, who was known for his justice, indicates that he considered Pliny's action a proper one.[37]]

They [those accused of being Christians] affirmed, however, the whole of their guilt, or their error, was, that they were in the habit of meeting on a certain fixed day before it was light, when they sang in alternate verses a hymn to Christ, as to a god, and bound themselves by a solemn oath, not to any wicked deed, but never to commit a fraud, theft or adultery, never to falsify their word, nor deny a trust when they should be called upon to deliver it up; after which it was their custom to separate, and then reassemble to partake of food—but food of an ordinary and innocent kind. Even this practice, however, they had abandoned after the publication of my edict, by which, according to your orders, I had forbidden political associations. I judged it so much more necessary to extract the real truth, with the assistance of torture, from two female slaves, who were styled deaconesses [*ministrae*]: but I could discover nothing more than depraved and excessive superstition. I therefore adjourned the proceedings, and betook myself at once to your counsel . . .[38]

50. St. Jerome. Letter LXXVII. To Oceanus on the Death of Fabiola (Written 399)

[St. Jerome, or Eusebius Hieronymus, the great Christian scholar, and Father of the Church, was born in 345 in Dalmatia and died in 420. His literary works, aside from his *Letters,* are voluminous and include Bible translations, commentaries, books on scriptural subjects, and Church history as well as general history. His *Letters* are sometimes grouped with three other outstanding collections of letters in Latin—those of Cicero, Seneca, and Pliny.[39] Many of them were written in praise of certain Roman matrons who performed many charitable deeds, including the care of the sick, and who lived lives of extreme asceticism. This and Reading No. 51 are two of his letters.]

Today you give me as my theme Fabiola, the praise of the Christians, the marvel of the gentiles, the sorrow of the poor, and the consolation of the monks. Whatever point in her character I choose to treat of first, pales into insignificance compared with those which follow after. Shall I praise her fasts? Her alms are greater still. Shall I commend her lowliness? The glow of her faith is yet brighter. Shall I mention her studied plainness in dress, her voluntary choice of plebian costume and the garb of a slave that she might put to shame silken robes? To change one's disposition is a greater achievement than to change one's dress.

Yet it was then that she put on sackcloth to make confession of her error. It was then that in the presence of all Rome . . . she stood in the ranks of the penitents and exposed before bishop, presbyters, and people—all of whom wept when they saw her weep—her dishevelled hair, pale features, soiled hands and unwashed neck. . . . That face by which she had once pleased her second husband she now smote with blows; she hated jewels, shunned ornaments and could not bear to look upon fine linen.

Restored to communion before the eyes of the whole church, what did she do? In the days of prosperity she was not forgetful of affection; . . . she broke up and sold all that she could lay hands on of her property (it was large and suitable to her rank), and turning it into money she laid out this for the benefit of the poor. She was the first person to found a hospital, into which she might gather sufferers out of the streets and where she might nurse the unfortunate victims of sickness and want. Need I recount the various ailments of human beings? Need I speak of noses slit, eyes put out, feet half burnt, hands covered with sores? Or of limbs dropsical and atrophied? Or of diseased flesh alive with worms? Often did she carry on her own shoulders persons infected with jaundice or with filth. Often too did she wash away the matter discharged from wounds which others, even though men, could not bear to look at. She gave food to her patients with her own hand, and moistened the scarce breathing lips of the dying with sips of liquid. I know of many wealthy and devout persons who, unable to overcome their natural repugnance to such sights, perform this work of mercy by the agency of others, giving money instead of personal aid. I do not blame them and am far from construing their weakness of resolution into a want of faith. While however I pardon such squeamishness, I extol to the skies the enthusiastic zeal of a mind that is above it . . .

> Not with a hundred tongues or throat of bronze
> Could I exhaust the forms of fell disease

which Fabiola so wonderfully alleviated in the suffering poor that many of the healthy fell to envying the sick. However she showed the same liberality towards the clergy and monks and virgins. Was there a monastery which was not supported by Fabiola's wealth? Was there a naked or bedridden person who was not clothed with garments supplied by her? Were there ever any in want to whom she failed to give a quick and unhesitating supply? Even Rome was not wide enough for her pity. Either in her own person or else through the agency of reverend and trustworthy men she went from island to island and carried her bounty not only round the Etruscan Sea, but throughout the district of the Volscians, as it stands along those secluded and winding shores where communities of monks are to be found.

Suddenly she made up her mind, against the advice of all her friends, to take ship and come to Jerusalem. Here she was welcomed by a large concourse of people and for a short time took advantage of my hospitality.

51. St. Jerome. Letter CVIII. To Eustochium (Written 404)

In what terms shall I speak of her [Paula's] distinguished, and noble, and formerly wealthy house; all the riches of which she spent upon the poor? How can I describe the great consideration she showed to all and her far reaching kindness even to those whom she had never seen? What poor man, as he lay dying, was not wrapped in blankets given by her? What bedridden person was not supported with money from her purse? She would seek out such with the greatest diligence throughout the city, and would think it a misfortune were any hungry or sick person to be supported by another's food. So lavish was her charity that she robbed her children; and when her relatives remonstrated with her for doing so, she declared that she was leaving to them a better inheritance in the mercy of Christ.

Not long afterwards, making up her mind to dwell permanently in holy Bethlehem, she took up her abode for three years in a miserable hostelry; till she could build the requisite cells and monastic buildings, to say nothing of a guest house for passing travellers where they might find the welcome which Mary and Joseph had missed.

She never entered a bath except when dangerously ill. Even in the severest fever she rested not on an ordinary bed but on the hard ground covered only with a mat of goat's hair; if that can be called rest which made day and night alike a time of almost unbroken prayer . . .

Besides establishing a monastery for men, she divided into three companies and monasteries the numerous virgins whom she had gathered out of different provinces, some of whom were of noble birth while others belonged to the middle or lower classes.

How shall I describe her kindness and attention towards the sick or the wonderful care and devotion with which she nursed them? Yet, although when others were sick she freely gave them every indulgence, and even allowed them to eat meat; when she fell ill herself, she made no concessions to her own weakness, and seemed unfairly to change in her own case to harshness the kindness which she was always ready to shew to others.[40]

52. St. Basil. Letter XCIV. To Elias, Governor of the Province (Written 372)

[St. Basil, known as Basil the Great, lived from about 330 to 379. He came of a distinguished family which included his brother, Gregory of Nyssa, and his sister, St. Macrina. He became Bishop of Caesarea in 370. Among his writings are three hundred letters,[41] extracts from four of which, referring to the hospital which he founded in Caesarea, are quoted here in the three following readings.]

Still possibly it might be urged that I have done damage to the government by erecting a magnificently appointed church to God, and round it a dwelling house, one liberally assigned to the bishop, and others underneath, allotted to the officers of the Church in order, the use of both being open to you of the magistracy and your escort. But to whom do we do any harm by building a place of entertainment for strangers, both for those who are on a journey and for those who require medical treatment on account of sickness, and so establishing a means of giving these men the comfort they want, physicians, doctors, means of conveyance and escort?

53. St. Basil. Letter CXLII. To the Prefect's Accountant (Written 373)

I assembled all my brethren the chorepiscopi at the Synod of the blessed martyr Eupsychius to introduce them to your excellency. On account of your absence they must be brought before you by letter. Know, therefore, this brother being as worthy to be trusted by your intelligence, because he fears the Lord. As to the matters on behalf of the poor, which he refers to your good will, deign to believe him as one worthy of credit, and to give the afflicted all the aid in your power. I am sure you will look favourably upon the hospital of the poor which is in this district, and consent to exempt it altogether from taxation. It has already seemed good to your colleague to make the little property of the poor not liable to be rated.

54. St. Basil. Letter CXLIII. To Another Accountant (Written 373)

Had it been possible for me to meet your excellence I would have in person brought before you the points about which I am anxious and would have pleaded the cause of the afflicted, but I am prevented by illness and the press of business. I have therefore sent to you in my stead this chorepiscopus, my brother, begging you to take him into counsel, for his truthfulness and sagacity qualify him to advise in such matters. If you are so good as to inspect the hospital for the poor, which is managed by him (I am sure you will not pass it without a visit, experienced as you are in the work; for I have been told that you support one of the hospitals at Amaseas out of the substance wherewith the Lord has blessed you), I am confident that, after seeing it, you will give him all he asks. Your colleague has already pronounced me some help towards the hospitals. I tell you this, not that you may imitate him, for you are likely to be a leader of others in good works, but that you may know that others have shown regard for me in this matter.

55. St. Basil. Letter CL. To Amphilochius in the Name of Heraclidas (Written 373)

I was lately at Caesarea in order to learn what was going on there. I was unwilling to remain in the city itself, and betook myself to the neighboring hospital [built by Basil], that I might get there what information I wanted.[42]

56. *The Ecclesiastical History of Eusebius*

[Eusebius of Caesarea (c. 263–339?), bishop of Caesarea in Palestine but better known as a historian, wrote from a moderate point of view on the events of his day. He wrote theological treatises, histories, and a biography of Constantine. His *Ecclesiastical History,* written between 323 and 325,[43] in ten books, is one of the few contemporary records of the events of the early Christian Church.[44]]

For most of our brethren were unsparing in their exceeding love and brotherly kindness. They held fast to each other and visited the sick fearlessly, and ministered to them continually, serving them in Christ. . . . And many who cared for the sick and gave strength to others died themselves, having transferred to themselves their death.[45]

57. *The Ecclesiastical History of Sozomen*

[Sozomen, a fifth-century church historian, without doubt drew his material from the church history of Socrates Scholasticus, his contemporary, who, in turn, probably used the work of his predecessor, Eusebius. Sozomen's work was written between 439 and 450.[46] Among matters touched on are the founding of hospitals, laws of Theodosius relating to the deaconesses, and the work of certain individuals in nursing the sick. The following extracts refer to the work of St. Ephrem and of Nicarete.]

III, 16. Concerning St. Ephraim.

The city of Edessa being severely visited by famine, he quitted the solitary cell in which he pursued philosophy, and rebuked the rich for permitting the poor to die around them, instead of imparting to them of their superfluities. . . . The rich men, revering the man and his words, replied, "We are not intent upon hoarding our wealth, but we know of no one to whom we can confide the distribution of our goods, for all are prone to seek after lucre, and to betray the trust placed in them." "What think you of me?" asked Ephraim. On their admitting that they considered him an efficient, excellent, and good man, and worthy, and that he was exactly what his reputation confirmed, he offered to undertake the distribution of their alms. As soon as he received their money, he had about three hundred beds fitted up in the public porches; and here he tended those who were ill and suffering from the effects of the famine, whether they were foreigners or natives of the surrounding country. . . . He attained no higher clerical degree than that of deacon . . .

.   .   .   .

Among the zealous men and excellent women . . . was Nicarete, a lady of Bithynia. She belonged to a noted family of the nobility, and was celebrated on account of her perpetual virginity and her virtuous life. She was the most modest of all the zealous women that we have ever known, and was well ordered in manner and speech and in behavior, and throughout her life she invariably preferred the service of God to all earthly considerations. She showed herself capable of enduring with courage and thought the sudden reversals of adverse affairs; she saw herself unjustly despoiled of the greater part of her ample patrimony without manifesting any indignation, and managed the little that remained to her with so much economy that although she was advanced in age, she contrived to supply all the wants of her household, and to contribute largely to others. Since she loved a humane spirit, she also prepared a variety of remedies for the needs of the sick poor, and she frequently succeeded in curing patients who had derived no benefit from the skill of the customary physicians. With a devout strength which assisted her in reaching the best results, she closed her lips. To sum up all in a few words, we have never known a devoted woman endowed with such manners, gravity, and every other virtue. Although she was so extraordinary, she concealed the greater part of her nature and deeds; for by modesty of character and philosophy she was always studious of concealment. She would not accept the office of deaconess nor of instructress of the virgins consecrated to the services of the Church, because she accounted herself unworthy, although the honor was frequently pressed upon her by John.[47]

58. *The Ecclesiastical History of Theodoret*

[Theodoret, church historian, became bishop of Cyrrhus, in Syria, in 423.[48] He was a lifelong friend of Nestorius, and held that the Nestorians, who opposed certain orthodox Church teachings, were misunderstood.]

Yet other opportunities of improvement lay within the emperor's [Theodosius'] reach, for his wife [Placilla or Flacilla] used constantly to put him in mind of the divine laws in which she had first carefully educated herself. In no way exalted by her imperial rank she was rather fired by it with greater longing for divine things. The greatness of the good gift given her made her love for Him who gave it all the greater, so she bestowed every kind of attention on the maimed and the mutilated, declining all aid from her household and her guards, herself visiting the houses where the sufferers lodged, and providing every one with what he required. She also went about the guest chambers of the churches and ministered to the wants of the sick, herself handling pots and pans, and tasting broth, now bringing in a dish and breaking bread and offering morsels, and washing out a cup and going through all the other duties which are supposed to be proper to servants and maids.[49]

59. *Procopius*

[Procopius, Byzantine historian, lived in the fifth century, although the exact date is uncertain. His histories are thought to have unusual merit, showing industry in collecting facts and in describing events which he witnessed, but carelessness in the use of sources.[50] He describes in detail the chief public works of Justinian, of which the hospitals are of especial interest.]

He made provision likewise for the poor of the place [Antioch] who were suffering from maladies, providing buildings for them and for all the means for the care and cure of their ailments, for men and women separately, and he made no less provision for strangers who might on occasion be staying in the city.

[At Pythia] ... he enlarged and made much more notable both the Church of the Archangel and the infirmary for the sick.

[In Jerusalem] ... he ... built two hospices. ... One of these is destined for the shelter of visiting strangers, while the other is an infirmary for poor persons suffering from disease.[51]

60. William, Archbishop of Tyre. *A History of Deeds Done Beyond the Sea*

[William, Archbishop of Tyre, the author of this account, is generally regarded as having written with meticulous care the first comprehensive history of the Crusades. He was archbishop of Tyre from 1175 until his death in 1184 or 1185.[52] His detailed history of the founding of the Hospital of the Latins in Jerusalem in the sixth century is of great interest. Although written in a time much later than the early centuries of the Christian Era, it is included here because it describes a hospital built in Jerusalem at a very early date.]

In the time of the Roman Emperor Heraclius [c. 575–642], according to ancient histories ... the kingdom of Jerusalem, with all Syria and Egypt and the adjacent provinces, because of our sires fell into the hands of the enemies of the Christian faith and name. Nevertheless, although the holy places were thus under the power of the enemy from time to time, many people from the West visited them for the sake of devotion or business, possibly for both. Among those from the West who ventured at that time to go to the holy places for the purpose of trade, were certain men from Italy who were known as Amalfitani from the name of their city ...

Faithful to the traditions of their fathers and the Christian profession, these merchants were in the habit of visiting the holy places whenever opportunity offered. They had no house of their own at Jerusalem, however, where they might remain for a while. ... They [therefore] ... presented a petition in writing [to the caliph of Egypt, for a place where they might build a church].

In accordance with the caliph's command, a place sufficiently large for the necessary buildings was set aside for the people of Amalfi. Offerings of money were collected from the merchants, and before the door of the church of the Resurrection of the Lord, barely a stone's throw away, they built a monastery in honor of the holy and glorious mother of God, the Ever Virgin Mary. In connection with this there were suitable offices for the use of the monks and for the entertainment of guests from their own city.

When the place was finished, they brought an abbot and monks from Amalfi and established the monastery under a regular rule as a place of holy life acceptable to the Lord. Since those who had founded the place and maintained it in religion were men of the Latin race, it has been called from that time until this the monastery of the Latins.

Even in those days it often happened that chaste and holy widows came to Jerusalem to kiss the revered places. Regardless of natural timidity, they had met without fear the numberless dangers of the way. Since there was no place within the portals of the monastery where such pilgrims might be honorably received, the same pious men who had founded the monastery made a suitable provision for these people also, that when devout women came they might not lack a chapel, a house, and separate quarters of their own. A little convent was finally established there, by divine mercy, in honor of that pious sinner Mary Magdalene, and a regular number of sisters placed there to minister to women pilgrims.

During these same perilous times there also flocked thither people of other nations, both nobles and those of the middle class. As there was no approach to the Holy City except through hostile lands, pilgrims had usually exhausted their travelling money by the time they had reached Jerusalem. Wretched and helpless, a prey to all the hardships of hunger, thirst, and nakedness, such pilgrims were forced to wait before the city gates until they had paid a gold coin, when they were permitted to enter the city. Even after they finally gained admission and had visited the holy places one after another, they had no means of resting even for a single day, except as it was offered in a fraternal spirit by the brothers of this monastery . . .

Since there was no one to offer shelter to the wretched pilgrims of our faith, thus afflicted and needy to the last degree, the holy men who dwelt in the monastery of the Latins, in pity took from their own means and, within the space allotted to them, built a hospital for the relief of such pilgrims. There they received these people, whether sick or well, lest they be found strangled at night on the streets. In addition to offering shelter in the hospital, they arranged that the fragments remaining from the food supplies of the two monasteries, namely, of the monks and of the nuns, should be spared for the daily sustenance of such people.

Furthermore, they erected in that place an altar in honor of St. John the Almoner. This John was a native of Cyprus . . . called *Eleymon*, which being interpreted, is "merciful."

This venerable foundation which thus stretched out the hand of charity to its fellowmen had neither revenues nor possessions; but each year the citizens of Amalfi, both those at home and those who followed the business of trading abroad, collected money from their own number as a voluntary offering. This they sent to the abbot of the hospital, whoever he might be at the time, by the hands of those who were going to Jerusalem. From this money food and shelter were provided for the brethren and sisters and the remainder was used to extend some assistance to the Christian pilgrims who came to the hospital . . .[53]

61. *Of the Holy Places Visited by Antoninus Martyr*

[Little is known of the Antoninus who wrote this account. The title "Martyr" is assumed to have arisen from a confusion with an earlier pilgrim. There seems to be no reason to question that he really made the journey. It is believed that the date was about A.D. 530. He may have been a member of a religious group of some sort.[54] He tells his tale in simple language without any literary pretensions, with some inaccuracies, and with a strong belief in magic. It is of interest in its reference to the monastery of St. John, and of the hospices.]

Above the Jordan, and not far from the river where our Lord was baptised, is the Monastery of St. John, a very large building, in which are two hospices.

From Sion we came to the Basilica of the Blessed Mary, where is a large congregation of monks, and where are also hospices (for strangers, both) for men and women. There I was received as a pilgrim; there were countless tables, and more than three thousand beds for sick persons.

Setting out from the city of Elath [Elua or Eluaha] we entered the desert. Twenty miles on the road there is a castle, where is a hospice of St. George, in which travellers find shelter and hermits an allowance.[55]

62. Epitaphs on the Tombs of Two Deaconesses

[The epitaphs quoted below are of interest and value as evidence concerning the female diaconate. Each gives the name of the deaconess. The first is of the sixth century, and was found at Pavia in northern Italy. The second, of the eleventh century, was discovered at Hellespontus, a province of Asia Minor (modern western Turkey).]

Epitaph on the tomb of a deaconess, in Pavia, Italy

HERE · RESTS · IN · PEACE
THEODORA · THE · DEACONESS
OF · BLESSED · MEMORY
SHE · LIVED · IN · THE · WORLD
FORTY · EIGHT · YEARS · MORE · OR · LESS
AND · WAS · LAID · TO · REST
ON · THE · TWENTY · SECOND · OF · JULY
IN · THE · YEAR
FIVE · HUNDRED · AND · THIRTY · NINE [56]

Epitaph on the tomb of a deaconess at Hellespontus, Asia Minor

HERE · RESTS
THE · EVER · TO · BE · REMEMBERED
HANDMAID · OF · CHRIST · AERIA
WHICH · WAS · DEACONESS · OF · THE · SAINTS
THE · FRIEND · OF · ALL
SHE · PASSED · TO · REST
THE · THIRD · OF · JANUARY · 1086 [57]

63. Charles Kingsley. *Hypatia*

[Charles Kingsley (1819–1875), English clergyman and novelist, is perhaps best known for his historical novels. In the preface of *Hypatia,* he states, "I have in my sketch of Hypatia and her fate closely followed authentic history." In a letter to a friend in January, 1851, he says that his idea in writing the novel was to set forth Christianity as the only really democratic creed and philosophy.[58] The scene of the following excerpt from the novel is laid in Alexandria. It describes the work of the *parabolani,* a minor group of attendants on the sick in that city.]

So Philammon went out with the parabolani, a sort of organized guild of district visitors. . . . And in their company he saw that afternoon the dark side of that world whereof the harbor panorama had been the bright one. In squalid misery, filth, profligacy, ignorance, ferocity, discontent, neglected in body, house and soul by the civil authorities, proving their existence only in aimless and sanguinary riots, there they starved and rotted, heap on heap, the masses of the old Greek population, close to the great food-exporting harbor of the world. Among these, fiercely perhaps, and fanatically, but still among them and for them, labored those district visitors night and day. And so Philammon toiled away with them, carrying food and clothing, helping sick to the hospital, and dead to the burial; cleaning out the infected houses —for the fever was all but perennial in those quarters—comforting the dying with the good news of forgiveness from above, till the larger number had to return for evening service. He, however, was kept by his superior watching at a sick bedside, and it was late at night before he got home, and was reported to Peter the Reader as having acquitted himself like "a man of God," as, indeed, without the least thought of doing anything noble or self-sacrificing, he had truly done, being a monk.[59]

CONCLUDING STATEMENT

Having before it the teachings of Christ as expressed in the four Gospels of the New Testament, directing the disciples to be concerned for and actively engaged in the care of the sick and unfortunate, the

Church set about providing for this in various ways. Among the earliest regulations were the *Apostolical Constitutions* and the *Didascalia Apostolorum,* which were crystallizations of the moral and ecclesiastical instructions of the Church; and the canons of the early Church, which represented the decisions of Church councils. These writings set forth the characteristics and duties of early Church officers such as the deacons and deaconesses, widows, and virgins. Among the important functions was the ministration to the sick. These documents are sometimes contradictory with reference to the status of these individuals, as in the case of the ordination of deaconesses.

Monastic rules, the first developed by St. Benedict in 528, specify that the sick of the religious community were to be cared for by the other brethren or sisters. Whether the monks and nuns went outside the walls of the monastery to minister to the sick is not indicated by the rules quoted. Other writings of the Church Fathers mention the nursing done by various individuals, whether as deacons and deaconesses or in the capacity of other officials of the Church. In these, the distinction is not always clear between "visiting the sick" and "ministering" to them.

St. Jerome, the great historian of the Roman matrons, distinctly states that certain women of his day nursed the sick. The ascetic aspect of the lives of these women is clearly indicated.

Our knowledge of the nursing of the workers of the early Christian Church is also increased by the histories of the ecclesiastical historians who relate the stories of some contemporary deacons and deaconesses and others who ministered to the sick as an expression of their deep religious devotion. The epitaphs of two Christian deaconesses give the names of these women, and the dates on the inscriptions indicate the length of time when these officers continued to be recognized by the Church. The lessening of their importance seems to coincide to some extent with the growing importance of the monastic movement. Of less significance, but indicative, is the story of the young monk of Alexandria, who observed and participated in the work of the *parabolani,* a minor order which included nursing among its duties.

This work of the Church, begun in the first centuries of the Christian Era and carried on by various officers of the Church and by groups devoted to human welfare, continued to, and beyond, the period known as the Middle Ages, and up to the present time. In the span of approximately a thousand years, following the early Christian Era, great social movements of historical importance occurred.

The two main developments of interest in the history of nursing were the Crusades and the rise of certain orders in the Church, characterized by democratic and secular tendencies. These provided a number of outstanding individual workers as well as great institutions where the sick were cared for more effectively than formerly. These will be the subject of the next chapter, which seeks to present certain sources of the period of the Middle Ages that illustrate developments in nursing history.

Chapter 3

Nursing in the Literature
of the Middle Ages

INTRODUCTION

THE term "Middle Ages" is usually used to denote the period of history which occurred between the middle of the fifth century and the middle of the fifteenth century, or between ancient and modern times. Like other terms of a similar nature, it is erroneous in that history is progressive rather than static. Since the term has been employed by historians and others for a long period, its use becomes almost inevitable. It is a useful term because, for most practical purposes, it is fairly well understood.

In the history of the evolution of nursing, the period known as the Middle Ages is represented by two fairly distinct developments, occurring almost simultaneously. The two movements were different in that the one, the growth of militarism, was of a distinctly aristocratic nature, while the other, the rise of democracy, tended to be characterized by a spirit of equality. Both were associated with the Church in some measure. These great changes in social life fostered the foundations of groups known in the history of nursing as, first, the military nursing orders, chiefly the Knights of St. John, the Knights of St. Lazarus, and the Teutonic Knights; and second, the democratic or secular orders, first among which were the three orders of St. Francis of Assisi, the Brothers Minor, the Poor Clares, and the Tertiaries, in Italy, and of the Beguines in Flanders. The military nursing orders were an outcome of the Crusades to the Holy Land, and occurred, in point of time, approximately a century before the founding of the first Franciscan Friars. Both, however, arose in the period known as the Middle Ages, and continued side by side in their development. Both will be considered in this chapter, beginning first with the military nursing orders.

Pilgrimages to the tomb of Christ started soon after the crucifixion. In the beginning these journeys were undertaken by the inhabitants of the Holy Land itself. Later, as the gospel spread through the countries near Judea, they were engaged in by the faithful from more distant lands, as acts of Christian devotion. The ideal of Christian chivalry, characteristic of feudal society, stimulated more extensive expeditions in the Middle Ages, in which the avowed purpose was to conquer the Holy Land which had been in the hands of the Mohammedans for several centuries. Combined with this religious motive were others: political ambition, economic gain, and the desire for adventure. Thus, those participating included the clergy and pious folk, adventurers, and others who used the Crusades as an opportunity to satisfy many motives.

Next to participating in the pilgrimage as a combatant, the greatest virtue in the eyes of the faithful was devoting oneself to the service of the pilgrims. This gave rise to the formation of groups which were dedicated in various ways to this service: in the building of hospitals along the routes of the Crusades—upon banks of rivers, upon mountains, in cities, and in desert places—and in the giving of personal care to the patients in these hospitals. The military religious orders which combined the characteristics of religion and chivalry, militarism and charity, were an expression of the desire for service to the pilgrims.

The chief knightly orders of the Middle Ages were the Hospitallers and the Templars. The latter were devoted entirely to military purposes, while the former originated for the sole purpose of nursing the sick and wounded and affording shelter and aid to pilgrims visiting the Holy Sepulcher. Military duties were added by the Hospitallers at a later date.

The Crusades of the Middle Ages represented aristocratic and military ideals in social life, and the extension of Christianity by means of war— a holy war. On the other hand the work of the orders, founded in this same period by St. Francis of Assisi and others, exemplified the democratic and secular tendencies which developed almost side by side with the military orders, and the extension of Christianity by peaceful means. Many devout people took part in this movement. Those leaders best known to us include, among others, St. Francis of Assisi, St. Clare of Assisi, St. Elizabeth of Hungary, and St. Catherine of Siena. These individuals are of interest to those who seek to understand nursing history. All participated personally in the care of the sick of their communities and otherwise promoted measures which contributed to their care.

The place of St. Francis of Assisi in the history of nursing rests on his personal care of the lepers and the founding of the secular orders which were charged with the responsibility of caring for the sick and unfortunate. The life of St. Francis has been interestingly told many times. His care of the lepers in the beginning of his career of devotion, and his promotion of the three orders—the first, the Brothers Minor, or Little Poor Brothers, the second, the Poor Clares, and the third, the Tertiaries—did much to spread democratic ideals in social life and, in particular, in the care of the sick.

The life of St. Clare of Assisi was interwoven with that of St. Francis, first as a friend and later as the co-founder of the Poor Clares to whom St. Francis is believed to have given a rule in 1253. It would probably be a mistake to ascribe to the Poor Ladies any widespread activity in the care of the sick. Their chief preoccupation seems to have been with the contemplative life. They did, however, care for their own members in the monastery, as have many other orders. It is said, also, that they cared for those who were brought to them.

The virtues of St. Elizabeth of Hungary have been set forth in prose, in poetry, and in music. Her claim to a place in nursing history rests on her personal care of the sick, particularly children and lepers, and the promotion of hospital building in Hungary. Both she and her relatives built hospitals.

St. Catherine of Siena, although remembered chiefly for her political influence, was also a hospital nurse during times of pestilence in Italy. Her nursing of individuals suffering from leprosy and other diseases is of interest also.

These four "nursing saints" but exemplify the many men and women who, in this era, lived lives of devotion to the sick and needy of their communities, and whose influence was felt widely in succeeding ages. In northern Europe, at this time, another group of workers with secular characteristics began caring for the sick of Flanders. These women were known as the Beguines and antedated the Franciscans. An order of men, the Beghards, was of short duration.

In addition to the work of the increasingly important secular groups, nursing by the regular orders continued. At the same time it is interesting to note the occasional reference to nursing in the home, which, it may be assumed, went on as before, aided by the work of the members of religious groups. This period was also a time of activity in hospital building by individuals, as in the case of St. Elizabeth of Hungary.

The literature of the Crusades has been fully and adequately dealt with by many scholars. Each Crusade found its chroniclers, both Eastern and Western. The purposes of this book will be best served by reference chiefly to those sources which hold special interest for the student of nursing history. For a full understanding of the role of the Crusades in the care of the sick, it is necessary to consult not only the writers of the West but also those of the East.

The most interesting and instructive sources for the study of the

Crusades themselves include eyewitness accounts, chronicles, narratives, and histories written from the original sources by contemporary and later historians. The crusaders themselves sometimes kept diaries, and historians of the times, mainly in the Church, wrote accounts from those documents coming to their hands. These have value because they constitute almost the first pictures of contemporary life in Europe after the fall of the Roman Empire in the fifth century. Rich in military history, they, however, yield few direct references to nursing. Excerpts from three of these will be included: Thomas Fuller's *The Historie of the Holy Warre,* written in 1639 (64); *The Alexiad* of Anna Comnena, written from the Eastern point of view (65); and *Memoirs of the Crusades,* by Villehardouin and de Joinville, the so-called "Joinville's Chronicle" (66).

Another source of information is found in contemporary official documents, such as the bulls of popes relative to the military orders, and rules adopted by the knights. Pilgrim travelers who followed in the wake of the crusaders aid our knowledge, particularly with reference to the hospitals in the Holy Land, and in other countries occupied by the crusaders. Contemporary documents, recognizing the orders officially, gave importance to the work of the latter. Among those quoted here are the following: the bull of Pope Paschal II (67); the bull of Alexander IV (68); the charter given by Richard Coeur-de-Lion to the commandery of Villedieu-les-Pöeles (69); the rules of Raymond du Puy (70), Roger des Moulin (71), and Nicholas le Lorgue (72); and the regulations of Malta Hospital in the eighteenth century (73). *The Old and New Statutes of the Order of St. John of Jerusalem,* dated 1676, give many points concerning the qualifications and duties of the knights (74).

Accounts of pilgrim travelers who followed the crusaders include those of Saewulf (75), Fetullus (76), John of Würzburg (77), Theodorich (78), and von Suchem (79). All refer in their narratives to the hospitals of the knights. Later travelers such as John Howard (80), Sir Richard Colt Hoare (81), and the Comte de Saint Priest (82), speak of the hospitals of the military orders and indicate the changes which had taken place after the lapse of centuries.

Information concerning the activities of the so-called democratic and secular orders of the Middle Ages is more plentiful than in the case of the military nursing orders. This is especially true of the sources on St. Francis of Assisi and the groups founded by him. Criticism of the sources on St. Francis engages the interest of scholars even today. The chief ones of interest include the *Rules* of the Franciscans, and the *Testament* of St. Francis, both among the writings of the saint himself (83); the lives of the saint by Brother Thomas of Celano (84); the

68

official biography, the *Legenda Maior S. Francisci,* by St. Bonaventura (85); the *Legend of S. Francis by the Three Companions* (86); the *Mirror of Perfection of St. Francis of Assisi* (87); and the *Fioretti* or *Little Flowers of St. Francis* (88). Authorities differ about the genuineness and value of the last three of these works. However, as pictures of the supposed activities, they give the student of nursing history a feeling of the tradition of the saint.

With reference to materials on St. Clare of Assisi, the situation is somewhat different. Sabatier states that the greater number of the documents concerning St. Clare have disappeared.[1] Some are available, however. The Rule of 1253 (89) indicates that the Poor Clares cared for their own members, but whether their care extended to the surrounding community is uncertain.

For St. Elizabeth of Hungary, one of the earliest lives is that of Theodorich of Thuringen, or Dietrich of Apolda, which, as far as is known, has not been translated into English. A short excerpt is included here (90). Another is by Montalembert, published in 1836 (91). St. Elizabeth has been the subject of many later works, among which is *The Saint's Tragedy* (92) by Charles Kingsley.

The sources for the life and deeds of St. Catherine of Siena include the original life, called the *Legenda;* the *Process;* the *Supplementum* to the *Legenda;* an abridgment of Raimondo's *Legenda,* the *Legenda Abbreviata;* and finally a few letters of Catherine, which have been preserved. The sources quoted in this chapter include the original *Life* by Raimondo, or Raymond of Capua (93), and a modern one by Augusta Theodosia Drane, who purportedly compiled it from the sources mentioned above (94).

For information concerning the Beguines, the present compilation has relied on modern accounts by English travelers in Flanders in the nineteenth century. Among these visitors, Robert Southey (95), Dr. Robert Gooch (96, 97), and Elizabeth De Bunsen (98), were much impressed by the work of the Beguines, and advocated similar orders for England.

A few references to nursing by members of regular orders indicate that this was done, either in the monastery or in the homes of the patients; the point is not clear. It is assumed that nursing was carried on in both places. The regulations of medieval religious orders included provisions for an "infirmaress," who was to care for the sick of the religious community. Such an order was that of Syon Monastery in Middlesex, England (99). Occasionally a recorded will in England is instructive. The will of Sir Roger Salwayn, knight of York, shows that a nun had cared for him at one time (100). The ballads of Robin Hood's death picture him as being cared for by a prioress, his cousin (101).

Nursing in the home is also mentioned in some references; for example, "Joinville's Chronicle" of the Crusade of St. Lewis speaks of "ladies who were tending him." In the Paris Tax Roll of 1292, ten "nourrices" are listed, while two are to be found as recipients of public alms in 1462 (102).

References to the building of hospitals sometimes stated in detail the purpose of their founding (103). Except in rare instances, no mention is made specifically of nurses for the patients of those hospitals, until a later date. That there were individuals charged with that responsibility is assumed. The gifts to hospitals by individuals occasionally included the provision, in return, that the person should be permitted to live in the hospital and render service as a sister or nurse. The charter of Isabella of Bray to St. Bartholomew's Hospital included such a provision (104). The will of William Gregory, Mayor of London from 1451 to 1452, included bequests to several hospitals and mentioned a "suster" in Elsyng Spitell (105).

THE SOURCES

The Military Nursing Orders

64. Thomas Fuller. *The Historie of the Holy Warre*

[Thomas Fuller (1608–1661) was an English divine and historian. After graduation from Cambridge he became the curate of St. Benet's, Cambridge, and later prebend of Broadwindsor. While at Broadwindsor he wrote *The Historie of the Holy Warre* (1639). He was author of a well-known church history also. He was known as a witty orator and preacher, with a keen sense of humor which made him moderate in his religious views.[2]]

About this time [1099] under Gerald their first master, began the order of Knights-hospitallers. Indeed more anciently there were Hospitallers in Jerusalem; but these were no knights: they had a kind of order, but no honour annexed to it; but were pure Almsmen, whose house was founded and they maintained by the charity of the merchants of Amalphia a citie in Italy ...

To make one capable of the highest order of this knighthood (for their servitours and priests might be of an inferior rank) the party must thus be qualified: Eighteen years old at the least; of an able body, not descended of Jewish or Turkish parents; no bastard, except bastard to a Prince, there being honour in that dishonour, as there is light in the very spots of the moon. Descended he must be of worshipfull parentage. They wore a red belt with a white crosse; and on a black cloke the white crosse of Jerusalem, which is a crosse crossed, or five crosses together, in memorie of our Saviours five

70

wounds. Yet was there some difference betwixt their habit in peace and in warre. Their profession was to fight against Infidels, and to secure Pilgrimes coming to the Sepulchre; and they vowed Poverty, Chastity, and Obedience . . .[3]

65. Anna Comnena. *The Alexiad*

[This Byzantine account of the First Crusade, by Anna Comnena, the daughter of the Emperor Alexius I (1081–1118), is regarded as the most important Eastern source because of Anna's position which gave her firsthand knowledge of public affairs. Though thought to be weak in chronology and geography, it represents one of the few detailed sources for events written from the point of view of the East.[4]]

Moreover since many of the women were with child and many of the men afflicted with disease, whenever a woman's time for bringing forth came, a trumpet was sounded at a nod from the Emperor and made all the men stop and the whole army halted on the instant. And when he knew the child was born a different call, not the usual one, but provocative of motion, was sounded and stirred them all up to continue the journey . . .

And when it was the Emperor's time for lunch he invited the men and women who were labouring under illness or old age and placed the greater part of the victuals before them and invited those who lunched with him to do the same.[5]

66. "Joinville's Chronicle"

[Jean Sire de Joinville (1224–1319) was head of a noble family of Champagne. He followed King (St.) Louis IX on the Seventh Crusade, and as an old man wrote in simple and reverent style the chronicle of the exploits of the king and of the Crusade. The following brief passage from the text mentions nurses who were caring for the king.[6]]

St. Lewis falls ill, and takes the Cross in 1244.

After the things related above, it happened, as God so willed, that a very grievous sickness came upon the king in Paris, and brought him to such extremity, so it was said, that one of the ladies who were tending him wished to draw the cloth over his face, saying he was dead; but another lady, who was on the other side of the bed, would not suffer it, and said the soul was still in his body.[7]

Official Documents Relating to the Care of the Sick by the Knights of St. John of Jerusalem

[Certain contemporary official documents are of interest in connection with the Hospitallers, and give some information concerning their activities in caring for the sick. The first, the bull of Pope Paschal II, confirming the foundation of the order, is dated February 15, 1113, and mentions the Blessed Gerard, the first head of the order. The habit of the knights was granted officially in 1259 in the bull of Alexander IV. Richard Coeur-de-Lion refers to the nursing activities of the knights in a eulogy given them when he granted a charter to a commandery of the order in Normandy in 1192.]

67. Bull of Pope Paschal II. Confirming the Foundation of the Order
Dated 15 *February* 1113

Paschal, Bishop, Servant of God, to his venerable son Gerard, founder and Provost of the Hospital in Jerusalem, and to his lawful successors in perpetuity. The request of a devout desire ought to meet with a corresponding fulfilment. In as much as of thine affection thou hast requested, with regard to the Hospital which thou hast founded in the city of Jerusalem, near to the church of the Blessed John Baptist, that it should be supported by the Apostolic See, and fostered by the patronage of the Blessed Apostle Peter. We therefore much pleased with the pious earnestness of thine hospitaller work do receive thy petition with our paternal kindness, and do ordain and establish by the authority of the present decree, that that house of God the Hospital, shall now be placed and shall forever remain under the protection of the Apostolic See and the guardianship of the Blessed Peter.... Amen. Amen.

> (signed) Paschal, Bishop of the Catholic Church [and other Bishops and Cardinals]...
>
> Given at Benevento by the hand of John, Cardinal of the Holy Roman Church and Librarian, on the 15th day before the Calends of March, in the 6th Indiction in the year 1113 of the Incarnation of Our Lord and in the fourteenth year of the Pontificate of our Lord Pope Paschal II.[8]

68. Bull of Alexander IV. Granting a Distinctive Dress to the Knights
Dated 11 *August* 1259

Alexander, Bishop, servant of the servants of God, to our beloved sons the Master and Brethren of the Hospital of St. John of Jerusalem, greeting and apostolic benediction...

Since it has come to our knowledge that amongst the brethren of your Order, both Knights and others, there is no distinction or diversity of dress, contrary to the usual custom in most other similar institutions,...we...do hereby grant to you by the authority of these presents, permission to decree unanimously and hereafter to maintain inviolate this rule, that the Knights, who are brethren of your Order, shall wear black mantles, in order that they may be distinguished from the other brethren of the said Order. In war however and in battle they shall wear jupons and other military surcoats, which shall be of a red colour, having sewn upon them a white cross, exactly as upon your standard, so that thus by the uniformity of outward signs the identity of your souls may be easily apparent, and that in consequence the safety of your persons may be ensured. Therefore let no one infringe upon this statute of our concession. For if anyone shall presume upon such an attempt, let him know that he will fall under the indignation of Almighty God, and of his blessed apostles, Peter and Paul.

Given at Angnia, on the 3rd day before the Ides of August, in the 5th year of our Pontificate.

69. The Eulogy to the Knights of St. John of Jerusalem Given by Richard Coeur-de-Lion, When He Gave a Charter to the Commandery of Villedieu-les Pöeles, in Normany [Given at Spire, 1192]

The grandeur and extent, not only of the renown of their organization, but also of the experience of it, has brought to our knowledge how magnificent and how great are the works in which this very holy House of the Hospital of Jerusalem abounds; all of which both by experience and testimony, we have seen with our own eyes, which have assured us of it. For besides the ordinary aid which the Masters and Brothers of Jerusalem give and render to the poor paupers, and over and above the efficiency and well-being of their House, they have also, both on this side and on the other of the sea, succoured, aided and entertained us with so great devotion and magnificence, that the extent of their aid and great benefits oblige our conscience not to pass it over in silence, but to be grateful for it.[9]

70. The Rule of Raymond du Puy

[Raymond du Puy succeeded Gerard, the first head of the hospital, probably in 1120, as Grand Master of the Order of Knights of St. John of Jerusalem.[10] Gerard, as founder, had established the strictly eleemosynary character of the order, which it retained during his lifetime. It is thought that Raymond was the first to institute military duties for the brothers, when it was necessary for them to defend the kingdom against the invaders from the East.[11] The date of the adoption of the rule is unknown but was, of course, between 1120 and 1160, when the name of Raymond's successor appears in the annals.]

This is the Constitution Ordained by Brother Raymond.—

In the name of God I, Raymond Servant of Christ's poor and warden of the Hospital of Jerusalem with the advice of all the Chapter, both clerical and lay brethren, have established these rules and statutes in the house of the Hospital of Jerusalem.

1. How the Brethren should make their Profession.—

Firstly I ordain that all the brethren engaging in the service of the poor shall keep with God's help the three promises that they have made to God, that is to say, chastity, obedience which is anything that is commanded them

73

by their masters, and to live without any property of their own, because God will require of them at the Last Judgment the fulfilment of these three promises.

.   .   .   .

16. How our Lords the Sick Should be Received and Served.—

And in that obedience where the master of the Hospital shall have permitted, when a sick person shall have come there, let him be received thus: firstly, having confessed his sins to a priest of the Religion (i.e., of the Order), let him partake of holy communion, and afterwards let him be carried to bed and there just as if he were the Lord let them be charitably entertained every day of the best the house can provide, before the brethren shall break their fast . . .[12]

71. The Rule of Fr. Roger des Moulin

[Roger des Moulin was elected in 1179 to fill the vacancy left by the death by wounds of the Master Joubert. Roger des Moulin thus became the seventh master. He lost his life in a battle with the Saracens under Saladin.[13] He was said to have been a valorous knight.[14] It is assumed that the following is an adaptation or a paraphrase rather than a literal translation of the rules.]

And secondly, it is decreed with the assent of the brethren, that for the sick of the Hospital of Jerusalem there should be engaged four wise doctors, who are qualified to examine urine, and to diagnose different diseases, and are able to administer appropriate medicines.

And thirdly, it is added that the beds of the sick should be made as long and as broad as is most convenient for repose, and that each bed should be covered with its own coverlet (*couvertour*) and each bed should have its own special sheets.

4. After these needs is decreed the fourth command, that each of the sick should have a cloak of sheepskin (*pelice a vestir*), and boots for going to and coming from the latrines, and caps of wool.

It is also decreed that little cradles should be made for the babies of women pilgrims born in the House, so that they may lie separate, and that the baby in its own bed may be in no danger from the restlessness of its mother.

.   .   .   .

The seventh clause commands that wheresoever there are hospitals for the sick, that the Commanders of the houses should serve the sick cheerfully and should do their duty by them, and serve them without grumbling or complaining, so that by these good deeds they may deserve to have their reward in the glories of heaven.

.   .   .   .

Moreover guarding and watching them day and night, the brethren of the Hospital should serve the sick poor with zeal and devotion as if they were their lords, and it was added in Chapter-General, that in every ward (*rue*) and place in the Hospital, nine serjeants [15] should be kept at their service who should wash their feet gently, and change their sheets, and make their beds, and administer to the weak necessary and strengthening food, and do their duty devotedly, and obey in all things for the benefit of the sick:

The Holy House of the Hospital is accustomed to receive sick men and women, and is accustomed to keep doctors who have the care of the sick, and who make syrups for the sick, and who provide the things that are necessary for the sick. For three days in the week the sick are accustomed to have fresh meat, either pork or mutton, and those who are unable to eat it have chicken.

And two sick persons are accustomed to have one cloak of sheepskin (*pelice de brebis*), which they use when going to the latrines (*chambres*), and between two sick persons, one pair of boots. Every year the House of the Hospital is accustomed to give to the poor one thousand cloaks of thick lamb skins.

And all the children abandoned by their fathers and mothers, the Hospital is accustomed to receive and to nourish. To a man and woman who desire to enter into matrimony, and who possess nothing with which to celebrate the marriage, the House of the Hospital is accustomed to give two bowls (*escules*) or the ration of two brethren.[16]

72. Statutes of Fr. Nicholas le Lorgue

[Nicholas le Lorgue was elected by the Knights of St. John to replace de Revel in 1278. Vertot says of him that he was "a knight of good natured and insinuating temper, who used his utmost endeavours, during his administration, to put an end to the divisions between the knights of his own order and those of the temple." [17]]

3. Concerning Black Mantles.—Item, it is decreed that all the brethren of the Hospital should wear black mantles with the white cross [worn originally by knights only].[18]

73. Regulations of Malta Hospital, 1725

The Wards

The proper separation of the diseases and conditions of the sick is observed in the Holy Infirmary, and therefore every room has its particular use, viz.:

The ward for the knights and persons of the habit (*persone dell' abito*), which is most comfortable (convenient), and there are two good rooms set apart for the wounded. An old ward for the laity, religious orders, and pilgrims. A large ward for those with fevers and other slight ailments. A small ward for serious cases and the dying, with a room adjoining. A new ward for those suffering from dysentery (*flussanti*), with two rooms for those who undergo lithotomy. A ward for the wounded, with two rooms. A very large ward for galley-slaves and two rooms. A room for the insane and their warder. Two wards for those undergoing mercurial inunction, separate from the Infirmary. A ward for those who take the hot baths, outside the Infirmary, to avoid any chance of *mal'aria*. Every ward in the Infirmary has its chapel well fitted for the Mass; and besides these, there is a chapel of the Most Holy Sacrament, the door of which opens towards the ward for the dying, for the convenience of the viaticum. The ordinary number of the sick is from 350 to 400, who remain until they are convalescent.

The Beds, Sheets, and Coverlets

The beds of the sick are changed from time to time for requisite cleanliness, and they are remade every morning by the warders, whose duty it is to keep them clean . . .

The beds used by persons suffering from consumption and similar complaints are burnt, with all the sheets and other things belonging without any reservation . . .

The sheets are changed, without exception, according to the needs of the sick, even though they should require changing several times a day . . .

The Silver Plate

It contributes greatly to the dignity of the Infirmary and to the cleanliness of the sick, their being served night and morning with covers (*posate*), bowls (*scodelle*), and plates (*tondini*) of silver; even the small boilers (*calderoni*), from which the soup is served, and the large dishes for the meat, and other things, are of silver . . .

The Quality of the Food

The *Prodomi*, above everything, look after the good quality of the supplies used in the preparation of the food, selecting the best of everything always; and therefore the sick are given the best soups made of chicken, herbs, vermicelli, rice, and minced meat which have been ordered for them, such as chicken, pigeons, fowls, beef, veal, game, hashes, fricassees, stews, forced meats,—in such quantities as are necessary; besides milk of almonds, fresh eggs, plums and raisins, and every kind of refreshments allowed sick people, such as restoratives, cakes, apples, pomegranates with sugar, and other kinds of confectures, according to the wants of each one. The Knights and Persons of the Habit receive double portions.

The Hangings and Pictures

For the greater comfort of the sick in winter, the walls of the rooms are hung with woolen curtains. . . . In summer the rooms are ornamented with pictures, which are properly dispersed about the walls—many of them representing the history of the Holy Religion. . . .

Regulations for the Sick Poor of Malta. Supplement to Regulations for
the Holy Infirmary, 1725

In order that the sick poor living in the four towns, Valetta, Borgo, Isola and Brumola, and in the island of Malta should receive proper assistance, two professed knights of different *langues* are nominated by the Most Eminent Grand Master, who are called Commissioners of the Sick Poor. They perform their duties for a month each in turn, and are entrusted with making a list, at the beginning of each week, of the sick poor in the four towns, in order to give them proper assistance. They superintend the physicians, to see that they perform their duty and visit each day the poor whose names are on the list, noting the remedies for those who require them, with due charity. To effect this, they are accustomed frequently to visit the poor at their homes, to relieve the wants of each, with the assistance of the supernumeraries, and to see that they are given the portions allowed them from the *Pitanziera,* and also that the Surgeons attend properly to the wounds and infections . . .

There are, moreover, four elderly women, known as *Pitanziere,* for the four towns aforesaid, who are charged with dispensing, day by day, the succor accorded the sick poor by the commissioners, and every week they must bring them the lists, all duly signed by physicians, to take the necessary orders.

They must accompany the commissioners whenever desired by them, in their visits, in order to show them the homes of the sick poor. These women have under them four other paid women, to carry the bread.

There are four paid maid-servants to wait on the poor, and who make the beds and do anything else that may be necessary.

There is likewise another woman to look after the *mancia,* and heat the food that may be needed. She must always keep a good soup in readiness for anyone who may need it at any time.

There is a man employed to look after the mercurial inunctions, and to wait on the incurables as may be required.[19]

74. *The Old and New Statutes of the Order of St. John of Jerusalem,* Edition of Borgoforte, A.D. M, DC, LXXVI

By Order of the Chapter of the Great Priory of France
Of the Habit of the brothers of the hospital of Jerusalem

Br. Raimon du Puy [1118?–1160]

3. 'Tis becoming our profession, that all the brothers of the hospital be obliged to wear a black robe or mantle with a white cross.

Br. Nicholas de Lorgue [1278–1289]

We enact likewise, that in the exercise of arms (i. e. when they are making a campaign) they wear over their cloaths red subreveste or military cassock, with the white cross strait.

Of the qualifications required in such as are admitted to make profession in our Order

Br. Hugh Revel [1259–1278]

5. We enact that no body shall from henceforward be admitted to profession, if he be not born in lawful wedlock, or if his father be a bastard, excepting however the sons of counts and persons of higher rank and quality.

Br. John de La Valetta [1557–1568]

6. And that such sons of counts and persons of higher quality, be descended from a father, whose father and grandfather by the father's side (the 13th article of this title adds great grandfather) were counts or lords of greater rank and degree.

Br. Claude de la Sengle [1553–1557]

7. And be born likewise of a mother that was a gentlewoman by birth.

Br. Anthony Fluvian [1421–1437]

12. Neither can any body that hath committed murder, or led a wicked and debauched life in the world.

Br. Philip de Villers de Lisle-Adams [1521–1534]

13. The habit of the order shall not be given to any body under eighteen years of age . . .

Br. Philip de L'Isle Adam

16. Let no body be admitted but who has good health, a strong constitution, and a body fit for fatigue, and is likewise in his right wits, and regular in his life and conversation.

Of the proofs necessary to be made before a knight is admitted

Br. Hugh Revel

17. Such as desire to be admitted knights, must prove by authentick evidence that they are born of parents noble both by name and arms.

Br. John de la Valette

18. Though our regulations do not insist on a noble descent, with regard to such as are to be admitted in quality of brother chaplains, or servants of arms, yet they ought not to be taken out of the rabble, and without any choice, which would be a ready way to make them contemptible: And therefore we enact, that for the future no body shall be admitted a brother chaplain, or servant of arms, either within or without the convent, not even by the special grace of the languages or priories, till he has first duly proved, that besides the necessary qualifications required by our statutes, he is born of genteel and creditable parents; that he never followed any mean and servile art or business; that he never was engaged under any body in any

vile or base employment; that neither he nor his parents ever followed any handicraft business, or practised any mean mechanical trade: provided, however, that this regulation do not extend to such as have signalized themselves in military actions, or by any eminent services that they have done to the order.

.   .   .   .   .   .

That the director of the infirmary visit the sick every night

Br. John de Lastic [1437–1454]

13. The director of the infirmary ought to be very careful of the sick, that no accident happen by his negligence. We enjoin him therefore to go attended by a faithful servant, to visit them with prudence and discretion at the hour of compline and day break, speak to them, exhort them, encourage them and assist them all he can. The comptrollers, when they go thither in the morning, shall enquire whether he has done his duty; if he has failed in any respect, they shall give him a severe reprimand, and order him to be more exact for the future; in failure of which, they must provide somebody else. The director of the infirmary shall take care to give the sick none but the best and most delicate sorts of food, as pullets and chickens, good bread and good wine, to supply them with good nourishment: the comptrollers are likewise ordered to take care that the sick be so treated.[20]

Hospitals of the Military Orders, as Described by Pilgrim Travelers and Others

75. The Travels of Saewulf

[The earliest of a new group of writers following the Crusades, Saewulf, came from England. He was probably not the first pilgrim traveler of this time, but he was the first to leave a record of his journey. In his old age, Saewulf became a monk in the Abbey of Malmesbury. It was as a merchant, in the years 1102 and 1103, that he undertook the pilgrimage to Jerusalem.[21]]

Without the gate of the Holy Sepulchre, to the south, is the church of St. Mary, called the Latin. . . . Adjoining to this church is another church of St. Mary, called the Little, occupied by nuns who served devoutly the Virgin and her Son. Near which is the Hospital, where is a celebrated monastery founded in honour of St. John the Baptist.[22]

76. *Fetullus*

[This narrative, under the name of Fetullus, Archbishop of Antioch, was written about 1200. It may have originated at an earlier date.[23] It is not known who the author really was, but it is said that the Archbishop was not the writer. It is so named because he executed one of the best-known editions of the work.[24]]

In Jerusalem is a Xenodochium, or Muscomion. Xenodochium is the Greek for a reception-house for strangers and the poor; Muscomion, i. e., a hospital where the sick are gathered from the streets and the villages and taken care of. Outside the walls of Jerusalem, between the Tower of Tancred and the Gate of St. Stephen, is a station for lepers. Myrcanus, the prince of the Jews, is said to have been the first to institute Xenodochia with money which he abstracted from the Sepulchre of David.[25]

77. *Description of the Holy Land by John of Wurzburg*

[John was priest of the Church of Wurzburg and, afterward, bishop of the city. He probably visited Jerusalem between 1160 and 1170, and wrote his description soon after 1200. He dedicated it to Theodorich.[26] In the narrative he complains that no one but the Germans help to support the hospice and church of St. Mary.]

Over against the Church of the Holy Sepulchre, . . . is a beautiful church built in honour of John the Baptist, annexed to which is a hospital, wherein in various rooms is collected together an enormous multitude of sick people, both men and women, who are tended and restored to health daily at a very great expense. When I was there I learned that the whole number of these sick people amounted to two thousand, of whom sometimes in the course of one day and night more than fifty are carried out dead, while many other fresh ones keep continually arriving. What more can I say? This same house supplies as many people outside it with victuals as it does those inside, in addition to the boundless charity which is daily bestowed upon poor people who beg their bread from door to door and do not lodge in the house, so that the whole sum total of its expense can surely never be calculated even by the managers and stewards thereof.

As you descend the same street beside the gate which leads to the Temple, on the right hand side, there is a kind of passage through a long portico, in which street is a hospice and a church, which has been newly built in honour of St. Mary, and which is called the House of the Germans, upon which hardly any men who speak any other language bestow any benefactions.[27]

78. *Theodorich's Description of the Holy Places*

[This Theodorich may be the one to whom John of Wurzburg dedicated his record, or he may have been the one who became Bishop of Wurzburg in 1223. His narrative is that of an intelligent eyewitness. The evidence points to the conclusion that he visited the Holy Land between 1169 and 1173.[28]]

Here, in front of the church [of the Latins], stand six columns, with arches above them; and here, on the south side of the church, stands the Church and Hospital of St. John the Baptist. As for this, no one can credibly tell another how beautiful its buildings are, how abundantly it is supplied with rooms and beds and other material for the use of the poor and sick people, how rich it is in the means of refreshing the poor, and how devotedly it labours to maintain the needy, unless he had the opportunity of seeing it with his own eyes. Indeed, we passed through this palace, and were unable by any means to discover the number of sick people lying there; but we saw that the beds numbered more than a thousand.

At the gate itself [St. Lazarus] stands a venerable hospice, which in Greek is called a *xenodochium*.

Many towers and large houses are possessed there [at Bethany] by the power of the Templars, whose practice, as also that of the Hospitallers is to escort pilgrims who are going to the Jordan, and to watch that they be not injured by the Saracens either in going or returning, or while passing the night there.[29]

79. *Ludolph von Suchem's Description of the Holy Land and of the Way Thither*

[The German priest who wrote this narrative dedicated it to Baldwin of Steinfurt, Bishop of Paderborn from 1340 to 1361. It has been described as "detailed," "legendary," and "amusing." [30] It is not always mythical, however. This account makes reference to the method of payment for care in the hospital of St. John of Jerusalem.]

Near the Church of the Holy Sepulchre once dwelt the brethren of St. John of Jerusalem, and their palace is now the common hospital for pilgrims. This hospital is so great that one thousand men can easily lie therein, and can have everything that they want there by paying for it. It is the custom in this palace, or hospital, that every pilgrim should pay two Venetian pennies for the use of the hospital. If he sojourns therein for a year he pays no more, if he abides but for one day he pays no less. In my time there dwelt in this palace, or hospital, a matron named Margaret of Sicily, who had a brother a canon of the Holy Sepulchre, named Nicholas. This Margaret was of great use and service there, and to my certain knowledge suffered much misery and trouble for love of the Christians, and was always viewed by the Soldan with especial favour because of her usefulness.[31]

80. John Howard. *An Account of the Principal Lazarettos in Europe*

[John Howard (1726–1790), the English prison reformer, was instrumental in securing the amelioration of conditions in prisons in England

and, indirectly, in America. His interest in plague prevention led him
to visit European hospitals. During his journeys he even caused himself
to be imprisoned in a Venetian lazaretto in order to learn at first hand
what the conditions were.[32] On one of his journeys he visited the hospital
of St. John of Jerusalem. This account, of a later time than the preceding
ones, indicates that some changes may have occurred in the care given
in this medieval military hospital.]

The *Hospital* (de S. Jean de Jerusalem) for men, is situated near the
water. The three principal wards are in the form of a T, which communicate
with one another, having an altar in the center. By additional buildings the
ward on one side is made longer than that on the other. Their breadth is
thirty-four feet and a half, but the cross ward is only twenty-nine feet and
four inches wide. These three wards connected are called the hall. The pave-
ment is of neat marble (or stone) squares. The ceiling is lofty, but, being
wood, now turned black; the windows being small, and the walls hung round
with dusty pictures, this noble hall makes but a gloomy appearance. All the
patients lie single. One ward is for patients dangerously sick or dying; another
for patients of the middle rank of life; and the third for the lower and poorer
sort of patients. In this last ward (which is the largest) there are four rows of
beds; in the others, only two. They were all so dirty and offensive as to create
the necessity of perfuming them; and yet I observed that the physician, in
going his rounds, was obliged to keep his handkerchief to his face . . .

.   .   .   .   .   .

The patients are twice a day, at eight and four, served with provisions;
one of the knights, and the under-physician constantly attending in the two
halls, and seeing the distribution. From the kitchen (which is darker and
more offensive than even the lower hall, to which it adjoins) the broth, rice
soup and vermicelli are brought in dirty kettles first to the upper hall, and
there poured into three silver bowls, out of which the patients are served.
They who are in the ward for the *very* sick, and those of the *middle* rank of
life, are served in plates, dishes and spoons of silver; but the other patients
(who are far the most numerous) are served in *pewter*.

The number of patients in the hospital during the time I was in Malta
(March 28th to April 19, 1786) was from five hundred and ten to five
hundred and thirty-two. These were served by the most dirty, ragged, unfeeling and unhuman persons I ever saw. I once found eight or nine of them
highly entertained with a delirious *dying* patient. The governor told me that
they had only twenty-two servants, and that many of them were debtors or
criminals, who had fled thither for refuge. . . . I cannot help adding, that in
the center of each of [the] . . . stables, there was a fountain out of which
water was constantly running into a stone basin; but that in the hospital,
though there was indeed a place for a fountain, there was no water.

.   .   .   .   .   .

In the *Hospital* for *Women* there were two hundred and thirty patients, who had all separate beds. The governess attended me through every ward, and was constantly using her smelling bottle; in which she judged very properly, for a more offensive and dirty hospital for women I never visited.[33]

81. Sir Richard Colt Hoare. *Recollections Abroad During the Year 1790*

[Sir Richard Colt Hoare, British historian and antiquarian, was born in 1758 and died in 1838. He traveled extensively both in the British Isles and in other countries of Europe. He explored thoroughly Rome and its vicinity. He wrote many books, most of which he himself illustrated.[34]]

Friday, June 11 [1790].

The public hospital [in Valetta] is a handsome edifice, and the institution itself is noble and charitable. Two extensive galleries, besides smaller apartments, are destined for the reception of the sick, who are treated with the utmost attention. A few devout, and perhaps penitent, knights still observe the ancient custom of attending the sick in person, which was one of the duties incumbent on the Order, while it preserved its original spirit and character. At present the prophecy of Fazellus seems fast approaching its full accomplishment. *Ubi et remisso priscae veritatis vigore, inertiam prope secantur; propediem (ni falso auguror) defecturi.*[35] Besides the Hospital, there are other charitable institutions, both for male and female inhabitants.[36]

82. François Emmanuel Guignard, Comte de Saint Priest. *Malta by a French Traveler*

[The Comte de Saint Priest (1735–1821) was a French statesman who became a member of the Order of Malta at the age of five and entered the army at fifteen. As a member of the French court, he spent considerable time in other countries.[37] His account of Malta, published in 1791, includes a brief description of the hospital of the knights.]

The hospital has several large wards, well aired and spacious storerooms in which one can easily put a fourfold line of beds. In this refuge, open to the downtrodden of all lands, of every religion, of every creed one lavishes on the sick every care, every remedy, every consolation. The knights superintend not only the different departments of the administration in which the chief position is held by a great dignitary of the Order, but they all go in person to the hospital to serve the sick. The dishes in use are mostly all of silver the simplicity of its design being less a matter of luxury than a means of cleanliness.[38]

83

Nursing by Medieval Saints '

ST. FRANCIS OF ASSISI

83. The Writings of St. Francis

[Modern critics agree almost unanimously upon what may be regarded as the authentic writings of St. Francis (1181 or 1182–1226). These include the three referred to in the next three quotations: the *Regula Prima* of 1221, the first rule; the *Regula Secunda,* or *Regula Bullata* of 1223, or the second rule; and the *Testament.* In each of these there is reference to the care of the sick by the Little Poor Brothers, or the Friars Minor, the first order founded by St. Francis. It is generally agreed that the Rule of 1221 is but an amplification or extension of an earlier rule which has been called the *Regula Primitiva.* This rule was formulated in 1210 and confirmed orally by Pope Innocent III. When the Rule of 1221 became obsolete, the Rule of 1223 became the official rule of the Order. Shortly before his death, the saint formulated the *Testament,* perhaps between 1224 and 1226; critics differ as to the date. It is simple and moving, and in the very first paragraph St. Francis speaks of his care of the lepers in his early days in religion.[39]]

The *Regula Prima*

Chapter X. Concerning Sick Brethren:

Whenever a Brother may fall sick, let care be taken that there be enough Brethren to tend him as one would wish to be served oneself. If, however, nothing else can be arranged, let him be confined to the care of one person who is charged to care for him.[40]

The *Regula Secunda*

6. And if any of them [the brothers] fall into sickness, the other brothers ought to serve him, as they would wish themselves to be served.

The *Testament*

1. While I was still in my sins, the Lord enabled me to begin to do penance in the following manner: It seemed to me bitterly unpleasant to see lepers, but the Lord led me among them and gave me pity for them . . .[41]

84. *The Lives of St. Francis of Assisi* by Brother Thomas of Celano

[In 1228, at the time of the ceremonies of canonization of St. Francis, Pope Gregory IX delegated to Brother Thomas of Celano the writing of the first life of the saint. Brother Thomas was a man of good education, a good writer, who had joined the Brothers in 1215, and was thus one of the first companions of St. Francis. He was later chosen as one of the first band of friars to go to Germany. He was regarded as a man

of moderate views who would give to the world an unbiased portrait of
St. Francis. While there are obvious omissions and imperfections in the
two *Lives of St. Francis,* written in 1228 and 1248,[42] critical opinion
seems to be coming to the view that Brother Thomas' works are among
the best available sources for an understanding of this beloved saint.[43]]

I. Cel. VII, 17.

And then the holy lover of all humility betook him to the lepers, and was
with them, serving them all most zealously for God's sake, washing all foul-
ness from them and even wiping away the matter from the ulcers; even as he
says himself in his Testament, "For when I was in sin it seemed to me exceeding bitter to look on lepers, but the Lord brought me among them, and I
showed mercy unto them."

I. Cel. XV, 38, 39.

But the chief matter of our discourse is the Order which as well from
charity as by profession he took upon him and maintained. What then shall
we say of it? He himself first planted the Order of Friars Minor (Lesser
Brethren) and on that very occasion gave it that name; since (as is well
known) it was written in the Rule: "And be they lesser:" and in that hour,
when those words were uttered, he said: "I will that this brotherhood be
called the Order of Lesser Brethren" (Friars Minor). And truly they were
"lesser," for, being subject to all, they ever sought for lowly dwellings, and
for occupations in the discharge of which they might appear in some sort to
suffer wrong, that they might deserve to be so founded on the solid bases of
true humility, that in happy disposition the spiritual building of all the
virtues might arise in them ...

For when as often happened, they lacked a lodging in the coldest weather,
an oven sheltered them, or, at least, they lay hid by night humbly in under-
ground places or in caves. And by day those who knew how to, worked with
their hands, and they stayed in lepers' houses, or in other decent places,
serving all with humility and devotion.

I. Cel. XXIX, 83.

He was of middle height, inclining to shortness; his head was of moderate
size, and round; his face somewhat long and prominent, his forehead smooth
and small; his eyes were black, of moderate size, and with a candid look; his
hair was dark, his eyebrows straight; his ears upright, but small; his temples
smooth. His words were kindly, [but] fiery and penetrating; his voice was
powerful, sweet-toned, clear and sonorous. His teeth were set close together,
white, and even; his lips thin and fine, his beard black and rather scanty; his
neck slender; his shoulders straight, his arms short, his hands attenuated,
with long fingers and nails; his legs slight, his feet small, his skin fine, and
his flesh spare. His clothing was rough, his sleep very brief, his hand most

beautiful. And, for that he was most humble, he showed all meekness to all men, adapting himself in profitable fashion to the behaviour of all ...

II. Cel. CXXXIII, 175, 176.

175. Great was his compassion for the sick, and great his care for their needs. If ever the kindness of lay folk sent him electuaries he gave them to the other sick though he needed them more than they. He entered into the feelings of all the sick, and gave them words of sympathy when he could not give words of help. He would himself eat on fast-days that the sick might not be ashamed to eat, nor to be ashamed of begging for meat through the streets of a town for a sick brother. Yet did he admonish the ailing to bear their wants patiently, and not to cause scandal by their discontent, though everything might not be done to their satisfaction ...

176. He once took into a vineyard a sick man whom he knew to be longing to eat grapes, and, sitting down under a vine, himself began to eat first, to encourage the other to eat.[44]

85. St. Bonaventura. *Legenda Maior S. Francisci*

[The writer of this, the "official" biography of St. Francis, was the eighth minister general of the Friars Minor, from 1257 to 1274.[45] He belongs to the second generation of Franciscans. The *Legenda* was finished about 1262 and is essentially a transcription of the two *Lives* of Thomas of Celano.[46]]

Ch. II, 6.

Thence that lover of utterest humility betook himself unto the lepers, and abode among them, with all diligence serving them all for the love of God. He would bathe their feet, and bind up their sores, drawing forth the corrupt matter from their wounds, and wiping away the blood; yea, in his marvellous devotion, he would even kiss their ulcerated wounds, he that was soon to be a Gospel physician.[47]

86. *The Legend of S. Francis by the Three Companions*

[Like all the other writings about St. Francis, the *Legenda Trium Sociorum* has been the subject of critical attack. It is a compilation of simple stories and legends, supposedly written by Brothers Leo, Angelo, and Rufino, the saint's companions, in 1246. It has 74 chapters prefaced by an introductory letter. It may be only a fragment of the original document.[48]]

A few days later, he took much money, and went into the spital of the lepers, and gathering all together, did give unto each an alms, kissing his hand. Then as he departed, in very truth that which had aforetime been bitter unto him, to wit, the sight and touch of the lepers, was now changed into sweetness. For, as he confessed, the sight of lepers had been so grievous unto him that he had been minded to avoid not only seeing them, but even going nigh their dwellings. And if at any time he chanced to pass their abodes, or to see them, albeit he was moved to compassion to do them alms through another person, yet always would he turn aside his face, stopping his nostrils with his hand. But through the grace of God he became so intimate a friend of the lepers that, even as he recorded in his will, he did sojourn with them and did humbly serve them.[49]

87. *The Mirror of Perfection of St. Francis of Assisi*

[Recent critical analysis of the Franciscan literature has ascribed the compilation of the *Speculum Perfectionis,* not to Brother Leo, in 1227, as was formerly believed, but to an unknown scribe at the Portiuncula in 1318. Apart from a few chapters, practically all of it is taken from the *Legenda Antiqua* of Perugia. The latter document was compiled a few years earlier and was based on the writings of Brother Leo. *The Mirror of Perfection* is a study of character rather than a chronological account.[50]]

Ch. XLIV.

Whence, at the beginning of the Religion, he would that the brethren should abide in the hospitals of the lepers to wait upon them, and there lay the foundation of holy humility. For sithence that both gentle and simple did come into the Order, among other things that were declared unto them, it was said that needs must they humbly be as servants unto the lepers and abide in their houses; as is contained in the first Rule: "Willing to have naught under heaven save only holy poverty, whereby they are nourished in this world by bodily and spiritual food, and in the world to come shall obtain their heavenly heritage."

Ch. LVIII.

Now when the Blessed Francis returned to the church of the Blessed Mary of the Little Portion, he found brother James the Simple with a certain leper that had many sores. For the Blessed Francis had commended this leper and all other lepers unto him, for as much as he was, as it were, their leech and did willingly tent and cleanse and bind up their wounds, for at that time the brethren abode in the hospitals of the lepers.

Ch. XC.

And especially did he admonish them [the Sisters of St. Clare] that out of such alms as the Lord might give them they should discreetly make provision for their bodies with cheerfulness and thanksgiving, and most of all, how they that were heal in their toils that they did undergo on behalf of their sick sisters, and they themselves that were sick should also be patient in their infirmities.[51]

88. *The Little Flowers of St. Francis*

[The *Actus S. Francisci* and its Italian translation, the *Fioretti di San Francesco,* have been called the most exquisite of all the Franciscan documents. The *Little Flowers* is not a biography but a collection of stories about the saint himself or his followers. There seems to be no manuscript containing all the chapters, which suggests the possibility that it was compiled from the common stock of legends. It was probably compiled between 1322 and 1328. Though said, in some ways, to be the least reliable of all the sources, containing mistakes and accounts of events the historical truth of which is open to question, it seems to be peculiarly in keeping with the tradition of the St. Francis who is known and loved by the modern world. Various names have been suggested for the original translator, but it is not known who he was; it is thought, however, that he was a Franciscan.[52]]

And he [Francis] not only served lepers gladly, but had also ordained that the friars of his Order, as they went about the world, should serve lepers for love of Christ, who for our sakes was willing to be accounted a leper. Now it befell on a time, in a friary nigh unto where St. Francis then was dwelling, that the friars were serving lepers and other sick folk in a lazarhouse, among them was a leper, so froward, so intolerable, and so insolent, that all believed of a surety he was possessed of the devil; and so in sooth it was, for he reviled so shamefully with words, and belaboured whosoever was tending him; and, what is worse, did foully blaspheme the blessed Christ and His most holy Mother the Virgin Mary, so that in no wise could one be found willingly or able to serve him. And albeit the friars strove to bear patiently the injuries and insults heaped upon themselves, their consciences were unable to endure those uttered against the Christ and His Mother: So they resolved to forsake the said leper, but would not until they had signified all things in due order to St. Francis, who was then dwelling in a friary hard by. And when they had signified these things to him, St. Francis came to this perverse leper, and drawing nigh, gave his salutation, saying, "God give thee peace, my dearest brother." The leper answers, "What peace can I have from God, who hath taken peace from me and all good things, and hath made me all rotten and stinking?" and St. Francis said, "My son, have patience, for the infirmities of the body are given to us by God in this world for the salvation of souls; inasmuch as they are of great merit when they are endured patiently." The sick man answers, "And how can I bear patiently this continual pain that afflicts me day and night? and not only am I afflicted by my sickness, but the friars thou gavest to serve me do even worse, and serve me not as they ought?" Then St. Francis, knowing by divine revelation that this leper was possessed of the evil spirit, went aside and betook himself to prayer, and devoutly prayed God for him. His prayer ended, he returns to the leper and bespeaks him thus, "My son, I will serve thee, even I, since thou art not content with the others." And the leper answers, "So be it; but what canst thou do more than the others?" St. Francis answers, "Whatsoever thou wilt, that will I do." Says the leper, "I will that thou wash me all over, for I stink so foully that I cannot abide myself." Then St. Francis made quickly water boil, with many sweet-smelling herbs therein; then did strip the leper and began to wash him with his own hands, while another friar poured water over him . . .[53]

ST. CLARE OF ASSISI

89. The Rule of 1253

[Four rules were observed by the Second Order of St. Francis, the Poor Clares, before the death of St. Clare. The first rule is regarded by critics of the sources as one of the "lost writings" of St. Francis. Clare speaks of it in the rule which was approved in 1253, and Thomas of Celano refers to "a manner of living and way of life" which Francis gave "to either sex." [54] Clare, to the end of her life, fought for the privilege of living in that absolute poverty which she regarded as the chief distinguishing mark of the order established by St. Francis.[55] Writings of, and about, St. Clare are few. The *Life of St. Clare,* from which the following excerpt of the Rule of 1253 is taken, has been attributed most recently to Brother Thomas of Celano. Whether the members of the Poor Clares cared for the sick outside the community is not specified in the text of this rule.]

VIII. As to the Sisters who are ill, the Abbess is strictly bound either by herself or by other Sisters to make solicitous inquiry as well in respect of counsel as of food and of other necessaries which their infirmity requires, and to provide for them charitably and compassionately according to the possibility of the place. For all are obliged to serve and care for their Sisters who are ill even as they would wish to be treated if taken down by an illness themselves. Let each disclose with confidence her needs to another. And if a mother love and nurture her daughter according to the flesh, how much the more ought a Sister to love and nurture her Sister according to the Spirit. Those who are ill may lie on sacks filled with straw and may have feather pillows for their heads. And those who need them may use woolen socks and mattresses. The aforesaid Sisters who are ill may, when they are visited by those who enter the monastery, answer each one speaking any good words to them . . .[56]

ST. ELIZABETH OF HUNGARY

90. Theodoric of Thuringen. *The Life of Saint Elizabeth*

[This, the original life of St. Elizabeth (1207–1231) was written by Theodoric (Dietrich) of Apolda, born in Thuringia, near the place where Elizabeth lived, a few years before her death. In preparation for the writing of the biography, Theodoric conversed with many persons who knew Elizabeth, and drew information also from the best writings of the times. He visited monasteries, castles, and towns, interviewing many trustworthy persons, seeking completeness and truth. His work was published in 1725 in Basnage's *Canisius*. From it, several succeeding biographies have been written. Dietrich died two years before the canonization of St. Elizabeth.[57]]

Although she could never endure bad air anywhere else, nevertheless, even in warm weather, she herself, without any show of repugnance, put up with the foul smells of the sick, which the servants complained about bitterly and scarcely tolerated; handling them cheerfully, she wiped with her veil the saliva and spittle from their faces, and the catarrhal discharge from ears and nose. Besides these, she cared for little poverty-stricken boys in the same house. To them she manifested such a gentle spirit that they all called her mother and ran to meet her when she entered the house, gathering about her with filial affection. Among these she showed preference for the unkempt, the sickly, those more ragged than the others, and particularly the deformed, stroking their heads with her hands and holding them in her lap.

She busied herself with works of charity and mercy, and those whom poverty, sickness, or infirmity had oppressed more than others and were thereby more deserving of care she placed in her hospital and most humbly ministered to their wants with her own hands.

She arranged their baths, put them to bed, and covering them, saying to her servants: "How well it is for us, that thus we bathe and cover our Lord." [58]

91. Count de Montalembert. *Life of Saint Elizabeth of Hungary, Duchess of Thuringia*

[Count de Montalembert was born in London in 1810. His mother came from an old Scottish family.[59] His *Life of Saint Elizabeth* is based on the *Life* by Theodoric, and other contemporary and later writers. In his "Introduction," he states, "Thanks to the many invaluable monuments of the life of St. Elizabeth, which are found in the great historical collections of Germany as well as in the manuscripts of its libraries. Thanks to the numerous and minute details transmitted to us by biographers, some of them contemporaries of St. Elizabeth ..." In another place he says, ... "in this little book I have not inserted anything but what I gathered from correct manuscripts, or heard from religious persons of unquestionable veracity." [60] The *Life* has been called not so much a history as a religious manifesto.[61] In it, St. Elizabeth's care of the sick is described in detail.]

But it was not alone by presents or with money that the young princess testified her love for the poor of Christ; it was still more by personal devotion; by those tender and patient cares which are, assuredly, in the sight of both God and of the sufferers, the most holy and most precious alms. She applied herself to those duties with simplicity and unfailing gaiety of manner. When the sick sought her aid, after relieving their wants, she would inquire where they lived, in order that she might visit them.

And then, no distance, no roughness of road, could keep her from them. She knew that nothing strengthens feelings of charity more than to penetrate into all that is positive and material in human misery. She sought out the huts most distant from her castle, which were often repulsive, through filth and bad air, yet she entered these haunts of poverty in a manner at once full of devotion and familiarity. She carried herself what she thought would be necessary for their miserable inhabitants. She consoled them, far less by her generous gifts than by her sweet and affectionate words. When she found them in debt and unable to pay, she engaged to discharge their obligations from her privy purse.

Poor women in childbed were particularly the object of her compassion. Whenever she could, she used to go sit by their bedsides to assist and encourage them. She used to take their new-born children in her arms with a mother's love, and cover them with clothes made by herself.

·   ·   ·   ·   ·   ·   ·

Amongst the unfortunate who particularly attracted her compassion, those who occupied the chief place in her heart were the lepers; the mysterious and special character of their malady rendered them, throughout the middle ages, objects of a solicitude and affection mingled with fear.

·   ·   ·   ·   ·   ·   ·

Having one day met one of these unfortunates, who suffered besides from a malady in the head, and whose appearance was repulsive in the highest degree, she led him to a retired part of the orchard, cut off his matted hair, laid his head on her knees and washed and cleansed it; her maids of honour having surprised her at this strange occupation, she smiled, but said nothing.

·   ·   ·   ·   ·   ·   ·

91

Another time, the Landgrave having gone to spend some days at his castle of Naumberg, which was situated in the center of his southern possessions, and near Saxony, Elizabeth remained at Wartburg and employed herself during her husband's absence in redoubling her zeal and care of the sick and poor, in washing and clothing them with garments, the work of her own hands, notwithstanding the discontent testified by the Duchess-mother, Sophia, who had remained with her son since the death of her husband. But the young Duchess did not heed the complaints of her mother-in-law.

Among the sick there was a poor little leper named Helias, whose condition was so deplorable that no one would take charge of him. Elizabeth, seeing him thus abandoned by all, felt herself bound to do more for him than for any other; she took and bathed him herself, anointed him with a healing balm, and then laid him in the bed, even that which she shared with her royal husband.

Elizabeth . . . erect[ed] an almshouse midway up the rocky height crowned by the castle of Wartburg, on the site since occupied by a convent of Franciscans. She therein maintained, from that time, twenty-eight sick and infirm poor persons, chosen from amongst those who were too feeble to ascend to the castle. Every day she went to visit them, and carried with her meat and drink for their use.

She established two almshouses in the city of Eisenach, one for poor women, under the invocation of the Holy Spirit, near the gate of St. George; another under that of St. Ann, for the sick in general. The latter exists to this day. Twice every day without fail, at noon and at eventide, the young Duchess descended and reascended the toilsome road from Wartburg to these houses, regardless of the fatigue she thereby endured, in order that she might visit her poor ones, and carry to them all that would be useful for their wants. When arrived at these asylums of misery, she used to go from bed to bed, asking all what they wished for, and performing for each services the most repulsive, with a zeal and tenderness which the love of God and his special grace alone could inspire. She fed with her own hands those whose maladies were most severe; she made their beds, raised and carried them on her back, or in her arms, to lay them on their couches; she washed their faces with her own veil, and did all with a gaiety and amenity that nothing could alter . . .

Elizabeth founded in one of these hospitals an asylum for deserted children or orphans . . .

About this time she founded the hospital of St. Mary Magdalene, at Gotha, which she had planned during her husband's life-time, and which she completed at her return to her possessions.

After having for a long time considered upon what manner of life would be most pleasing to God, and having examined the different rules of the Monastic Orders then existing, and even the solitary life of the recluses, the remembrance and example of the glorious seraph-saint of Assisium, whose child she was already, as a Penitent of the Third Order, gained the mastery of her heart. . . . [She then entered the] order of St. Francis [and] assumed the habit of the Third Order . . .[62]

92. Charles Kingsley. *The Saint's Tragedy*

[Charles Kingsley (1819–1875), the English clergyman and novelist, was but twenty-three when he wrote the work which proved to be his first to be published, *The Saint's Tragedy*.[63] It was originally written as a prose history and was illustrated with his own pen-and-ink drawings. It was intended, at the time of its writing, not for publication but "as a gift book to his wife on his marriage-day, if that day should ever come." [64] It was later reworked into a drama and published. Its principal characters are Lewis, Landgrave of Thuringia, betrothed as a child to Elizabeth, daughter of the King of Hungary; the saint herself; and Conrad of Marburg, papal commissioner for the suppression of heresy and Elizabeth's confessor. It has been said of it that the facts are in accepted history and legend, but that the delineation of Elizabeth's state of mind (not shown in this quotation) is Kingsley's own interpretation.[65] The extract quoted outlines briefly Elizabeth's well-known care of the sick and unfortunate of her own community, when, after renouncing all rights to the regency, she lived in seclusion, doing penance and ministering to the sick.]

Act IV. Scene II.   Open space in a suburb of Marpurg, near Elizabeth's hut.

Con. How now? Who more than she, in faith and practice, a living member of the Communion of Saints? Did she not lately publicly dispense in charity in a single day five hundred marks and more? Is it not my continual labour to keep her from utter penury through her extravagance in almsgiving? For whom does she take thought but for the poor, on whom, day and night, she spends her strength? Does she not tend them from the cradle, nurse them, kiss their sores, feed them, bathe them, with her own hands, clothe them, living and dead, with garments, the produce of her own labour? Did she not of late take into her own house a paralytic boy, whose loathesomeness had driven away every one else? And now that we have removed that charge, has she not with her a leprous boy, to whose necessities she ministers hourly, by day and night? What valley but blesses her for some school, some chapel, some convent, built by her munificence? Are not the hospices, which she has founded in divers towns,

93

the wonder of Germany?—Wherein she daily feeds and houses a multitude of the infirm poor of Christ? Is she not followed at every step by the blessings of the poor? Are not her hourly intercessions for the souls and bodies of all around incessant, world-famous, mighty to save? While she lives only for the Church of Christ, will you accuse her of selfish isolation? [66]

ST. CATHERINE OF SIENA

93. Blessed Raymond of Capua. *Life of Saint Catherine of Sienna*

[This is the first American edition of the *Life of Saint Catherine* by the confessor of St. Catherine, Raymond of Capua. It is taken from the text of the Bollandists, dated Siena, April 29, 1853. Raymond in his close relation to Catherine, had ample opportunity to become acquainted with her actions and motives. He was himself a well-educated man, who had held various important offices in the Order of St. Dominic, of which he was a member. He accompanied Catherine on her journeys to France and Italy. He died in the midst of his work in 1399. The *Life* is based on testimony of living witnesses. Raymond wrote, in addition to this *Life,* several other works on religious subjects. Catherine was born in 1347, one of twin daughters of Lapa and Jacomo Benincasa, the latter a dyer. She died on April 29, 1380.[67]]

Catherine was wonderfully compassionate to the wants of the poor, but her heart was even more sensitive to the sufferings of the sick. To relieve them, she accomplished things apparently incredible. . . . I have, for proof, the written and verbal testimony of Friar Thomas, whom I have already named, of St. Dominic of Sienna, doctor of divinity, and prior provincial of the Roman Province. I could also cite Lapa and Lysa with several respectable ladies who have affirmed the same things to me.

There was at Sienna a poor sick woman named Tecca; her indigence was so extreme, that she was forced to seek in a hospital the remedies she needed, and which she was unable to procure. The hospital in which she entered was barely able to furnish what was strictly necessary. Her disease grew worse and worse, so that the leprosy covered her whole body; the smell arising from her disease repelled every one, so that no person had courage to take care of her, and preparations were made to remove her outside of the city, as is customary in such maladies. When Catherine heard this, her charitable heart was touched; she hastened to the hospital, visited the leper, kissed her, and offered not only to supply all her necessities, but also to become her servant during the remainder of her life. Catherine literally fulfilled her promise; every morning and every evening, she visited the patient in person and gave her whatever was necessary; she contemplated in this poor leper, the spouse of her soul and assisted her in every possible way, and with an indescribable respect and love.

The exalted virtue of Catherine, however, only inspired the leprous woman with pride and ingratitude; ... Catherine's charity and humility rendered Tecca arrogant and irritable. When she saw Catherine so solicitous in serving her, she considered the charitable attentions due to her, and scolded her benefactress with injurious words, when every thing did not conform to her wishes. Often the servant of our Lord, prolonged her morning devotions in the Church and hence came later than usual to the hospital. On such occasions Tecca would display her ill-temper, in phrases like this: "Good morning, my Lady, Queen of Fonte-Branda (this was the name of the section of the city in which Catherine resided;) Your Majesty takes pleasure in staying the livelong day in the Church of the Friars; it is *there* you have wasted all this forenoon I am sure, my fine lady: you are never weary of the *dear* Friars!" She strove to irritate her by such words; but Catherine always calm, appeased her in the best way she could, and answered with as much meekness and humility as if she had been her own mother—begging her to be quiet for the love of our blessed Lord: "I have been a little late it is true, but soon all your little wants shall be attended to"—and quickly lighting the fire and putting on water, she would prepare her food, and arrange everything with such promptitude that the ill-tempered sick woman herself would be in surprise. This continued a considerable time, her patience and zeal never diminishing.

.   .   .   .   .

There was at that time a Sister of Penance of St. Dominic, called Andrea, who was extremely ill with a cancer in the breast which consumed and gnawed away gradually her whole chest; the odor from this wound was so disgusting that it was impossible to approach her without closing firmly the nostrils, and there was scarcely any one to be found that was willing to pay this unfortunate Sister a friendly visit. Directly Catherine knew this, she comprehended that God reserved to her this poor forsaken one; she hastened to comfort her with a cheerful countenance, and offered to assist her so long as that dreadful illness might last. The Sister accepted her offer the more easily as she found herself neglected by all others.

Behold, therefore, the Virgin serving the widow, youth succouring old age, and she who languished with the love of God, devoted to one who languished with sorrows of earth. Catherine omits no attention, although the stench becomes more and more insupportable; she remains by the bedside continually, using no precautions, uncovers the wound, cleanses it and changes the linens, and never exhibits the slightest repugnance, whatever be the length of time required or the difficulty in the dressing.[68]

94. Augusta Theodosia Drane. *The History of St. Catherine of Siena and Her Companions*

[The writer of this biography, known also as Mother Francis Raphael, was born near London in 1823. She was a converted Catholic and belonged for over forty years to the Third Order of St. Dominic. Bishop

Ullathorne said of her that she was "one of those many-sided characters who can write a book, draw a picture, rule an Order, guide other souls, superintend a building, lay out grounds, or give wise and practical advice with equal facility and success." [69] The material for her life of St. Catherine was drawn from the chief recognized sources, which included *Vita della Serafica Sposa di Gesu Christo, Sta. Caterina de Siena,* or the *Legend,* the original *Life,* written (1384–1395) by Raymond of Capua, the saint's confessor; *La Legenda Minore,* an abridgment, written by Caffarini (d. 1434); *Supplemento allo Leggenda di Santa Catherina,* also written (1414) by Caffarini; and *Lettere di Santa Caterina,* first published in Venice in 1500.[70]]

[In 1374, during the plague.]

Once more, therefore, was Catherine to be seen in the hospitals, and the most infected parts of the city, assisting all no less with her charitable services than with her prayers. "Never did she appear more admirable than at this time," says Caffarini; "she was always with the plague-stricken; she prepared them for death, she buried them with her own hands. I myself witnessed the joy with which she tended them, and the wonderful efficacy of her words, which effected many conversions. Not a few owed their lives to her self-devoted care, and encouraged her companions to perform the like services." [71]

THE BEGUINES

[The origin of the name Beguine has been the subject of much difference of opinion. The most widely accepted theory is that the institution derived its name from Lambert le Bègue, a priest of Liége, who conceived the idea in 1170 of establishing an association of women who would devote themselves to the religious life without taking monastic vows. The order spread rapidly in Belgium, France, Germany, Holland, and northern Italy. The members engaged in various activities, including nursing in the hospitals and in the towns.[72] Among the most famous of the Beguinages, the one at Ghent aroused the greatest admiration on the part of nineteenth-century English travelers, some of whose accounts are quoted below to indicate the characteristics as they appeared at a later date. In this connection, it has been assumed that the basic character of the institutions had changed little in the time which had elapsed since their founding.]

95. Robert Southey. *Journal of a Tour in the Netherlands in the Autumn of 1815*

[Robert Southey (1774–1843), English poet and historian, was made poet laureate in 1813. He was a prolific writer not only of history and poetry but also on religious and political subjects, the latter appearing in periodical publications such as the *Quarterly Review*. His letters afford many side lights on his sympathies. The charitable works of the Beguines and the Sisters of Charity excited his interest, and he advocated the promotion of similar orders in England under the auspices of the Established Church.[73] The information given in the book from which the following extract is taken is given also in a letter to John Rickman, Esq., from Brussels, October 2, 1815.[74]]

But the most interesting object in Ghent to me, and indeed the most remarkable, is the Beguineage, which is the principal establishment of the order, and very much the largest. It is at one end of the city, and entirely enclosed, being indeed a little town or world of itself. You enter thro' a gateway, where there is a statue of St. Elizabeth of Hungary, the patroness of the institution. The space enclosed cannot be less than the area of the whole town of Keswick; but the Beguineage itself is unlike almshouse, college, village or town. It is a collection of contiguous houses of different sizes, each with a small garden in front, and a high, well-built brick wall inclosing them all. Upon every door is the name, not of the inhabitants, but of the Saint under whose protection the house is placed; but there is no opening in the door thro' which anything can be seen. There are several streets thus built, with the houses on both sides; the silence and solitude of such streets may easily be imagined, and the effect is very singular upon coming from the busy streets of Ghent. You seem to be in a different world. There is a large church within the enclosure; a burying ground in which there are no monuments; a branch from one of the many rivers or canals wherewith Ghent is intersected, in which the washing of the community is performed from a large boat, and a large piece of ground planted with trees where the clothes are dried.

We were at length courteously accosted by a sister who proved to be the second personage in the community . . .

According to this lady, there are about 6000 Beguines in Brabant and Flanders, in which countries they are confined: there are 620 resident in the Beguineage. They were rich before the Revolution; then in the general spoliation their lands were taken from them and they were commanded to lay aside their distinctive dress, but this mandate was only obeyed in part, because public opinion was strongly in their favour, and they were of such manifest utility to all ranks that very few were disposed to injure them. They receive the sick who come to them for succour, and they support as well as attend them as long as the case requires; they go out also to nurse the sick where their services are requested. They are bound by no vow, and M. Devolder (this was the name of our obliging informant) assured us with an air of becoming pride that no instance of a Beguine leaving the establishment had ever been known. The reason is obvious: the institution is in itself reasonable and useful as well as religious; no person is compelled to enter it, because there is no clausure, and no person can be compelled to stay, and I suppose their members are generally, if not wholly, filled up by women who, when their youth is gone by, seek a retirement or need an asylum from the world. M. Devolder herself entered after the death of her husband. The property which a Beguine brings with her reverts to her heirs-at-law.... The Sisters dine in the Refectory if they please, but anyone who prefers it may have dinner sent from thence to her own apartments. We were taken into three of these chambers; they are small, and furnished with little more than necessary comforts, but these comforts they had, and they were remarkably clean ...

The dress of the Beguines is not inconvenient, but it is abominably ugly, as the habits of every female order are, I believe, without exception.[75]

96. Dr. Robert Gooch, "Protestant Sisters of Charity," *Blackwood's Edinburgh Magazine*, July-December, 1825, pp. 732–735

[Dr. Robert Gooch, the author of the articles from which this and the next extract are taken, was born at Yarmouth, Norfolk, in 1784, the son of a sea captain. After graduating from the University of Edinburgh in 1807, he was elected to the lectureship of midwifery at St. Bartholomew's Hospital. He became very much concerned about the nursing care of the sick, especially in country towns. While traveling on the continent, he observed the work of the Beguines and the Sisters of Charity, about which he corresponded with Robert Southey. His articles, in the form of letters, urging reform, if possible under the auspices of the Church, were published in *Blackwood's Edinburgh Magazine* (1825), and in the *London Medical Gazette* (1827). The letters were also reprinted in the Appendix of Southey's *Sir Thomas More or; Colloquies on the Progress and Prospects of Society,* published in 1829.[76]]

When I was in Flanders a short time ago, I saw at Bruges and Ghent some of this singular and useful order of nuns—they are all of a respectable station in society, and I was told, that it is not uncommon for the females of the most wealthy, and even noble families, voluntarily to quit the world and its pleasures, enter this order, and dedicate themselves to the most menial attendance on the sick. I went one morning to the hospital at ———; all the nurses are "soeur de charité," and it was a striking sight to see these women, whose countenances, manners, and a something in the quality, or cleanness of their stiff white hoods, and black russet gowns, are expressive of a station superior to their office, one with a pail in her hand, another down on her knees washing the floor of the chapel. The physician of the hospital spoke in the highest terms of the humility and tenderness with which they nursed his patients.

97. Dr. Robert Gooch in *The London Medical Gazette*, Vol. 1 (1827), pp. 55–58

A few summers ago I passed through Flanders on my way to Germany, and at the hospital at Bruges saw some of the Beguines, and heard the physician, with whom I was intimate, speak in strong terms of their services; he said "there are no such nurses." I saw them in the wards attending on the sick, and in the chapel of the hospital on their knees, washing the floor. They were obviously a superior class of women, and the contrast was striking between these menial offices, and the respectability of their dress and appearance; but the Beguinage at Ghent is one of their principal establishments . . .

The beguinage, or residence of the Beguines at Ghent, is a little town of itself, adjoining the city, and enclosed from it. The transition from the crowded streets of Ghent, to the silence and solitude of the Beguinage is very striking. The houses in which the Beguines live are contiguous, each having its small garden, and on the door the name not of the resident, but of the protecting saint of the house; these houses are ranged into the streets. There is also the large church, which we visited, and a burial ground, in which there are no monuments. There are upwards of six hundred of these nuns in the Beguinage at Ghent, and about six thousand in Brabant and Flanders. They receive sick persons into the Beguinage, and not only nurse but support them until they are recovered; they also go out to nurse the sick. They are bound by no vows except to be chaste and obedient while they remain in the order: they have the power of quitting it and returning again into the world whenever they please, but this it is said they seldom or never do. They are most of them women unmarried, or widows past the middle of life. In 1244, a synod at Fritzlan decided that no Beguine should be younger than forty years of age. They generally dine together in the refectory; their apartments are barely yet comfortably furnished, and like all the habitations of Flanders, remarkably clean . . .

In one part of the hospital there was a large square court, bordered with galleries leading to apartments suitable to such [opulent] patients; when they quitted the hospital the donations which they left were added to its funds.

98. Mme. Elizabeth S. (Gurney) De Bunsen. *Elizabeth Fry's Journeys on the Continent, 1840–1841*

[Elizabeth Gurney De Bunsen was the niece of Elizabeth Fry, the English Quaker prison reformer and philanthropist. Together with her father, her aunt, and some others, she visited Holland, Belgium, Denmark, and Germany. The book from which the following quotation is taken consists of a diary and a journal kept by her on two journeys to the continent. The excerpt is from the diary.]

Feb. 29, 1840.

The Beguinage was a singular sight. Here 600 nuns reside *each* having her separate little house and establishment and a fine large chapel where all assemble for services morning and evening. I much regretted that our dinner hour prevented my going to the evening service as the chanting of so many female voices is said to be very fine. I went into one of their little houses. They appeared quite accustomed to strangers' visits. The old Soeur showed me over her rooms with apparent pleasure and was very full of their laws and regulations. The Beguins are bound by no vow. They may return to the world when they please but they boast that no Sister has ever yet been known to leave. They visit the sick in Private Houses or attend at the Hospitals and other Asylums. You walk thro' the streets of it like walking thro' a town. It is the effect of a small town more than anything else.[77]

The Regular Orders

99. *Additions to the Rules of Syon Monastery*

[Syon Monastery in Middlesex, England, was founded and endowed in 1415 by King Henry V. The "Monastery of St. Saviour and St. Bridget of Syon" belonged to the order of St. Augustine. It was one of the few religious houses restored in Mary's reign.[78] The "Additions" alluded to here exist in duplicate. One copy relates to the nuns and the other to the monks. One copy of the rules relating to the nuns is preserved in the British Museum, and one, relating to the monks, is in the Library of St. Paul's Cathedral, London.[79]]

Ch. LVII.

Of the fermereye, parlour, and of the fermeres.

Sethe our Lord Ihesu Criste takethe that is done to the seke, as yf it were done to hymselfe, the abbes owethe to haue grete tendernes ouer them, that they be not forslewed of ther kepers. Wherfor, like as ther be dyuers infirmitees, so ther owen to be dyuers howses to kepe hem in. One for al maner sekenes, as is the comen fermery; another for them that be in recouerynge, as in the comen parlour; another for them that be distracte of ther mendes; another for lepres, stondyng fer from al other, so zet that the sustres may come to them and comforte hem. If any suster be so seke that sche may not be couered withe oute medycyne, sche schal be brought to the crates to the phisician; so that the phisician come not in to the monastery in any wyse, but for a very necessary cause. To kepynge of the seke in the fermery, schal be depute suche a suster by the abbes that dredethe God, hauyng a diligence aboute hem for hys loue, and kan skylle for to do servyse to them, stronge and myghty to lefte them up, and lede them from place to place whan nede is, to the chirche or fermery chapel, and kan exhorte, styrre, and comforte them to be confessed, and receyve the sacramentes of holy chirche. Ofte chaunge ther beddes and clothes, zeue them medycynes, ley to ther plastres,

100

and mynyster to them mete and drynke, fyre and water, and al other neces-
saryes, nyghte and day, as nede requyrethe, after counsel of the phisicians,
and precepte of the souereyne, not squaymes to wasche them, and wype them,
or auoyde them, not angry nor hasty, or unpacient thof one haue the vomet,
another the fluxe, another the frensy, which nowe syngethe, nowe cryethe,
nowe lawghethe, nowe wepethe, nowe chydethe, nowe fryghtethe, nowe is
wrothe, now wel apayde, ffor ther be some sekenesses vexynge the seke so
gretly and prouokynge them to ire, that the mater drawen up to the brayne
alyenthe the mendes. And therfor they owe to haue moche pacience withe
suche, that they may therby gete them an euerlastyng crowne.[80]

100. The Will of Sir Roger Salwayn, Knight of York, 1420

[This will, one of the fifty earliest wills in the Court of Probate of
London, is the only one of the group which mentions a nurse. Its provisions, in addition to the one concerning money for the nun who nursed
him, include gifts to four orders of Friars, gifts of household goods and
money to his wife, money for his son, marriage portions for his daughters,
payment of debts, leniency to poor tenants, sending a pilgrim to Jerusalem
at a cost of not more than £100, gifts of money and horses to relatives
and friends, gifts of armour, an annuity to a man, and selling of "furred
garments" for the testator's soul.]

Also I will pat p[e] Nonne pat kepid me in my seknes haue ij nobles, and
pat ther be zif in-to the hous pat she wonnes in, 'xx's' for to syng and pray
for me.[81]

101. Legends of Robin Hood's Death

[These legends contain reference to a prioress, a cousin of Robin
Hood, who bled him until he died of loss of blood. In spite of their
legendary character, they have value as indicating that members of
religious orders carried out some procedures used in the care of the sick.
Quotations from two early versions of the legend are given below.]

Robin Hood's Death

R. H. is ailing, and is convinced that the only course for him is to go to
Kirkless priory for blooding. Robin makes the prioress a present of twenty
pound, with a promise of more when she wants, and she falls to work with
her bleeding-irons.

R. Hoode his Death, Percy MS. p. 21; Hale and Furnivall I, 53.

> 14 And downe then came dame prioresse,
>   Downe she came in that ilke,
>   With a pair of blood-irons in her hands,
>   Were wrapped all in silke.

15 "Sett a chaffing-dish to the fyer," said dame prioresse,
   "And Stripp thou vp thy sleeue:"
   I hold him but an unwise man
   That will noe warning leeue.

16 Shee laid the blood-irons to Robin Hoods vaine,
   Alacke, the more pitye!
   And pearct the vaine, and let out the bloode,
   That full red was to see.

17 And first it bled, the thicke, thicke bloode,
   And afterwards the thinne,
   And well then wist good Robin Hoode,
   Treason there was within.

R. H's Death and Burial.

[This will, one of the fifty earliest wills in

   a. The English Archer, Paisley, John.
   b. Ditto, York, printed by N. Nickson in Feasegate, n. d.
   Bodleian Library, Douce, F. F. 71(4), p. 70.

3 Now Robin he is to fair Kirkly gone,
   As fast as he can win:
   But before he came there, as we do hear,
   He was taken very ill.

4 And when he came to fair Kirkly-hall,
   He knocked all at the ring,
   And none was so ready as his cousin herself
   For to let bold Robin in.

5 "Will you please sit doen, cousin Robin," she said,
   "And drink some beer with me?"
   "No, I will neither eat nor drink,
   Till I am blooded by thee."

6 "Well, I have a room, cousin Robin," she said,
   "Which you did never see,
   And if you please to walk therein,
   You blooded by me shall be."

7 She took him by the lily-white hand,
   And led him to a private room,
   And there she blooded bold Robin Hood,
   While one drop of blood would run down.

8 She blooded him in a vein of the arm,
   And locked him up in the room;
   Then did he bleed all the livelong day,
   Until the next day at noon.[82]

Nursing in Homes and Hospitals

102. Lists of Secular Nurses in France

[It is assumed that the individuals listed below were nurses who did not belong to a religious order but were secular nurses caring for patients in their homes.]

Nurses listed in the Paris Tax Roll in 1292.

Aalès. *Nourrice* of Guillaume, le perrier.

Alison. *Nourrice* of Guillaume, Rue Andri-Malet.

Avès. *Nourrice* of Andri l'Englais. Rue Neuve.

Erembourc. *Nourrice* of Oudart de Villers. Rue de Violette.

Héloyson. *Nourrice* of Guillaume Boncel. Rue de Arsis.

Jehanne. *Nourrice* of Gefrai Le Lorrain. Parish of Saint-Jehan-en-Grève.

Jourdenete. *Nourrice* of Guillaume Boncel. Rue de Arsis.

Mabile. *Nourrice* of Sedile de Falaise. Parish of Saint-Germain.

Perronele. *Nourrice* of Pierre de Fournay. Rue de Arsis.

Ysabian. *Nourrice* of Jehan de Fossez, *ferron*. La Ferronnerie.

Nurses listed in Poitiers as recipients of public alms in 1462.

Catherine (Nourrice).

Jehanne (Nourrice).[83]

103. Charters of Selected Hospitals

[The purposes of the founding of a number of English hospitals of this period are given in their charters. The following excerpts indicate these purposes. It will be noted that it is not specified who will care for the patients.]

Chichester, St. Mary's Statutes, 12th century

If anyone in infirm health and destitute of friends should seek admission for a time, until he shall recover, let him be gladly received and assigned a bed. . . . In regard to the poor people who are received late at night, and go forth early in the morning, let the warden take care that their feet are washed, and, as far as possible, their necessities attended to.

Bethlehem Hospital, 1247

A chyrche of Owre Lady that ye namyde Bedlam. And yn that place ben founde many men that ben fallyn owte of hyr wytte. And full honestely they ben kepte in that place; and sum ben restoryde unto hyr witte and helthe agayne. And sum ben a-bydyng there yn for evyr, for they ben fall soo moche owte of hem selfe that hyt ys uncurerabylle unto man.

God's House, Southampton, 1185

Thys Hospitale was foundyd by q Marchauntes beyng Bretherne [wherof] the one was caullyd Ge[rvasius] the other Protasius. . . . These 2 Brethern, as I lernid, dwellyd yn the very Place wher the Hospitale is now. . . . These

2 Brethern for Goddes sake cause[d] their House to be turned to an Hospitale for poore Folkes, and endowed it with sum Landes.

St. Bartholomew's Hospital, London, 1123

... he [Rahere] began to be uexed with greuous sykeness, and his douloures, litill and litill, takynge ther encrese, he drew to the extremyte of lyf.... Albrake owte in terys, than he auowyd yf helthe God hym wolde grawnte, that he myght lefully returns to his contray, he wolde make and hospitale yn recreacion of poure men, and to them so there i gaderid, necessaries mynstir, after his power.[84]

104. Charter of Isabella of Bray

[Isabella of Bray, the daughter of Edward of Bray and his wife Matillis, became a sister in St. Bartholomew's Hospital in the reign of Henry III (1207–1272). Her maternal grandfather, Adam Scott, was "warden of the chest of the fabric of St. Paul's Cathedral," and from the funds under his charge paid the workmen's wages when the choir was being rebuilt. He was a charitable man and paid a yearly rent of twelve shillings to St. Paul's. William de Sanctmerglise, Dean of St. Paul's in 1242, sanctioned his gift to Edward of Bray and Matillis, of the land in St. Gregory's parish which Isabella later granted to St. Bartholomew's Hospital. In return for what she brought to the hospital estate, she was entitled to a home and maintenance in the hospital, and to take part in its work. The terms of her charter indicate that she entered the hospital and became a sister, and perhaps ended her days there.[85]]

To all Christians to whom the present writing shall come, Isabella daughter of Edward of Bray hail. Be it known to you all that I in my full age and free power have given and granted, and by this my present charter confirmed, to the hospital of St. Bartholomew of London the whole of my holding with all its belongings altogether which I have in London in the parish of St. Gregory between the land and houses of Master Richard of Wendovre, canon of the church of St. Paul, and the land and house of Roger Albyn fishmonger: To have and to hold by the aforesaid hospital and the brethren and sisters ministering to the sick lying there, freely, quietly, well and in peace for ever. Returning every year to the lord king two pence of soccage on Easter eve; and to the chapter of the church of St. Paul every year twelve shillings, and to the hospital of the church of St. Giles of the lepers every year four shillings, and to the aforesaid church of St. Gregory every year twelve pence, at the regular and accustomed terms for all services, as is contained better and more fully in the charters which I have thence from my ancestors through whom the aforesaid holding comes hereditarily to me: which charters indeed with the present charter and with plenary seisin I have rendered to the brethren of the aforesaid hospital. For this my gift, grant, and for the confirmation of the present charter, the master and brethren gave me a sister's gown, receiving me as sister, and giving to me the profession of a sister and the office about the sick and the emolument of the house for my whole life. These being witnesses: Richard of Hadestoke, then alderman of the same ward: Adam of Basing, then warden of the said Hospital (i. e. of St. Giles): Henry Kingesson: Adam Bruning: Robert of Westmelne: Henry Wdemongere: Roger Albin: Alexander the Clerk, and Others.[86]

105. The Will of William Gregory

[William Gregory was mayor of London in 1451–1452. While in office he kept the city chronicle, in which he recorded the important events of the times. In his will, quoted below, he bequeathed money to Bedlam, or Bethlehem Hospital, the first "lunatic asylum in England," founded in 1247 as a priory for the sisters and brothers of the order of the Star of Bethlehem, and first located in Bishopsgate Street.[87] In addition to this bequest, Gregory mentions a "suster" in the "Elsyng Spitell," and leaves money to that hospital and two others.]

Also I bequeth to gyf among pouer folk liyng sike in the hospitall called Saint Mary Spitell without Bishoppesgate, xxs. And to the pouere seke people of the hospitall of Saint Mary of Bethelem, xlx. Also I bequethe to ye pouere people of Elsyng Spitell, to pray for my soule, xiijs. iiijd. Also to Richard Warners cosyn, beyng suster in the same Elsyng Spitell, vjs.viijd. Also I biqueth to the pouere people liying in the hospitall of Saint Thomas the Martir in Southwerk, xxs.[88]

CONCLUDING STATEMENT

The chronicles and histories of the Crusades relate little of how the knights cared for their sick and wounded as compared with their revelations concerning the military aspects of these great pilgrimages. Some information about the requirements, the habiliments, and the activities of the military nursing orders is given in early official documents, especially the rules of the orders themselves. These indicate that great hospitals were built and equipped and the patients nursed by the knights. One interesting development later (in the eighteenth century) was the provision of a kind of visiting nursing in the homes of the poor in Malta, under the supervision of the knights. The actual nursing in this instance seems to have been done by "four paid maid-servants."

Pilgrim travelers to the Holy Land briefly alluded to the hospitals noted in their travels. Some were favorably impressed with the care given, while others, like John Howard, indicated that the conditions had changed for the worse, in later centuries.

From the numerous materials about St. Francis of Assisi, it is clear that in his early life in religion the saint cared for the lepers. The histories and legends of St. Francis reiterate the stories of his care of this group. He also provided for the care of the sick by the brethren in the Franciscan orders. The rarer references on St. Clare of Assisi, St. Elizabeth of Hungary, and St. Catherine of Siena point to the certainty that they too tirelessly nursed the sick in their own communities with gentleness and consideration; St. Clare, perhaps only within the walls of the monastery.

The Beguines of Flanders included hospital and home nursing among their responsibilities, and their characteristics in later centuries much impressed various travelers from England, such as Robert Southey, Dr. Robert Gooch, and Mme Elizabeth De Bunsen. The work of the regular orders went on as is shown in history and legend, and patients were nursed in sectarian and nonsectarian hospitals and in their homes.

As the Middle Ages evolved into the modern era, changes in many areas of social life became apparent. The exchange of goods and ideas brought about by the Crusades produced not only new institutions but modifications of the old ones. In this transition no institutions were affected more, perhaps, than those having to do with the care of the sick. Promoted by the changing needs of society and the response of groups and individuals to these needs, reforms began to occur. These were very slow in coming in most instances, as is apparent from the sources.

Some of the sources illustrating the state of nursing in the hospitals and homes of England from the sixteenth to the eighteenth centuries are presented in the next chapter, together with some of those reflecting the efforts of St. Vincent de Paul to improve conditions in France in the seventeenth century.

Chapter 4

*Some References to European Nursing,
Sixteenth to Eighteenth Centuries*

INTRODUCTION

THE centuries immediately following the Crusades were marked by
great social changes, among which one, the Reformation, perhaps
more than the others, was to have a far-reaching effect on the care of
the sick. The Reformation was not only a religious movement; its results
were secular as well. The established institutions of the times were affected
by it. Among those institutions profoundly influenced were hospitals
and methods of caring for the sick. Up to this time, much of the care
had been the responsibility of the Church, either directly or indirectly.
When the results of the Reformation caused a closing of large numbers
of monasteries and hospitals, especially in those northern European
countries where the reform movement was most widespread, other provisions were, of necessity, instituted to meet the need. The era is marked
by the establishment of secular hospitals and the growth of the use of
secular nurses. At the same time, nursing under religious auspices continued and was itself the subject of attempts at reform.

The most important group of the latter type, whose work resulted in
improvement in nursing at about this time, was the Daughters of Charity,
or as they are known today, the Sisters of Charity. Founded by Mlle le
Gras and St. Vincent de Paul first in country districts of France, the
order spread not only in France but eventually to many other lands.
Their work through the centuries in peace and war has endeared them
to all groups. This beginning of reform in nursing care was to proceed
slowly through various stages and events for two centuries before the
establishment of professional nursing in England gave it new meaning.

The nursing of the Daughters of Charity in France was paralleled by
changes in the care of the sick in the hospitals and homes of England as
well as by other changes in France. In England, attention became focused
on hospitals by the writings of various individuals. One of the first of

these was Sir Thomas More, who in his *Utopia,* described what he considered to be an ideal hospital (106). This description, written in 1516, speaks of physicians and "the stewarde of the sicke" but does not mention nurses.

The care of the sick in hospitals is referred to in two books written by John Stow: *Annales of England* and *A Survay of London* (107, 108). Stow lists the hospitals which were in existence in London up to his own time (1525–1605) and describes, in some instances, the conditions in nursing. The minutes of committees administering the hospitals also are revealing with respect to nurses, as in the case of the Foundlings' Hospital, London, and the London Hospital (109, 110). The covenant between King Henry VIII and the people of London in the sixteenth century, regarding St. Bartholomew's Hospital, provided for nurses (111), while the orders of King Henry VIII and King Edward VI to the London Hospitals mentioned the duties of various attendants (112). Another official document, that of St. Thomas's Hospital, helps to fill in the story of nursing in this period (113).

Also of interest in understanding hospital nursing in the eighteenth century in England are three books, one written by a physician. Thomas Fuller, in 1730, described an ideal nurse for the care of smallpox patients (114), probably the first such detailed description in writing by an English physician. A book by William Nolan, *An Essay on Humanity,* tells of some of the evils existing in the nursing at St. Bartholomew's Hospital as seen by the writer himself (115). John Howard, the English philanthropist, made extensive visits to hospitals, lazarettos, and prisons in the latter part of the eighteenth century. His observations are found in *An Account of the Principal Lazarettos in Europe,* first published in 1789 (116).

Nursing in the home during these centuries was also described by some writers. Pictures of nursing under abnormal conditions are not infrequently part of the literature of the great plague in London in 1665. Examination of these materials indicates that one writer often drew his information directly from another, making the statements repetitious. For this reason a small selection has been made from among them for inclusion in this chapter, as follows: Nathaniel Hodges' *Loimologia* (117); *Shutting Up of Infected Houses Soberly Debated* (118); William Austin's *The Anatomy of the Pestilence, in the Year of Our Lord, 1665,* written in verse (119); Thomas Vincent's *God's Terrible Voice in the City* (120); and Daniel Defoe's *A Journal of the Plague Year* (121). *The Diary and Correspondence of Samuel Pepys* has a large number of references to the plague of 1665, one of which speaks of a nurse (122).

Primary sources for nursing in the home in relatively normal times in

England are few. Among those of interest are the *Diary of Lady Margaret Hoby,* which covers the years 1599 to 1605 (123), and the *Journal* of Lady Mildmay, 1570 to 1617 (124). The good works of Lady Letice, Viscountess Falkland, are described in 1653 in a letter written by a friend to Lady Letice's mother (125). Documents in the *Sussex Archeological Collections* not seldom give hints concerning nurses who cared for individual patients in England in the seventeenth and eighteenth centuries (126–128).

At about this time in France the work of the surgeon, Ambroise Paré, attracted much attention because of its outstanding success. *The Workes of that Famous Chirurgion Ambroise Parey* (129) describes in detail the care given by Paré to Monsieur le Marquis l'Auret, much of which will be seen to be the function of nurses of a later day.

Two references to deaconesses in Europe in this period, from the writings of the Pilgrims, are included. One of these is the catechism of John Robinson, the leader of the Pilgrims in Holland, which provides for deaconesses for the care of the sick, probably in the church in Leyden (130), and the other is found in *Chronicles of the Pilgrim Fathers of the Colony of Plymouth from 1602 to 1625,* which tells the virtues of a deaconess of Amsterdam in Holland (131).

As has been stated, the initiation of reform in nursing in France came through the work of St. Vincent de Paul and the Daughters of Charity. St. Vincent's *Rules of the Confraternity* (132–134), the latter a group of women first organized in Chatillon to care for the sick in their homes, are partly in the hand of St. Vincent. The record of his *Conferences* with the Daughters (135) is enlightening as an indication of his ideas on nursing. Of interest also are *Letters of St. Vincent de Paul* (136). His communications with Mlle le Gras, his co-worker and co-founder of the Daughters, reveal many of his thoughts in connection with the functioning of the organizations which he had established for community work. Excerpts from both letters and conferences present other information about this group of nurses (137). The vow taken by a Sister of Charity in 1642 (138) indicates the objective of the Daughters, while St. Vincent's announcement of the Archbishop's approbation of the organization bespeaks the feeling with which St. Vincent viewed the privilege which was the Daughters' in their work among the sick (139).

THE SOURCES

106. Sir Thomas More. *Utopia*

[Sir Thomas More (1478–1535) is best known for his *Utopia,* a classic picture of an ideal state, which was first published in 1516 in

Latin. Because of his disapproval of the divorce of Henry VIII from Catherine of Aragon, he incurred the disfavor of the king, was finally imprisoned in the Tower of London, and was beheaded. He was canonized by Pope Pius in 1935.[1] He is described by most writers as a man of noble character, a gentleman and a scholar, qualified in the practice of law and interested in music and painting.]

But first and chieflie of all, respect is had to the sycke, that be cured in the hospitalles. For in the circuite of the citie, a little without the walles, they have iiii hospitalles, so bigge so wyde so ample, and so large, that they may seme iiii little townes, which were devised of that bignes partely to thintent the sycke, be they never so many in numbre, shuld not lye to thronge or strayte, and therefore uneasely and incommodiously: and partely that they which were taken and holden with contagious diseases, suche as be wonte by infection to crepe from one to another, myght be layde apart ferre from the company of the residue. These hospitalles be so wel appointed, and with al thinges necessary to health so furnished, and more over so diligent attendaunce through the continual presence of cunning phisitians is geven, that though no man be sent thether against his will, yet notwithstandinge there is no sicke persone in al the citie, that had not rather lye there, then at home in his owne house. When the stewarde of the sicke hath received suche meates as the phisitians have prescribed, then the beste is equallye devided among the halles, according to the company of everyone, saving that there is had a respect to the prince, the byshop, the tranibours, and to ambassadours and all straungers, if there be any, which be verye fewe and seldome.[2]

107. John Stow. *Annales, or A Generall Chronicle of England*

[John Stow (1525–1605), the son and grandson of tailors, lived throughout the whole reign of Elizabeth and into that of James the First. He may have practiced his occupation for a few years, but his patriotic interest in the annals of his native land caused him to be remembered for a far different reason. He began at about the age of thirty to delve into the history of the past, and to collect books to aid him in his research. He is regarded as one of the most reliable of sixteenth-century chroniclers. Among his published works, the best known are *A Summarie of Englysh Chronicles,* published in 1561,[3] *Annales of England,* published first in 1592,[4] and *A Survay of London,* published in 1598.[5] In the *Annales* he mentions the founding of a hospital by Thomas Sutton, his contemporary, the son of an official of the city of London.]

Thomas Sutton Esquier, borne at Snaith in Lincolnshire, in his youth trained up in all good learning, then travailed into forraine nations, where he attained perfection of sundry Languages, hee was a student in Lincolnes Inne . . .

And namely in the Creating and founding of a most goodly and royall Hospitall, instituted, the Hospitall of King James, founded in Charter-house in the countie of Middellsex, at the humble petition, & only cost and charges of the above named Thomas Sutton Esquire who endowed the same with above three thousand pound of yearly rentes.

In this bounteous Hospitall, there is maintained fourescore poore men with sweete Lodging, wholsome diet, and allowance in money for apparell, therein is also maintained fortie poore children, with competent diet, Lodging and apparell, and a grammer Schoole, over which there is a Master and an Other to teach those boyes, for the which they have their diet, and lodging and faire stipends . . .

And for the orderly government of this most worththy hospital, the founder ordained y forever there should bee a discreet learned man chosen to be the master of the household, over which hee is to have the inward government. And also a learned devine to teach and instruct them, &c. besides these and all other necessarie officers for so great a familie, they likewise have allowed them a Phisitition and a Chirurgian.[6]

108. John Stow. *A Survay of London*

[The *Survay* lists the hospitals in existence in Stow's day, together with their purposes and contemporary status. It includes the rules established for nurses in St. Bartholomew's Hospital.]

Hospitals in this City, and Suburbs thereof, that have been of old Time, and now presently are, I read of these as followeth:

Hospital of St. Mary, in the parish of Barking Church, that was provided for poor priests and others, men and women of the city of London, that were fallen into frenzy of loss of their memory, until such time as they should recover, was since suppressed and given to the hospital of St. Katharine, by the Tower.

St. Anthony's, an hospital of thirteen poor men, and college, with a free school for poor men's children, founded by the citizens of London, lately by John Tait, first a brewer and then a mercer, in the ward of Broad Street, suppressed in the reign of Edward VI., the School in some sort remaining, but sore decayed.

St. Bartholomew, in Smithfield, an hospital of great receipt and relief for the poor, was suppressed by Henry VIII., and again by him given to the city, and is endowed by the citizens' benevolence.

St. Giles in the Fields was an hospital for leprous people out of the city of London and shire of Middlesex, founded by Matilda the queen, wife of Henry I., and suppressed by King Henry VIII.

St. John of Jerusalem, by West Smithfield, an hospital of the Knights of Rhodes, for maintenance of soldiers against the Turks and infidels, was suppressed by King Henry VIII.

St. James in the Field was an hospital for leprous virgins of the city of

London, founded by citizens for that purpose, and suppressed by King Henry VIII.

St. John, at Savoy, an hospital for relief of one hundred poor people, founded by Henry VII., suppressed by Edward VI., again new founded, endowed, and furnished by Queen Mary, and so remaineth.

St. Katharine, by the Tower of London, an hospital with a master, brethren, and sisters, and alms women, founded by Matilda, wife of King Stephen; not suppressed, but in force as before.

St. Mary within Cripplegate, an hospital founded by William Elsing, for a hundred blind people of the city, was suppressed by King Henry VIII.

St. Mary Bethlehem, without Bishopsgate, was an hospital, founded by Simon Fitzmary, a citizen of London, to have been a priory, and remaineth for lunatic people, being suppressed and given to Christ's Hospital.

St. Mary, without Bishopsgate, was an hospital and priory, called St. Mary Spittle, founded by a citizen of London for relief of the poor, with provision of one hundred and eighty beds there for the poor; it was suppressed in the reign of King Henry VIII.

St. Mary Rouncevall, by Charing Cross, was an hospital, suppressed with the priories aliens in the reign of King Henry V.; then was it made a brotherhood in the reign in the 15th of Edward IV., and again suppressed by King Edward VI.

St. Thomas of Acres, in Cheap, was an hospital for a master and brethren, in the record called Militia; it was surrendered and sold to the mercers.

St. Thomas, in Southwark, being a hospital of great receipt for the poor, was suppressed, but again newly founded and endowed by the benevolence and charity of the citizens of London.

An hospital there was without Aldersgate, a cell to the house of Cluny, of the French order, suppressed by King Henry V.

An hospital without Cripplegate, also a like cell to the said house of Cluny, suppressed by King Henry V.

A third hospital in Oldborne, being also a cell to the said house of Cluny, suppressed by King Henry V.

The hospital or almshouse called God's House, for thirteen poor men, with a college, called Whittington College, founded by Richard Whittington, mercer, and suppressed; but the poor remain, and are paid their allowance by the mercer.

Christ's Hospital, in Newgate Market, of a new foundation in the Grey Friars Church by King Henry VIII.; poor fatherless children be there brought up and nourished at the charges of the citizens.

Bridewell, now an hospital, or house of correction, founded by King Edward VI., to be a work house for the poor and idle persons of the city, wherein a great number of vagrant persons be now set-a-work, and relieved at the charges of the citizens. Of all these hospitals, being twenty in number, you may read before in their several places, as also of good and charitable provisions made for the poor by sundry well-disposed citizens.[7]

Some References to European Nursing

[Rules for the governance of the Sisters of St. Bartholomew's Hospital, during the reign of Edward VI (1537–1553).]

Your charge is, in all Things to declare and shew yourselves gentle, diligent, and obedient to the Matron of this House, who is appointed and authorised to be your chief Governess and Ruler. Ye shall also faithfully and charitably serve and help the Poor in their Griefs and Diseases, as well by keeping them sweet and clean, as in giving them their Meats and Drinks, after the most honest and comfortable Manner. Also ye shall use unto them good and honest Talk, such as may comfort and amend them; and utterly to avoid all light, wanton, and foolish Words, Gestures, and Manners, using Yourselves unto them with all Sobriety and Discretion, and above all Things, see that ye avoid, abhor, and detest Scolding and Drunkenness as most pestilent and filthy Vices. Ye shall not haunt or resort to any manner of Person out of this House, except ye be licensed by the Matron; neither shall ye suffer any light Person to haunt or use unto you, neither any dishonest Person, Man or Woman; and so much as in you shall lie, ye shall avoid and shun the Conversation and Company of all Men. Ye shall not be out of the Woman's Ward after the Hour of Seven of the Clock in the Night, in the Winter, Time, nor after Nine of the Clock in the Night in the Summer: except as ye shall be appointed and commanded by the Matron so to be, for some great and special cause that shall concern the Poor, (as the present Danger of Death or extreme Sickness), and yet so being commanded, ye shall remain no longer with diseased Person than just Cause shall require. Also, if any just Cause or Grief shall fortune unto any of you, or that ye shall see Lewdness in any Officer, or other Person of this House, which may sound or grow to the Hurt or Slander thereof, ye shall declare the same to the Matron, or unto one or two of the Govenours of this House, that speedy Remedy therein may be had; and to no other Person neither shall ye talk or meddle therein any farther. This is your Charge, and with any other Thing you are not charged.

. . . .

[The matron was instructed to] ... have also Charge, Governance & Order to all the Sisters of this House ... that every of them ... do their Duty unto the Poor, as well in making of their Beds, and keeping their Wards, as also in washing and purging their unclean Cloaths, and other Things. And that the same Sisters every night after the Hour of seven of the Clock in the Winter, and nine of the Clock in the Summer, come not out of the Woman's Ward, except some great and special cause (as the present Danger of Death, or needful Succour of some poor Person). And yet at such a special time it shall not be lawful for every Sister to go forth to any Person or Persons (not tho' it be in her ward) but only for such as you shall think virtuous, godly, and discreet. And the same Sister to remain no longer with the same sick Person than needful Cause shall require. Also at such times as the Sisters shall not be occupied about the Poor, ye shall set them to spinning or doing some other Manner of Work, that may avoid Idleness, and be profitable to the Poor of this House. Also ye shall receive the Flax ... the same being spun by the Sisters, ye shall commit to the said Governors. . . . You shall also . . . have special Regard to the good ordering & keeping of all the Sheets, Coverlets, Blankets, Beds, and other implements committed to your Charge, . . . Also ye shall suffer no poor Person of this House to sit and drink within your House at no Time, neither shall ye so send them drink into their Wards, that thereby Drunkenness might be used and continued among them.[8]

109. Minutes of Daily Committee, Foundlings' Hospital, London

[Thomas Coram (1668–1751), the founder of the Foundlings' Hospital, was a Dorset man who became a sea captain. In 1693 he crossed the Atlantic to Boston with a cargo of merchandise and was married in Boston in 1700. His idea of founding the hospital may have arisen from his concern over the abandoned infants he saw on his journeys to London. The Royal Charter for the incorporation of the hospital was given in 1739, when Coram was seventy-one years of age.[9]]

March 29, 1741.
Sarah Clarke one of the Nurses was Discharged for Disobedience and Sawciness to the Chief Nurse.

"Ackworth Dec[r]. 5th 1760
"Instructions to Nurse Greenwood
"She is to go to Doncaster on Saturday y[e] 6th Inst to meet Mat. Lee's y[e] Newcastle Waggon & travel in it from Thence to Newport Ragnal Wooburn or Dunstable. The Driver of the Waggon has Orders to receive Her & send Her on a Double Horse to Aylesbury from one of the above Places & give Her Directions in writing when the Waggon returns thro those Places, that She may be sure to meet it in due Time. When She gets to Aylesbury She is to enquire for y[e] Master of the Hospital & to desire Him to provide for Her while She stays there. She is to tell Him that She comes from D[r] Lee for Ten boys according to y[e] Directions of T. White Esq[r]. She has in Strict Charge to behave decently & take y[e] greatest Care to keep the Children warm as they come down." [10]

110. Minutes of the London Hospital

[The first London Hospital was a house in Featherstone Street, "near the Dog Bar," which was taken for £16 per annum, "with liberty to quit the same at six months' notice." It was opened as an infirmary in 1740. The first nurse appointed was known only by the name of "Squire." She was paid 5s. a week, and "lived out!" [11]]

[1752] Squire was reported to have taken money from patients; she was not dismissed however, as it was not in the rules that she should *not* do so. She promised not to do so again.[12]

111. Deed of Covenant between King *Henry* VIII and the Mayor, Commonalty, and Citizens of *London*, Respecting the Hospitals. 27 Dec. 38 *Hen.* VIII., 1546

[Although the title specifies "hospitals," it will be noted that this portion applied specifically to St. Bartholomew's Hospital. It provided for nurses and their payment.[13]]

This Indenture, made the twenty-seventh day of December in the thirty-eighth year of the reign of our Sovereign Lord *Henry* the Eighth, by the grace of God, King of *England France* and *Ireland,* Defender of the Faith and of the Church of *England* and also of *Ireland* in earth the Supreme Head, between the same our Sovereign Lord the King on the one part and the Mayor and Commonalty and Citizens of the City of *London* on the other part, witnesseth, that our said Sovereign Lord the King, considering the miserable state of the poore aged sick low and impotent people, as well men as women.

... further covenanting and granting to the King's Highness, his heirs and successors, shall make and provide at the scite of the said late hospital of Saint *Bartholomew's,* hereafter to be called the House of the Poore as is aforesaid, sufficient lodging for 100 poor men and poor women, and for one matron and twelve women under her to make the beds and wash and attend upon the said poor men and women there; and that the said Mayor and Commonalty and Citizens and their successors shall find perpetually to the said 100 poor folks, and to the said matron and twelve women under her, sufficient meat drink bedding cloathing wood coal and all other things mete convenient and necessary for them, and to give to the said matron in ready moneys 3 1.5s.8d. yearly, and to every of the said 12 women 40s. yearly ...

In witness whereof to the one part of this indenture, remaining with the said Mayor and Commonaltie and Citizens, our said Sovereign Lord the King hath caused his great seale of *England* to be put to, and to the other part of the same indenture, remaining with our said Sovereign Lord the King, and said Commonaltie and Citizens have put to their common seale, the day and year first above written.[14]

112. *The Order of the Hospitalls of K. Henry the viij and K. Edward the vith*

[The following order refers to four London Hospitals, namely, St. Bartholomew's, Christ's, Bridewell, and St. Thomas's, and provides for the duties of the matron, the nurses, and the keepers of the wards.]

115

By the Maior, Cominaltie, and Citizens of London, Governours of the Possessions, Revenues and Goods of the Sayd Hospitalls. 1557.

The Ordinances and Rules for the Governors of the Hospitalls in the Citie of *London*.

To be redd in every of the Said Hospitalls at a full Courte once every Quarter, either xiiij days before, or after the Quarter-day.

The Matrons Charge

Your office is an office of great charge and credite. For to you is committed the governance and oversight of all the women and children within this hospitall.

And also to yow is given authoritie, to commaunde, reproue and rebuke them or any of them; and if any shall hapen to disobey, whom you shall not be able to correct, yow shall from time to time make such knowen unto the almoners and governors of the howse; that they may take order with them, as shalbe thought meete by their wisdomes.

Your charge is also to searche and enquire whether the women doe their duetie, in washing of the childrens sheets and shirts, and in keeping cleane and sweet those that are committed to their charge; and also in the beddes, sheets, coverlets, and apparraile, (with keping cleane their wards and chambers) mending of such as shalbe broken from time to time. And specially yow shall geue diligent heede, that the said washers and nurses of this howse be alwaies well occupied and not idle. And that their linnen be wholsomly and cleanly washed; and the same first receued from the kepers be (after the washing thereof) quietly deliuered unto them.

You shall also once every quarter of the year, examine the inventorie which shalbe delivered unto you, of the implements of the howse; as of beddes, bolsters, mattresses, blanquets, coverlets, shets, pallads, shirts, hosen, and such other; whether any of the same be purloyned, embezeled, spoiled, or otherwise consumed; and to make such lacke and faults, as by yow shalbe espied, knowen unto the almoners of this howse for the time beinge, that they may take order therein.

You shall also geue great charge unto all the nurses of euery warde, that no child be received by them, before the name of the same childe be entred into the ward-booke; nor that any be deliuered to nurse or otherwise, but that they be also entred, and to whom they are delivered, with the day and month when the same was done.

You shall also neither receive nor deliver anythinge that is in the wardrop, unles yow cause the same to be written by them that are appointed thereunto. And be suer to receaue from the nurses in the country, when any children die, their apparaile.

You shall take such order among the nurses or otherwise, that the hall be kept swete and cleane; and suffer non of the children to be there after their meales, except it be of seruice time, and when it shall please the governors to appoint them.

You shall twise or thrise in euery weke arise in the night, and goe aswell into the sick warde as also into euery other ward, and ther se that the children be couered in the beddes, wherby they take no colde.

And laste of all, if yow shall perceave that any officer or officers of this howse doo abuse themselves, either in woorde or deede, yow shall admonishe the governors of the same, and not medle any further therin, neither to have to doo with any officer or officers, other than appertaineth to your owne office and charge as aforesaid.

102 *The Charge of the Nurses and Keepers* of the *Wardes.*

Your charge is faithfully and truely to serve in this howse, to obey the matron thereof.

Ye shall also flie and eschue all rayling, skoldinge, swearinge, and drunkennes.

Ye shall in your behauiour and doings be vertuous louinge and diligent.

Ye shall also carefully and diligently oversee, keepe, and governe all those tender babes and yonglings that shalbe comitted to your charge, and the same holesomly, cleanely, and sweetly noorishe and bringe up.

And in like maner shall ye keepe your wardes and every parte thereof swete and cleane.

Ye shall also, to avoid all idleness, when your charge and care of keping the children is paste, occupie your selves in spinninge, sewing, mending of shets and shirts, or some other vertuous exercise, such as you shalbe appointed unto.

Ye shall not resort, or suffer any man to resort to you, before ye have declared the same to the almoners, or matron of this howse, and have obtayned their lycence and favor so to doe.

Ye shall at lawfull times, according to such order as is and shalbe taken in this howse, be within your wardes and places of lodginge, and se that all your children before they be brought to bed, be washed and cleane, and imediately after, every of yow quietly shall goe to your bed, and not to sit up any longer; and once euery night arise, and se that the children be couered, for taking of colde.

Theis are the especial partes of your charge, whiche ye shall endeuour every of your selues, with all your powers to obserue and kepe; or els ye shall not only remaine under the corection and punishment that shall be thought meete, by the discretion of the governors, but also to be expulsed and banished this howse for ever. And whatsoeuer faults ye shall perceaue by any other officers in this howse, the same ye shall declare unto the governours, and not otherwise medle or make but in your owne busines.[15]

113. From the Records of St. Thomas's Hospital

[Of the foundation of St. Thomas's Hospital in London, it is impossible to be perfectly exact. It was probably founded in 1213, and was situated in Southwark. It was connected with the priory of Bermondsey.[16] Dissolved by Henry VIII, it was later re-established.[17]]

[April 19, 1563. The matron reported Margaret Allen, a sister]: For that she wolde not do her dutie in her office but ronne to the taverne and neglect her office, wherefore the masters gave her warning to amende her faults or elles to leave his service and forther punyshment.

[March 8, 1568] Yt is ordered that if any of the susters shall disorder themselves by brawlinge one with another, or other misdemeanour, that then upon complaynt made every suche suster to be removed her ward and sustership and discharged the house for ever.[18]

114. Thomas Fuller. *Exanthematologia; or a Rational Account of Eruptive Fevers*

[Thomas Fuller (1654–1734), physician, was educated at Queen's College, Cambridge, receiving his medical degree in 1681. He was a member of the College of Physicians of London and practiced all his life in Kent, acquiring a large practice and great popularity among the people. He published many books and was the first English writer to point out clearly how to distinguish the spots produced by flea bites from those seen in eruptive fevers. He was the first English physician to set forth in writing the qualifications necessary for a nurse in the care of smallpox patients.[19]]

Of a Nurse.

Though it is impossible to meet with a Nurse every way so qualify'd for the Business, as to have no Faults or Failings, yet the more she cometh up to the following Particulars, the more she is to be liked. It is therefore desirable that she be,

1. Of a middle Age, fit and able to go through with the necessary Fatigue of her Undertaking.
2. Healthy, especially free from Vapours, and Cough.
3. A good Watcher, that can hold fitting up the whole Course of the Sickness.
4. Quick in Hearing, and always ready at the first Call.
5. Quiet and Still, so as to talk low, and but little, and tread softly.
6. Of good Sight, to observe the Pocks, their Colour, Manner, and Growth, and all Alterations that may happen.
7. Handy to do every Thing the best way, without Blundering and Noise.
8. Nimble and Quick a going, coming, and doing every Thing.
9. Cleanly, to make all she dresseth acceptable.
10. Well-tempered, to humour, and please the Sick as much as she can.
11. Chearful and Pleasant; to make the best of Every Thing, without being at any time Cross, Melancholy, or Timorous.
12. Constantly careful, and diligent by Night and by Day.

13. Sober and Temperate; not given to Gluttony, Drinking, or Smoaking.

14. Observant to follow the Physician's Orders duly; and not be so conceited of her own Skill, as to give her own Medicines privately.

15. To have no Children, or others to come much after her.[20]

115. William Nolan. *An Essay on Humanity: or A View of Abuses in Hospitals with a Plan for Correcting Them*

[The book from which the following quotation is taken is dedicated to "John McNamara, Esq.; Member of Parliament for the City of Leicester." It is apparent from the context that William Nolan was interested in hospital conditions in London, whether as a member of a committee or as an individual appointed to make the investigation is not clear. At the end of his report, he recommends the formation of a *Humane Committee* in hospitals to "correct" and "reform" them.[21]]

Curiosity led me to St. Bartholomew's Hospital on a taking-in-day, (as it is termed) when a patient was admitted into the ward where I was; and after passing through the extra-formalities necessary for such admission, he was introduced by one of the beadles to the sister of the ward, who at first received him with that affected cordiality and seeming tenderness which pecuniary expectations make low minds assume; after which she asked him—"Had he got his wardage?"—The unhappy man said, "He had no money—That the last six-pence he had in the world he gave to the beadle who shewed him into the ward." The *tender* hearted sister on this information flew into the most outrageous passion, and in an imperious elevation of voice, in which were blended insolence, ignorance, and barbarity, demanded, "how he dare come there without it? Did he not know it was customary? and that it was her due or perquisite?—with a number of other interrogatories equally divested of decency, and humanity. The trembling patient modestly replied, He believed it might be customary; but alledged his inability as his only reason for non-compliance to it. This affecting confession, so far from softening the heart of the inexorable sister, exasperated her still more, in so much, that she absolutely insisted on his turning out of the ward immediately, and actually proceeded to push him out: shock'd at such unexampled inhumanity, I arrested her in the execution of her unfeeling purpose.—"Hold, monster," said I, "here is your wardage, and may the gin you procure for it, rid human nature of so great a reproach on it!" This inveterate imprecation I could not restrain, in the moment of my indignant resentment and detestation, for such unparralleled insensibility of soul!

.   .   .   .

This perquisite of wardage operates variously to the disadvantage of patients;—It makes the sister look with the eye of anxiety on the patient in all the progressive situations and stages of his cure; not from a humane concern for the restoration of his health, but with an avaricious expectation of having him discharged, as she is to get 3s. from the person whom accident or

119

decease makes his successor; and as, perhaps, she has no other bed in her ward to accomodate such casual successor with, but that occupied by some half-cured patient. It is therefore very evident, that the number of cures effected in the ward committed to her *humane* superintendence, is not so much the object of her solicitude, as the number of patients admitted into it, as she has 3s. for each. It is very reasonable to infer, from this circumstance, that her tenderness will not be much exerted towards the patients; the very reverse is justly to be apprehended, as she must know from experience, that moroseness and brutality might induce some to quit the hospital before their cures were accomplished, though tenderness and humanity would be an additional inducement to them to stay for that very desirable purpose to be accomplished.

Another infamous practice of these wretches, to multiply their perquisites, is to prefer complaints to the steward against the unhappy patients; for if in the acuteness of their pains they are guilty of the least vehement expression, they are immediately represented to the steward as intolerably noisy and troublesome. Thus for not having the constancy to maintain an equality of temper in the extremity of pain, they are painted out as intolerable and for no other human reason, than that perhaps their agonies are so! and a dismission soon after, notwithstanding any pathetic remonstrance to the contrary, is frequently the consequence.

This despotic act of power in the *Lord Steward* is faithfully copied by the *Lady Matron* in her department, with this difference only, that the delicacy of the complaints, which females frequently labour under, will not dispense with so immediate a dismission, but in any circumstances where they will, her plenitude of arbitrary authority will be as severely, and as instantaneously exercised; and for the same iniquitous reason already mentioned.

Is it not a melancholy consideration that the health, or perhaps the life, a useful member of society should thus fall a sacrifice either to the avarice of the sister, or the caprice of the steward? and it amounts to more than a presumption, that this is frequently the case, when patients are turned out of the hospital before their cures are effected.

.   .   .   .   .   .

The number of evils arising from this pernicious perquisite of wardage, are as obvious as they are distressing to the poor afflicted part of the community; it is therefore hoped, the governors and subscribers to hospitals will apply a radical cure to the evil, by totally suppressing it, and substitute in its room an additional equivalent of salary to the sisters and nurses . . .

.   .   .   .   .   .

I am very well convinced from my observations on human nature in the melancholy stages of perturbation of spirit, and corporeal pain, that a patient's cure is as much accelerated by the tenderness and humanity of the nurse, as by the most obedient conformity to the prescriptions of the doctor; and that to effectuate a cure in the body, I hold it absolutely necessary to maintain peace in the mind. It is evident from this, how essential it is to the health of a patient, to have an affectionate tender nurse; and consequently how necessary the precaution here recommended for the admission of such— as also the rejection of such others, as do not fall under this denomination.

. . . .

It is a matter of no consequence to the unhappy patient, who loses his health for want of due care, whether his misfortune is attributable to the inhumanity of the nurse, or the inattention or ignorance of his doctor; and here I cannot avoid observing, that as much from these causes, as from any incurable obstinacy of his disorder, the patient's dissolution happens.

. . . .

Should the adoption of the foregoing hints of reformation be thought likely to conduce to the obtaining the ends proposed, *The Humane Committee* would in the exercise of their new-invested authority inavoidably be presented with numberless objects of correction and reformation at the same time.[22]

116. John Howard. *An Account of the Principal Lazarettos in Europe*

[John Howard (1726–1790), English prison reformer and philan- thropist,[23] published his book on European hospitals in 1789. He died the following year as the result of fever which he contracted while making a study of prison conditions in Russia.[24] The first two hospitals mentioned in the following quotations were infirmaries; the third was a hospital for "seafaring men."]

The *Infirmary* at Maryborough for *Queen's County* is an old house in which are four rooms for patients. The floor of the room below was dirt, and the walls were black and filthy; it had in it three patients. In two of the rooms above, there were thirteen beds and fifteen patients, and a little dirty hay on the floor, on which they said the nurse lay. This room was very dirty, the ceiling covered with cobwebs, and in several places open to the sky. Here I saw one naked, pale object, who was under the necessity of tear- ing his shirt for bandages for his fractured thigh. No sheets in the house,— and the blankets were very dirty. No vault: no water.—The diet is a three- penny loaf and two pints of milk; or rather, if my taste did not deceive me, of milk and water.... April 16th, 1788, 20 patients.

. . . .

The *County Infirmary* at Castlebar is an old ruinous house, very dirty, and the windows were stopt with straw. No linen; and no blankets but such as are found by the patients. Only one room (eighteen feet and a half by fifteen and a half) for kitchen, turf-house and wash-house, and for the nurse's lodging which is under the staircase. Diet is water pottage and one pint of milk a day; besides one sheep's head boiled for soup for all the patients on three days a week, and on three other days a pennyworth of bread for each patient (weight *8 oz.*). The court in this, as in many other infirmaries, is very dirty, and has no conveniences. March 31st, 1788, 16 patients.

. . .

The Royal Hospital at Haslar near Gosport
The following Regulations and Orders were Hung up in the Wards.
Regulations
Respecting the Nurses and other Servants of the Royal Hospital at Haslar.
Ordered,

I. That none of the nurses, or other servants in the hospital, do conceal the effects of any of the patients who may die therein; reports of such effects are to be made, immediately after the decease of the patients, to the agent, or his clerk, by the respective nurses of the wards.

II. That no bags, chests, or bundles of any kind, belonging to the patients, to be received, or kept in any of the wards, or nurses cabins, but carried to the bed-house.

III. That no dirt, bones, or rags, be thrown out of any window, or down the bogs, but carried to the places appointed for that purpose; nor are any cloaths of the patients, or others, to be hung out of any of the windows of the house.

IV. That no foul linen, whether sheets or shirts, be kept in the cabins, or wards, but sent immediately to the matron, in order to its being carried to the wash-house; and the nurses are to obey the orders of the matron in punctually shifting the bed and body linen of the patients, *viz.* their sheets once a fortnight, their shirts once in four days, their night caps, drawers and stockings once a week, or oftener if found necessary.

V. That no nurse or other person do wash in the water closets.

VI. That no hospital dress or any part of that dress, be carried out of the fever, flux, or small-pox wards into other wards, nor are the men to be permitted to wear any part of their own cloaths in these wards; and the patients are to be suffered to wear the hospital night caps out of their proper wards, but by permission of the physician or surgeon.

VII. That dead bodies be not left longer in the wards or lobbies than the precise time ordered by the physician or surgeon, at the expiration of which, and not before, they are to be carried into the dead-house.

VIII. That no nurse do admit any patients, on any pretence whatsoever, into her cabin, nor suffer any person to remain in it at night, not even her husband or child.

IX. That any nurse concealing the escape of any patient from her ward, or that has not made due report, at the agent's office, of her having missed such patient, be discharged the hospital, upon proof thereof.

X. That all nurses who disobey the matron's order, get drunk, neglect their patients, quarrel or fight with any other nurses, or quarrel with the men, or do not prudently and cautiously reveal, to the superior officers of the house, all irregularities committed by the patients in their wards (such as drinking, smoking tobacco in the wards, quarrelling, destroying the medicines, or stores, feigning complaints and neglecting their cure) be immediately discharged the service of the house, and a note made against their names, on the books of the hospital, that they may never more be employed.

XI. That the nurses take care to prevent the patients from lying down in their beds with their cloaths on, or having their wearing apparel on their beds or cradles, or any bread, butter, or provisions of any kind, upon the heads of their cradles, or about their beds, and that no vituals be dressed in the wards.

XII. That if any men are taken ill in the recovery ward, so as to be obliged to take to their beds, the nurses do acquaint the assistant in waiting therewith, that they may be immediately removed, if that shall be judged necessary.

XIII. That the nurses provide themselves always with a sufficient quantity of such drinks for the patients as are ordered, and when they cannot be got, that they acquaint the physician or surgeon therewith. In the fever, flux, and small-pox wards, gruel and panado are constantly to be kept ready, a small chink of the upper part of some one or more of the windows is constantly to be kept open, so as at night gently to move the flame of a candle when standing on the table, unless otherwise ordered by the physician. The proper patients only are to come into these wards, and no others whatever.

XIV. That no cards, or gaming of any kind, be permitted in the hospital.

XV. That such nurses as can be spared by the matron, go to chapel every Sunday; and that the nurses take care, that such patients as are able do attend divine service whenever it is performed; and report to the physician or surgeon, such persons as neglect going there.

XVI. That no person whatever be permitted to sell wine, brandy, strong beer or other liquor, nor any article whatsoever, either within the hospital or its bounds.

XVII. That no will be made for any patient, without leave first had in writing, from the physician or surgeon; and that no officer, assistant, clerk, matron, nurse or any person whatsoever belonging to the hospital, shall accept a will made in their favour.[25]

117. Nathaniel Hodges. *Loimologia; or, an Historical Account of the Plague in London in 1665*

[The writer was a physician, a Fellow of the College of Physicians.[26] The *Oxford Dictionary* (1903) states that "Loimologia" refers to the "study of, or a treatise on the plague or pestilential diseases." This book was written in the plague year, 1665.]

But what greatly contributed to the Loss of People thus shut up, was the wicked Practices of Nurses (For they are not to be mentioned but in the most bitter Terms): These wretches, out of Greediness to plunder the Dead, would strangle their Patients, and charge it to the Distemper in their Throats;

123

others would secretly convey the pestilential Taint from Sores of the infected to those who were well; and nothing indeed deterred these abandoned Miscreants from prosecuting their avaritious Purposes by all the Methods their Wickedness could invent; who, although they were without Witnesses to accuse them, yet it is not doubted but divine Vengeance will overtake such wicked Barbarities with due Punishment: Nay, some were remarkably struck from Heaven in the Perpetration of their Crimes, and one particularly amongst many, as she was leaving the House of a Family, all dead, loaded with her Robberies, fell down dead under her Burden in the Streets: and the Case of a worthy Citizen was very remarkable, who being suspected dying by his Nurse, was before-hand stripped by her; but recovering again, he came a second time into the World naked. And so many were the Artifices of these barbarous Wretches, that it is to be hoped, Posterity will take Warning how they trust them again in like Cases; and that their past Impunities will not be a Means of bringing on us again the like Judgment.

But the worst Part of the Year being now over, and the Height of the Disease, the Plague by leisurely Degrees declined, as it had gradually made its first Advances; and before the Number infected decreased, its Malignity began to relax, insomuch that few died, and those chiefly such as were ill managed; hereupon that Dread which had been upon the Minds of the People wore off; and the Sick chearfully used all the means directed for their Recovery; and even the Nurses grew either more cautious, or more faithful, insomuch that after some Time a Dawn of Health appeared, as sudden, and as unexpected, as the Cessation of the following Conflagration [the Great Fire of 1665]; wherein after blowing up of Houses, and using all Means for its Extinction to little Purpose, the Flames stopped as it were of themselves, for Want of Fuel, or out of Shame for having devoured so much.[27]

118. *Shutting Up of Infected Houses Soberly Debated*

[This pamphlet was written in 1665. The author is unknown. The subtitle, "By way of Address from the poor souls that are Visited to their Brethren that are free," indicates that those suffering from the plague were "shut up" in their houses, a practice causing great suffering, and some doubts as to its wisdom and humanity, even as a preventive against the infectiousness of the disease.]

Little is it conceived how careless most nurses are in attending the visited, and how careless (being possessed with rooking avarice) they are to watch their opportunity to ransack their houses; the assured absence of friends making the sick desperate on the one hand, and them on the other unfaithful: their estates are the Plague most die on, if they have anything to lose, to be sure those sad creatures (for the nurses in such cases are the off-scouring of the City) have a dose to give them; besides that it is something beyond a Plague to an ingenious spirit to be in the hands of those dirty, ugly, and unwholesome hags; even a hell itself, on the one hand to hear nothing but screetches, cries, groans, and on the other to see nothing but ugliness and deformity, black as night, and dark as melancholy. Ah! to be at the mercy of a strange woman is sad; but who can express the misery of being exposed to their rapine that have nothing of the woman left but shape? [28]

119. William Austin. *The Anatomy of the Pestilence, in the Year of Our Lord, 1665*

[This is a poem in three parts describing the deplorable conditions which prevailed in the City of London in 1665, during the great disasters of that year. Nothing is known about the composer except from his poem. The verses were published in 1666.]

> Her [the nurse's] Politicks are not from Aristotle,
> But from the grave, the purse, the bag and bottle.
> Her task is hard: therefore one must allow
> Her food as much as if he were her plough.
> Her danger being great, he cannot think,
> Her analeptick worse than Spanish drink.
> Though she take many a preservative,
> Quicksilver's that which keeps her best alive.
> Her daily pay as commonly is known,
> As hers that lover serves for half a crown.
> Her hands, to take, are nut-hooks, and her feet,
> As ready are to run for winding-sheet.
> She keeps the sick from want, which she does ward
> Off so, it can't touch her who is his guard.
> Narcoticks are the best things he can keep
> By him: for she thrives best when he's asleep.
> He never chides her: nor indeed is't reason
> He shared: for well he knows 'tis out of season.
> Passion uncurbed by fear is mastive dog,
> To raging fury left and freed from dog.
> The Pestilence like Frigot then will ride,
> Hard goaded in the poop with winde and tide:
> And soon his life's dear longing he may loose,
> Who for his Nurse is nice to pick and choose.
> Suppose such are as scarce as may be Tare
> In corn that's weeded well: one here, one there
> Discarded nurse may do him as much harm,
> As Devil sent away without a charm.
> For want of Nurses think as many sholes
> Of sick have died, as hops without their poles.

For her neglect or absence his content
Is patients, as best fitting patient.
He'l ne're give out she kill'd him: for 'tis said,
He's to be alwayes silent when he's dead.
And while he lives, Nurses he'l never curse,
Knowing few good, most bad, and many worse.
Quietly he'l conclude she's such a thing
About his person, as is plague-sore ring.[29]

120. Thomas Vincent. *God's Terrible Voice in the City*

[Thomas Vincent may have been the London Presbyterian minister with whom William Penn first entered into public controversy concerning the doctrines of Quakerism. Vincent's pamphlet was published in 1667. It contains two parts—the first on the plague in London in 1665, and the second on the great London fire in 1666.[30] A note on the flyleaf of the copy consulted says, "Died at Hoxlow in 1678."]

. . . we may imagine the hideous thoughts and horrid perplexity of mind, the tremblings, confusions, and anguish of spirit, which some awakened sinners have had, when the Plague hath broke in upon their houses, and seized upon near relations, whose dying groans sounding in their ears have warned them to prepare: When their doors have been shut up and fastned on the outside with an Inscription, *Lord Have Mercy Upon Us,* and none suffered to come in but a Nurse, whom they have been more afraid of, than the Plague it self . . .[31]

121. Daniel Defoe. *A Journal of the Plague Year*

[Daniel Defoe, journalist and novelist, was born probably in 1660 or 1661. He qualified for the ministry, but went into business and became a liveryman of the city of London. At one time he published works against the church and was imprisoned in Newgate.[32] Although only five or six years of age at the time of the great plague, he states that he "very particularly remember[ed] the last visitation . . . which afflicted this nation in 1665, and had occasion to converse with many other persons who lived in this city all the while. . . ."[33] Although the character of the nurses in this account is startling, as it is in the others, there is one difference. Defoe evaluated the stories which he heard and tended to discount them.]

Orders Conceived and Published by the Lord Mayor and Aldermen of the City of London, concerning the infection of the Plague; 1665 . . .

Nurse Keepers

If any nurse keeper shall remove herself out of any infected house before twenty-eight days after the decease of any person dying of the infection, the

126

house to which the said nurse keeper doth so remove herself shall be shut up until the said twenty-eight days shall be expired.

We had at this time a great many frightful stories told us of nurses and watchmen who looked after the dying people; that is to say, hired nurses, who attended infected people, using them barbarously, starving them, smothering them, or by other wicked means, hastening their end, that is to say, murdering them; and watchmen, being set to guard houses that were shut up when there had been but one person left, and perhaps that one lying sick, that they have broke in and murdered that body, and immediately thrown them out into the dead-cart! and so they have gone scarce cold to the grave.

I cannot say but that some such murders were committed . . . but I must say I believe nothing of its being so common a crime as some have since been pleased to say . . .

I could give you an account of one of these nurses, who, several years after, being on her death-bed, confessed with the utmost horror the robberies she had committed at the time of her being a nurse, and by which she had enriched herself to a great degree . . .

They did tell me, indeed, of a nurse in one place that laid a wet cloth upon the face of a dying patient whom she tended, and so put an end to his life, who was just expiring before; and another that smothered a young woman she was looking to when she was in a fainting fit, and would have come to herself; some that killed them by giving them nothing at all. But these stories had two marks of suspicion that always attended them which caused me always to slight them, and to look upon them as mere stories, that people continually frighted one another with. First, that wherever it was that we heard it, they always placed the same at the farther end of the town, opposite or more remote from where you were to hear it . . .

In the next place, of what part soever you heard the story, the particulars were always the same, especially that of laying a wet double clout on a dying man's face, and that of smothering a young gentlewoman; so that it was apparent, at least to my judgment, that there was more of tale than of truth in those things.

The women and servants that were turned off from their places were likewise employed as nurses to tend the sick in all places, and this took off a very great number of them.[34]

122. Diary and Correspondence of Samuel Pepys

[Samuel Pepys (1635–1703), English diarist, was an official of the Navy office for several years. He also sat in Parliament in 1679 and became the object of an attack because of his supposed betrayal of naval secrets to the French. For this he was imprisoned in the Tower, but was later released and reappointed Secretary to the Admiralty. At the same time he became president of the Royal Society. His diary was kept in cipher and provides a record of the daily life of a young man of the times.[35] It contains almost a hundred references to the plague of 1665 in London.[36]]

Aug. 3, 1665.

By and by met my Lord Crewe returning; Mr. Marr telling me by the way, how a maid servant of Mr. John Wright's who lives thereabouts, falling sick of the plague, she was removed to an out-house, and a nurse appointed to look to her; who, being once absent, the maid got out of the house at the window, and ran away. The nurse coming and knocking, and having no answer, believed she was dead, and went and told Mr. Wright so; who and his lady were in a great straight what to do to get her buried . . .[37]

123. *Diary of Lady Margaret Hoby*

[Lady Margaret Hoby of Hackness, Yorkshire, the writer of this diary, was the wife of Sir Thomas Posthumous Hoby, her third husband. She has been called "the earliest known British woman diarist." The original of the diary is in the British Museum. It covers the period from 1599 to 1605—a short period in the writer's life. It is written precisely, on paper watermarked with a kind of Greek vase with a bunch of grapes at one end. Few punctuation marks appear, and the spelling is inconsistent. It is, however, the writing of one well accustomed to the use of the pen.[38] The account is very revealing of the character and daily life of the writer, and is filled with allusions to the measures which she employed for the relief of the sick. One of these, in particular, is rather startling, unless understood in the light of the conditions existing at the time.]

(Wensday 15)

In the morninge at :6: a clock I praied priuatly: that done, I went to awiffe in trauill of child, about whom I was busey tell :1 a Cloke, about which time, She bing deliuered and I hauinge praised god, returned home and betook my selfe to priuat praier :2: seuerall times vpon occasion: then I wrett the most part of an examenation or triall of a christian; framed by Mr Rhodes . . .

. . . .

(Tewsday the 27)

After priuat praier I went to the church: after, I praied, then I dimed, then I walked and did se a secke man: when I Came home I received diuerse things from Londone: after that I went to priuat praier and medetation, and from thence to publecke praers, so to supper: after, I wrought, and hard Mr Rhodes read of Mr Grenhame, and so praied priuatly and then went to bed:

.   .   .   .

(*Ianur The* 3 *day of the week* 30: 1599)

After I had praied priuatly I dressed a poore boies legge that Came to me, and then brake my fast wth Mr Hoby: after, I dressed the hand of one of our seruants that was verie sore Cutt, and after I wrett in my testement notes vpon James: then I went about the doinge of some thinges in the house, paiynge of billes, and after I had talked with Mr Hoby, I went to examenation and praier, after to supper, then to the lector; after that I dressed one of the mens handes that was hurt, lastly praied, and so to bed:

.   .   .   .

(*The* 5 *day of the weke Feb* :1:)

After I was readie I went about the house and then praied, brake my fast, dressed a poore boyes leg that was hurt, and Jurdens hand: after took a lector, read of the bible, praied, and so went to dinner: after: I went down a whill, then wrought tell 4: a Cloke and tooke order for supper, and then talked a whill wth Mr Hoby, and after went to priuat praier and medetation: after to supper, then to publect praiers, and lastly to bed:

(*The* 6 *day of the weke* 2:)

After I had praied I dressed the sores that Cam to me: after, I dined and talked to som of my neighbours the afternone tell about 3 a Cloke: then I rede of the arball, went a bout the house, and returned to priuat praers: after, to supper, then to publect praier, and lastly to priuat

(*Feb. The Lordes day* :3:)

After priuat praers I did eate my breakfast, and then dresed the sores that I had vndertaken: after, I went to the Church; after, I praied priuatly and then dined: in the afternone I went again to Church: after I Came home I reed of the testament, and wrett notes in itt and vpon Perknes, and then went about the house, and, at my accustomed hower, Came to priuat examenation and praier, and then to supper: after, to the repeticion and, when I had dressed some sores, I went to priuat praier and so to bed:

(*The* :1 *day of the week* :4:)

After I had praied I went about and dispatched the former busines I was accustomed: after, I studed my lector and dined: after dinner I talked a whill with Mr Hoby and then all the after none, I was busie in the kitchen and about som other thinges: at 5 a cloke I dressed my patientes, and then returned to priuat praier and examenation, then to supper, after to the lector: after that, to my Closit, wher I praied and Writt som thinge for mine owne priuat Conscience, and so I went to bed

129

[For the next twenty days, there is a notation in the diary, "dressed my patients," sometimes twice a day.]

(*The Lordes day* :26)

After I was readie I went to the church, and, after praiers and sermon, I Came home and dressed Blackbourns foote: after I dined, and after I talked and reed to some good wiffes: after I praied and reed, and wrett notes in my bible—the morninge exercise: after, I went to church, and, after sarmon, I dressed a poore mans hand; and after that I walked a broad, and so Came to priuat examenation and praier

(*The* 27 *day*)

After priuat praier I was busie about the house, and dressed my saruants foot and another poore mans hand, and talked with others that Came to aske my Counsill . . .

(*The* 28 *day*)

After priuat praier I went to worke, and, before diner time, came my Cosine Iohn Bouser, with whom I kept companie vntell diner: after, we walked forth, and when he was gone, I dressed packeringes hand: after, I hard Mr Rhodes read of perkin, and after I went to priuat examenation and praier

(*The* :5 *day of May* 1601)

After praers, I went to the church, wher I hard a sarmon: after, I Came home and hard Mr Rhodes read: after diner I went abroad, and when I came home I dressed some sores . . .

(*The* 26: *day*)

this day, in the afternone, I had had a child brought to se that was borne at Silpho, one Talliour sonne, who had no fundament, and had no passage for excrementes but att the Mouth: I was ernestly intereated to Cutt the place to se if any passhage Could be made, but, although I Cutt deepe and seearched, there was none to be found.

(*The Lordes day* :6: *day:*)

After priuatt prairs I went to church: and after dinner I walked a whill with Mr Hoby: and, after I had againe binne att the church, I dressed Hilares finger, talked wth Anne Mathew about some abuse, and at my time went to priuatt praier

(The 13 *day)*

After I had praied I went to seamer, being sent for to my Cousine Bouchiers wiffe who was, that Morninge, brought to bed of A boye: and after I was retourned home againe I recieued a Letter from Mr Hoby

.   .   .   .

(The :4: day)
this day I had
a fatherly warninge
of god.

I was sent for to Trutsdall, to the trauill of my Cossine Isons wiffe, who that Morninge was brought to bed of a daughter: the same day, at night, I hard of a fish that was taken vp att Yarmoth, 53 foott Long and 23 broade [39]

124. The Journal of Lady Mildmay

[This journal, written from about 1570 to 1617, is unpublished. It was written in the old age of the writer, Grace (1552?–1620), the second of three daughters of Sir Henry Sherrington, of Laycock Abbey in Wiltshire, England. Through her marriage at fourteen years of age to Anthony, son of Sir Walter Mildmay, of Apethorpe, in Northampton-shire, she was introduced into a sternly Puritan household. In the district where she lived, she found a wide field of activity. It is said that in spite of her great charity, she was no indiscriminate Lady Bountiful. Much of her time and energy was devoted to compounding herbs with which to minister to the ills of those in her district.[40]]

Alsoe every day I spent some time in the Herball and books of phisick, and in ministering to one or other by the directions of the best phisitions of myne acquaintance; and ever God gave a blessing thereunto.[41]

125. John Duncon. *The Holy Life and Death of Lady Letice, Vicountess Falkland*

[The author of this religious biography was chaplain or confessor to Lady Letice, Vicountess Falkland, after her husband's death. The work was originally printed in 1648 as a letter to Lady Morison of Great Tew, Oxfordshire, Lady Falkland's mother, and went through several editions. Lady Falkland's husband was Sir Lucius Cary, Vicount Falkland, who had married her when he was only nineteen years of age, despite her lack of fortune, thus displeasing his father.[42] Vicount Falkland and Sir Henry Morison, Lady Falkland's brother, were dear friends, whose friendship has been commemorated in Ben Jonson's *Pindaric Ode*. Of Lady Letice little is known except what is given in Rev. Duncon's biography. Here we read that she was singularly beautiful, pious, wise, witty, discreet, with great judgment, sobriety, and gaiety of behavior.

131

The couple had three sons to whom they were devoted. Lady Falkland died in 1646 at the age of thirty-five.[43]]

Madam, . . .

But beyond all, *her mercifulnesse* towards the *sick,* was most laudable: *her* provision of *Antidotes* against *infection,* and of *Cordials* and other *severall* sorts of *Physick* for such of *her neighbours* as should need *them,* amounted yearly to very considerable summes: And though in distributing such *medicinall provisions, her hand,* was very *open,* yet it was *close* enough in applying them, her *skil* (indeed) was more then ordinary, and *her wariness* too.

When any of the poor neighbours were sick, *she* had a constant care, that they should neither want such *relief,* nor such *attendance,* as their weak condition called for, and (if need were) *she hired Nurses to serve them:* And *her* own frequent *visiting* of the poorest *Cottagers,* and *her* ready service to them, on their *sick-bed,* argued as great *humility,* as *mercifulness* in *her;* yet the Bookes of *Spirituall exhortations,* She carried in *her* hand to *these sick* persons, declared a further design she had therein, of promoting *them* toward *heaven,* by reading to *them,* and by administering words of *holy* counsell to them: . . .

Your servant in
Christ Jesus,

April 15.
1647.

J. D.[44]

126. *Hastings Documents, 1601*

[These documents are copies of records preserved in the church chest of the parish of All Saints, Hastings, Sussex, England, and are assembled in the *Sussex Archeological Collections,* housed in one of the towers of the old castle, supposedly built by King Alfred, in Lewes, Sussex.[45] The following reference to the employment of a nurse is dated 1601.]

Item, to Mother Middleton, for twoe nights watchinge with widow Coxe's child being sick . . . 6d.[46]

127. *Extracts from the Journal and Account Book of the Rev. Giles Moore*

[Little is known about the author of this manuscript. His patron was a Mr. Michelborne, a member of an ancient Sussex family. Mr. Moore had probably served as a soldier or as chaplain in the Royal Army. He was the rector of the parish of Horstead Keynes. The parish register states that he was buried on the third of October, 1679.[47]]

[1657–58] April 16th . . .

My mayde being sicke, I payd for opening her veine 4*d.*, to the widdow

Rugglesford, for looking to her, I gave 1ˢ., and to Old Bess, for tending on her 3 days and 2 nights, I gave 1ˢ., in all 2s. 4d., this I gave her.

[1666–67] 12th Feb.ʸ. Finding myselfe distempered, I sweated myselfe for 3 or 4 hours, and that day and most part of the next, I was tolerably well, but on the 14th, being Friday, I had a high feaver, and was very ill all that day, and the fore part of the night. On Sunday 16th I tooke physicke, and was mightily sicke, but about 4 p. m. I began to sweate, and grew a little better; on the 18th my feaver held mee strong from 3 in the morning till 1 in the afternoone, on which day I was purged by syrup of roses and greatly and frequently, and then the feaver did sensibly abate, and on Saturday I lost it altogether, Deo gratias! On the 9th of March my ague, being an each day ague, came againe, and held mee till the 19th. I payd Dr. Parker for coming over from Rotherfield to see mee £1. I gave Goodwyfe Ward, for being necessary to mee, 1ˢ., and I payed Mr. Duke, curate of Pricomb for preaching one whole Sunday, hee also staying 5 dayes in my house, 10ˢ.

[1674–75] July 8th. Between 1 and 2 o'clock Mat [48] was brought to bed of a daughter, which was baptised on the 21st by Mr. Bennett of Plumpton, Mistresse Springett and Mistress Storey answering for her with myselfe in the name of Mat; I then gave the mydwyfe, goodwyfe, and nurse 5ˢ., each.[49]

128. *Ancient Parochial Account Book of Cowden, 1704*

[This is an old manuscript in which are entered all the parochial accounts of Cowden, a border parish in Sussex, beginning in 1598 and ending in 1714. It contains not only the church warden's accounts but also all relief given to the poor, and other payments customarily made from the poor rates.[50]]

1701. For 100 faggots for Robert Still, 7s.; for a peck of wheat for him, 1s.; for going to the doctors for him, 1s.; to John Care, for a canary for him and his family, 1s. 7d. 1–2; to Goody Halliday, for nursing him and his family 5 weeks, £1 5s.; to Goody Nye, for assisting in nursing, 2s. 6d.; to Mr. Hayler, for journeys and physic for Robert Still, £2 12s. 6d.

1713. For expenses at Guilford in trying to remove Daniel Knight, £4 5s. 6d.; for a pair of pattens for Moll Colgate; for three pairs of leather breeches, 5s. 6d.; to Goody Peckham for nursing a beggar, 5s.

1714. For nursing Wickham's boy with the small-pocks, 12s.; for a pair of breeches for Thomas Still, 2s. 4d.; to Dr. Gainsford for curing John Humphrey's leg, 10s.; to the same for curing Goody Rose's hand, 17s.[51]

129. *The Workes of that Famous Chirurgion Ambroise Parey*

[This work was written by Paré in 1585, five years before his death. Ambroise Paré, who was born in what is now the city of Laval, France, probably in 1510, served an apprenticeship as barber-surgeon before being elected in 1554 to the College of St. Côme, thereby becoming a master surgeon. As a student he served as resident in the Hôtel-Dieu in Paris. In 1537 he began his career as a military surgeon, and on his first campaign discovered that boiling oil was not only useless but actually harmful in gunshot wounds.[52] The care given by Paré to Monsieur le Marquis l'Auret, described below, included not only surgical procedures but also details of good nursing care. The following translation is in the English of the seventeenth century.]

Monsieur the Duke of *Ascot* did not faile to send a Gentleman to the King with a letter, humbly to beseech him to doe him So much good and honour, as to permit and command his cheefe Chirurgion to come see the Marquesse of *Auret* his brother; who had received a Musket Shot neare the knee, with fracture of the bone, about seaven monthes since, which the Physitions and Chirurgions in those parts were much troubled to cure. The King sent for me, and commanded me to goe see the said Lord *Auret,* and to helpe him in all that I could for the cure of his hurt; I told him I would imploy all that little knowledge which it had pleased God to give me.

.   .   .   .

And to nourish and fatten the body, frictions must be made universally through the whole body, with warme linnen cloathes, above, below, on the right side, and left, and round about; to the end to draw the blood and spirits from within outward, and to resolve any fuliginous vapours retained betweene the skinne, and the flesh; therby the parts shall be nourished and restored ... and wee must then cease when we see heate and redness in the skinne. ... As for the Vlcer which he had upon his rumpe, which came through too long lying upon it without being removed, which was the cause that the spirits could not florish or shine in it; by the meanes of which there should bee inflammation, aposteme and then ulcer, yea with losse of substance of the subject flesh, with a very great paine; because of the nerves which are disseminated in this part. That wee must likewise put him into another soft bed, and give him a cleane shirt and sheets ...

.   .   .   .

Secondly, to looke into the great swelling and cold in his Legge, fearing least it should fall into a Gangreene; and that actuall heate must bee applyed unto him because the potentiall could not reduce the intemperature, *de potentia ad actam;* for this cause hot brickes must bee applyed round about, on which should bee cast a decoction of nervall herbes boyled in Wine and Vinegar, than wrapt up in some napkin, and to the feete an earthen bottle

134

filled with the Sayd decoction, stopt and wrapt up with some linnen clothes; also that fomentations must be made upon the thigh, and the whole Legge, of a decoction made of Sage, Rosemary, Time, Lavender, flowers of Camomile, Melilot, and red Roses boyled in white wine, and a *Lixivium* made with oake ashes with a little Vinegar, and halfe an handfull of Salt.

Thirdly, that there must be applyed upon the rumpe a great emplaster made of the red desiccative and *Vnguentum Comitisse* of each equall parts incorporated together, to the end to appease his paine and dry up the Vlcer, also to make him a little downe pillow which might beare his rumpe aloft without leaning upon it.

Also we must use good nourishment full of juice, as rere egges, Damaske prunes stewed in wine and sugar, also *Panado* made with the broth of the great pot . . . with the white fleshy parts of Capons.

Besides, one may cause it to raine artificially in pouring downe from some high place into a kettle, and that it make such a noyse that the patient may heare it, by meanes sleepe shall be provoked on him.

Then two or three houres after I caused a bed to bee made neare his owne, where there were cleane white sheets then a strong man lifted him into it, and rejoyced much in that hee was taken out of his foule stinking bed. Soon after hee demanded to sleepe, which hee did almost foure houres, where all the people of the house began to rejoyce, cheefely Monsieur the Duke of *Ascot* his brother.

The days following I made enjections into the bottome and cavities of the Vlcer, made with *Aegyptiacum,* dissolved sometimes in *aqua vitae,* and sometimes in wine. I applyed to mundifie and dry the spongie and loose flesh, bolsters, at the bottome of the sinusityes hollow tents of Lead, that the *Sanies* might have passage out; and upon it a great Emplaster of *Diacalcitheos* dissolved in wine: likewise I did rowle it with such dexterity, that he had no pains, which being appeased the fever began much to diminish.

Now I remained there about two month, which was not without seeing divers sicke people, as well rich as poore which came to me three or foure leagues about.[53]

130. *Works of John Robinson, Pastor of the Pilgrim Fathers*

[John Robinson (1576?–1624), the English nonconformist pastor of the Pilgrim Fathers in Holland, was educated at Cambridge. As leader of the Scrooby group who went to Amsterdam, he encouraged his flock to remove to America, although he did not accompany them and never reached American shores.[54] He has been called "the most learned, polished and modest spirit that ever that sect enjoyed." [55] The following quotation, which is an appendix to the "Six Principles of the Christian Religion" by William Perkins, a distinguished Christian minister in the time of Elizabeth, indicates that the deaconess was recognized as an important attendant of the sick of the congregation at that time in Europe.[56]]

Q. 12. How many are the offices of ministry in the church?

A. Five, besides the extraordinary offices of apostles, prophets, and evangelists, for the first planting of the churches, which are ceased, with their extraordinary gifts . . .

Q. 14. Show me which offices be, with their answerable gifts and works?

A. 1. The pastor (exhorter), to whom is given the gift of wisdom for exhortation. 2. The teacher, to whom is given the gift of knowledge for doctrine. 3. The governing elder, who is to rule with diligence. Eph. IV. II; 1. Cor. XII. 8; Rom. XII. 8; 1 Tim. V. 17. 4. The deacon, who is to administer the holy treasure with simplicity. 5. The widow or deaconess, who is to attend the sick and impotent with compassion and cheerfulness. Acts VI. 2–7; 1 Tim. III, 8, 10, &c. V. 9, 10; Rom. XVI. 1.[57]

131. *Chronicles of the Pilgrim Fathers of the Colony of Plymouth from 1602 to 1625*

[This volume contains eight early documents of the Pilgrim Fathers, including Governor Bradford's "Dialogue," from which the following excerpt is taken. The manuscript was found in the records of the First Church of Plymouth, into which it had been copied by Nathaniel Morton, Secretary of the Church before 1629. The full title of the dialogue is indicative of its character: "A Dialogue, or the Sum of a Conference Between Some Young Men Born in New England and Sundry Ancient Men That Came out of Holland and Old England Anno Domini 1648.[58] It was the first of three dialogues written by Bradford, this one written in defense of the Separatist movement. The Ancient Men (or Ancient Brethren) were the first congregation of consequence in the movement. They fled to Amsterdam in 1593, later becoming infamous because of their indefensible practices.[59] This dialogue is included here because it contains a description of a deaconess of Amsterdam in the sixteenth century.]

Truly there were in them many worthy men; and if you had seen them in their beauty and order, as we have done, you would have been much affected therewith, we dare say. At Amsterdam, before their division and breach, they were about three hundred communicants, and they had for their pastor and teacher these two eminent men before named [Smith and Robinson], and in our time four grave men for ruling elders, and three able and godly men for deacons, one ancient widow for a deaconess, who did them service many years, though she was sixty years of age when she was chosen. She honoured her place and was an ornament to the congregation. She usually sat in a convenient place in the congregation, with a little birchen rod in her hand, and kept little children in great awe from disturbing the congregation. She did frequently visit the sick and weak, especially women, and, as there was need, called out maids and young women to watch and do them other helps as their necessity did require; and if they were poor, she would gather relief for them of those that were able, or acquaint the deacons; and she was obeyed as a mother in Israel and an officer of Christ.[60]

Saint Vincent de Paul and the Sisters of Charity

[St. Vincent de Paul (1576–1660) is known as the founder of organized charity. Ordained in 1600, captured by pirates, and enslaved in Tunis, he converted his master to Christianity and escaped with him to Italy. He improved the condition of the galley slaves on the Mediterranean galleys, whose chaplain he became. Becoming interested in charitable work in the cities and towns of France, he founded first the Ladies of Charity, an organization or confraternity of women who cared for the poor and sick, while at the same time carrying on their home responsibilities. To supplement their work, St. Vincent and Mlle le Gras, his chief co-worker, instituted the Daughters of Charity (Sisters of Charity), who devoted their entire time and energies to the care of the sick in their homes and in hospitals.[61] The influence of St. Vincent de Paul has been widespread. His humanity, common sense, and wisdom are indicated in the provisions for the work of the Ladies and the Daughters.]

132. *The Rule of the Confraternity*

[As parish priest at Chatillon-les-Dombes, in 1617, St. Vincent saw the effect of well-intentioned but ill-regulated charity. As a result, the first confraternity was established. The idea spread to other parishes, and St. Vincent formulated regulations for them and for the Daughters who nursed patients in their homes, in the Hôtel-Dieu of Paris, and in other hospitals.[62] The original manuscript was discovered, in 1839, in the Mayoral Archives of Chatillon. Only a portion of it is in St. Vincent's handwriting.[63] It is dated 1617.]

The Confraternity of Charity is instituted for the honour of our Lord Jesus Christ and His Holy Mother, and to assist the sick poor of the places where it is established both in body and in soul: in body, by administering to them their food and drink, and the necessary medicines during the time of their illnesses: in soul, by obtaining for them the administration of the Sacraments of Penance, the Eucharist, and Extreme Unction; and by taking care that those who are dying shall leave this world in a right condition; and that those who are cured shall make a resolution to live well for the future.

The confraternity shall be composed of a certain limited number of women, married and unmarried: the latter with the consent of their parents, the former with that of their husbands: and they shall elect three of their number among themselves, in the presence of the clergyman of the parish by a majority of votes, every two years, on the day after Pentecost, who shall be their officers, the first of which shall be called Superior or Directress; the second, Treasurer or first Assistant, and the third, wardrobe-keeper or second Assistant. These three officers shall have the entire direction of the said Confraternity: under the advice of the clergyman they shall elect also a gentleman of the parish, one pious and charitable, who shall be their Agent.

The Superior shall take care that this present Rule is kept: that all the members of the Confraternity shall do their duty well: She shall receive the sick poor of the said parish who shall present themselves, and shall discharge them upon the advice of the other officers.

The Treasurer shall act as adviser to the Superior, shall keep the money of the Confraternity. . . . The wardrobe Keeper shall also advise the Superior, shall keep, wash, and mend the linen of the Confraternity, and from it shall provide the sick poor with what they need.

.   .   .   .

The Agent shall have the management of all the collections which shall be made at the church or at the people's houses. . . . In the . . . register he shall keep a catalogue of the ladies who shall be received into the Confraternity, . . . the names of the sick poor who shall have been assisted by the Confraternity. . . . The Sisters of the Confraternity shall in turns of a day each look after the sick poor who shall have been received by the Superior: they shall take to their houses their food and drink ready prepared: shall take it in turns to ask alms at church and at the houses on Sundays and on the principal solemn feast days: they shall hand over their collections to the Treasurer, and shall inform the Agent of the amount collected . . .

They shall be present in equally full force at the burial of the sick poor whom they shall have assisted . . .

There shall be given to each poor invalid for each meal as much bread as he can eat, five ounces of veal or mutton, soup, and half a bottle of wine (Paris measure). On fast days they shall be given, besides the bread, wine and soup, a couple of eggs, or a little butter, and for those who cannot take solid meat some broth and new-laid eggs four times a day, and a nurse for those who are in danger and have no one to look after them.[64]

.   .   .   .   .   .

They shall be very conscientious not to let them suffer in default of giving them precisely at the proper time and in the proper manner the assistance of which they have need, be it through negligence or culpable forgetfulness, be it because of some badly regulated attachment to their spiritual exercises, which they ought to postpone in favor of the necessary assistance of the poor sick.

And since ill regulated charity is not only displeasing to God, but also prejudicial to the souls of those who practice it thus, they shall not undertake to nurse or to physic any sick person against the will of those on whom they depend, nor against the order which has been given them paying no attention to the complaints which the discontented poor are accustomed to make.

... [the Daughters of Charity] shall render ... obedience in that which regards the service of the poor, ... to the Ladies of Charity of the Parishes, who are in charge.

She shall greet him gayly and kindly ... approaching his bed with a mien modestly cheerful ... shall raise the pillow for him, arrange the covers, place the small table near the bed, and on it arrange the napkin, the plate [and] the spoon, [and] rinse the gondola. She shall wash the hands of the sick, pour out the porringer and put the meat in a plate, arranging all on the said small table; then she shall kindly invite the sick person to eat for the love of Jesus and of His holy Mother: all with love as though she were treating her child, or rather God, Who ·considers done to Himself the good she does to this poor person, and she shall say to him some little word [of] holy joy and consolation for the purpose of cheering him. [She] shall cut the meat into morsels ... pour out the drink, [and] invite him anew to eat. Having thus set things going, if there is someone at hand [to continue], she shall leave him and go to find another whom she shall treat in like manner. [If, however, there is no one to continue the work she remains and] when he [the patient] has finished eating, having washed the dishes, folded the napkin and removed the table, [she] shall say grace for the sick and take leave of him immediately in order to go and serve another.[65]

133. *Special Rules for the Sisters of the Parishes*

[As the title indicates, these regulations were formulated for the Daughters working among the sick in the various parishes in France where they were organized at the time.]

Although they [the Daughters of Charity] ought not to be too yielding nor too condescending when they [the sick] refuse to take the remedies, still they shall be well on their guard not to ill-treat or slight them; on the contrary, they shall treat them with respect and humility, bearing in mind that the rudeness and the contempt one shows them, as well as the service and the honor which one renders them, are directed to our Lord himself . . .

In order to avoid serious objections that might arise, they [the Daughters of Charity] shall not undertake to sit up with the sick, nor with women who are laboring with child, anymore than to assist women of a bad life . . .

They [the Daughters of Charity] shall make it a matter of conscience not to fail in the slightest service which they ought to render to the sick, particularly as regards the remedies which they ought to give to them in the manner and at the hour prescribed by the physician, unless some great necessity obliges to use it otherwise; as for example, if their illness should become too bad, or if they were in a cold fit or in a sweat or some other like plight.

[The Daughters of Charity are forbidden] . . . to undertake the care of any sick or to give anything to any poor person contrary to the prescribed order or against the intentions of the lady officers.

Immediately after the morning's meditation, and in summer even before the reading of the subject, they [the Daughters of Charity] shall be solicitous to bring the medicines to the sick, and upon their return they shall go to Mass, during which they shall be able to make their meditation when they have not been able to do so at 4:30 o'clock. [After breakfast] . . . they shall repair at the usual hour, or sooner, if need be, to the house of the Lady where the kettle of the sick [has been left] . . . in order that the kettle be ready at exactly nine o'clock or later and that they be returned at 11:30 o'clock.

After dinner they shall have care to read the prescriptions of the physician and prepare the remedies to bring them to the sick at the necessary hour, and leave the kettle for the morrow at the home of the Lady whose turn it is. . . . After supper they shall prepare the medicines for the following morning.

If there be sick so abandoned that there is no one at hand to make their bed or to render them some other service still more abject, they [the Daughters of Charity] may do it according to the leisure they have, provided the Sister Servant [Superioress] find it proper; still they shall try to obtain, if possible, that some other person continues the same charity toward them for fear that this may retard the assistance of the other poor.[66]

134. *Rules for the Daughters of Charity of Hôtel-Dieu of Paris* [67]

[In 1634 St. Vincent yielded to the request of Mme Goussault to establish the Company of Ladies to visit the sick at Hôtel-Dieu of Paris. Mme Goussault was one of St. Vincent's most active co-workers, and had been in the habit of visiting the sick in the Hôtel-Dieu. It was her wish that the sick there might have some of the same benefits which had been afforded to others by the organization founded by St. Vincent. Some of the Daughters were delegated to assist the Ladies in this work.[68]]

At ten o'clock they shall all go to the infirmary and give dinner to the sick and serve them. The Superioress shall say the prayers aloud and shall invite the sick to join her, at least mentally. . . . [If order does not provide otherwise the meal shall consist of] a broth, veal and mutton with a little beef for dinner, and roast meat and boiled beef for supper.

[If no other provisions have been made] . . . the Sisters shall repair to the infirmary at exactly two o'clock in order to give some little sweetmeats to the said poor sick.

At four o'clock they shall give the medicines, change the sheets . . . adjust a little the beds of the sick.

At exactly five o'clock the Sisters shall go to the infirmary to give supper to the sick and serve them as at dinner.

[At seven o'clock they] shall order that there be some wine and some little sweetmeats to relieve the needs of the most sick.

She [the Sister] shall pass the night watching . . . reading and sleeping now and then while the poor are resting.

[St. Vincent admonishes the Daughters to] . . . represent to themselves the happiness of their state since they serve our Lord in the person of the poor . . . that it may please God to grant them the grace to accomplish all these things, they shall often pray to Him for it . . .[69]

141

135. *Conferences of St. Vincent de Paul with the Daughters of Charity*

[It was St. Vincent's practice to hold regular conferences with the Daughters. The records of these tell us much concerning his philosophy and the activities of the Daughters in nursing the sick in their homes.]

A community like yours, destined to so holy and noble an object, so agreeable to our Divine Savior, and so useful to our neighbor, could certainly have no other author but God himself; for until its commencement had anyone ever heard of such a work? Why has God done this? He did it to save the poor. We have seen, it is true, religious and hospitals for the assistance of the sick, but before your establishment there was never a community destined to go and serve the sick in their houses. If, in some poor family, anyone fell sick, he was sent to the hospital, and this separated the husband from his wife, and the children from their parents. Until now, O my God! you had not furnished the means of going to assist them in their houses, and it seemed in a manner as if Thy adorable providence, which never fails, did not extend its watchful care over them. Why, think you, my dear sisters, did God delay in granting this assistance to them? Oh! because it was to be reserved to you . . .

You should act, my sisters, with great respect and obedience towards the doctors, taking great care never to condemn or contradict their orders. Endeavour, on the contrary, to fulfil them with great exactitude, and without ever presuming to prepare the medicines according to your own way of thinking. Punctually follow what they have prescribed, both with regard to the quantity of the dose and the ingredients of which it is composed, because upon this fidelity and exactness depends nothing less, perhaps, than the life of the patient. Respect the doctors, not only because they are more learned and enlightened than you, but because God commands you in the Holy Scripture [Ecclus. 38. 1-2] to do so in the following words: *'Honour the physicians for the need thou hast of them. The kings likewise, and all the great ones of the earth, honour them.'* Why should you, my sisters, because you see and converse with them so frequently, fail to show them the honour and respect due to them? You are ignorant of the reasons they have for pursuing different methods in the treatment of maladies which seem to you to be the same. You must endeavour particularly to remember and observe their method of treating the sick, so that when you will be in the villages; or any other place in which there is no doctor, you may render yourself useful by applying their method. You ought therefore to instruct yourselves, so as to know in what case it is necessary to bleed in the arm or in the foot; what quantity of blood you should take on each occasion; when to apply the cupping-glasses. Learn also the different remedies necessary to be used in the various kinds of diseases, and the proper time and manner of administering them. All this is very necessary for you, and you will do a great deal of good when you are well instructed in it. I think it very essential that you should have some conferences with one another on this subject in the form of catechism.[70]

Encourage them [the sick] to suffer their ills patiently for the love of God, bear with their little whims, never become vexed with them nor speak rough words to them. Ah, they have enough to do to suffer their illness! Think, on the contrary, that you are their visible guardian angel, their father and their mother; do not contradict them except in what is harmful to them. . . . God has instructed you to be their consolation.

Your resolution ought therefore to be: I shall go out to serve the poor. I shall try to go with a mien modestly gay, I shall endeavor to console them and edify them. I shall speak to them as to my masters. There are some who are accustomed to speak roughly to me, I shall bear with it.

Be then very attentive, that nothing be wanting to them in all that you can [provide], whether it be for the health of the body or for the salvation of the soul.

It has not been the intention that one receive . . . those affected with dropsy, the consumptives, the epileptics, for what would one do if one received all these persons? . . . In Paris God has provided them with a hospital for the incurables.

Thus, my Sisters, you ought to be exact in doing all that the physicians prescribe, because if any accident happened to a sick person, you would be responsible, unless, as we have already said, some very remarkable change comes unexpectedly and such as those of which this rule speaks. Since I come to mention the physicians, I shall add that, besides the obedience you owe them, you must also show them great respect . . . for, if it should happen, as I have been told, that anyone [of you] had the intention of following her own judgment, or of doing something contrary to their intention, or of exceeding the orders she received, I should say to this Daughter that she committed a great fault. You ought, then to obey them in all that concerns the service of the sick and think that you are doing the will of God in doing theirs . . . [71]

136. *Letters of St. Vincent de Paul*

[Several editions of the letters of St. Vincent have appeared separately, while some letters are included in the *Letters and Conferences* quoted in

Reading No. 137. Many of his letters were written to Mlle le Gras, his helper and associate in founding the Daughters of Charity. They reveal his concern not only for Mlle le Gras but for the Daughters, and are of value in understanding the work of the Sisters of Charity.]

To Father Delville, a confrere (date not given).

If you meet with strong, healthy girls, inclined to join the Charity, who are of irreproachable life, fully determined to humble themselves thoroughly and to labour at the acquisition of virtue and to serve the poor for the love of God, you may give them hopes of admission.... They should be at least eighteen or twenty years old, bring sufficient clothing when they first come, as well as linen and their little wearing apparel, and some money for their return home, in case they may not be able to fall in with the mode of life of this little Company, or be judged unsuitable.[72]

To Mlle Le Gras, Dec. 30, 1636.

May God bless you, Mademoiselle, for your having gone and set your daughters to work in the Hôtel-Dieu, and for all that has resulted from it. But, in the name of God, take care of yourself, you see the need there is of your poor, little help.

To Mlle Le Gras (date not given).

Mon Dieu, Mademoiselle, how uneasy I have felt at seeing you remain so long from taking the air, and working so constantly as you do at the Hôtel-Dieu.[73]

To St. Louise de Marillac, May 27, 1636.

The grace of Our Lord be with you forever! I am sending this special messenger to obtain tidings of you, and I hope he will bring back good news. In the name of Our Lord, Mademoiselle, do everything in your power to that end. You have good reason to complain that I have not answered the letter you wrote to me when you went to Gournay. But what can you expect? It is one of my usual failings. I hope, if you have the charity to forgive me, that Our Lord will give me the grace to amend.... Your Daughters of the General Hospital are all doing well except Henrietta,[74] who is constantly depressed; Mary says it is on account of your absence. This prevented her from going to Saint-Nicholas, and Barbara from going to Saint-Sulpice. Isabella [75] is getting better.

From Saint-Lazare, this Tuesday morning, May 27, 1636.

I saw your daughters at the General Hospital yesterday; they are all quite well. If you require me, I will lay everything else aside; but I hope you may be able to get on without me.

Address: To Mademoiselle Le Gras.

To St. Louise de Marillac (October, 1638).

Mademoiselle,

The grace of Our Lord be ever with you! I very gladly implore Our Lord
to give His holy blessing to our dear Sisters, and also a share in the Spirit He
bestowed on the holy women who accompanied Him and who cooperated
with Him in assisting the sick poor and in teaching children. *Mon Dieu!*
Mademoiselle, what a happiness for these good girls to go about continuing,
wherever they may be, the work of charity which Our Lord wrought whilst
on earth! And who shall say, on seeing them together, those two bonnets
[an allusion to the head dress of the Sisters of Charity] in the coach, that they
were setting out on a work so wonderful in the eyes of God, and His angels,
that the God-Man considered it worthy of Himself and His Holy Mother? ...

On their arrival at Richelieu, they will first go and salute the Blessed
Sacrament, and then see Fr. Lambert and receive his orders; they will strive
to carry them out both in respect to the sick and the school children ...

V. D.[76]

137. *Letters and Conferences of Saint Vincent de Paul*

[In a supplementary edition of the *Letters and Conferences of Saint
Vincent de Paul,* many of the practices in training the Daughters are
given.]

Formerly in many houses, and particularly at the Hôtel-Dieu, it [the
training of Daughters] was done as follows: The newcomer was placed under
an older [Sister] that she might train her and have charge of her. But it was
found that the nieces bound themselves in such a manner to their aunts—so
they called them—that partialities were practised which put the houses in
disorder. Hence one thought it better to appoint a mistress who had care of
the novices, and they were all placed together.[77]

[Mlle le Gras employed some of the Daughters] to instruct the little girls
of the poor who came to School at her house; others to visit the sick of the
parish, bringing to them food or medicines, or nursing them; others to let
the blood and dress the sores of the poor who came to them from without
for this purpose; others to sew or to do similar work; others to learn to read
or write; others to perform the little household duties; all according to the
orders given them.[78]

It is for them [the Ladies] to order and for you [the Daughters] to obey.
... You must ... not encroach upon their authority in any way by ordering
things yourselves. They are as the head of a body and you are only the
feet.[79]

145

138. The Vow of a Sister of Charity

[St. Vincent was opposed to having his Daughters in a cloister where they would not be free to go out into the homes to nurse the sick. His oftenquoted statement emphasizes this: "Your monasteries are the houses of the sick; your cell, a hired room; your chapel, the parish church; your cloister, the streets of the city; your enclosure, obedience; your grille, the fear of God; your veil, holy modesty." [80] The vows taken by the Daughters were very simple, and reflect this philosophy. The following vow was taken by a Sister at St. Lazare in 1642.]

I, the undersigned, in the presence of God, repeat the promises made at my baptism, and make the vow of poverty, of chastity, and of obedience to the reverend Superior of the Priests of the Mission, in the Sisterhood of the Daughters of Charity, to give up myself during the whole of this year to the bodily and spiritual care of the sick poor, our veritable masters; to which end I pray God to help me for the sake of His Son Jesus Christ crucified, and through the prayers of the Blessed Virgin.[81]

139. Announcement of the Archbishop's Approbation of the Rule, November 20, 1646

[This announcement made on May 30, 1647, by St. Vincent, reveals the way in which he regarded what he considered to be the privilege which was the Daughters' in caring for the sick of the community.]

"The Confraternity of Charity of the servants of the parochial sick poor. . . ." Oh, what a lovely title, my Daughters! . . . O, Mon Dieu! What a lovely title and what a beautiful description! What have you done for God to have merited it? *Servants of the poor,* that is just the same as to say *Servants of Jesus Christ,* for He regards as done to Himself what is done to them, and they are His members. And what did He do whilst on earth but serve the poor? Oh! my dear Daughters, carefully preserve this characteristic for it is the most beautiful and most advantageous you could possibly have. . . . The Company is composed of maidens and widows who shall elect a Superioress from amongst themselves for three years . . . [adding that is to be understood as referring to what will take place after God has disposed of Mademoiselle] . . . remember . . . that to nurse the sick is to pray.[82]

CONCLUDING STATEMENT

In the early part of the sixteenth century in England, hospitals and hospital care claimed the attention of various writers. Among these, Sir Thomas More, in describing his *Utopia,* included a hospital as an important part of the ideal state and, while not mentioning nurses, spoke of a "stewarde" who may or may not have had some duties in nursing the sick. Meanwhile citizens, such as John Stow, listed the existing hospitals in London and gave their status at the time. Henry VIII, who suppressed many hospitals, established others, the deeds for a few of which included statements concerning the duties of nurses and matrons.

Scattered brief references in the literature mention payment to nurses for services rendered. These nurses seemingly cared for the sick in the home, but whether they pursued the occupation of nursing as a vocation, or only incidentally with other activities, is not clear. John Howard, the philanthropist of the eighteenth century who made a study of care in hospitals and lazarettos, quotes the rules of one Royal Hospital. These indicate that some of the chief problems in the hospital were keeping the hospital clean and orderly, and maintaining sobriety in the nurses. The literature of the great plague of 1665 in London is almost unanimous in expressing the view that nurses appointed to care for the victims of the disease were cruel, inhuman, and incompetent. There is considerable evidence that in writing these accounts one writer took his material from another, the same incidents being related over and over, in one or two instances in almost identical words.

In the seventeenth century in France, a beginning of reform of nursing was brought about by the organization by St. Vincent de Paul of the Ladies of Charity and the Daughters of Charity. The *Rules of the Confraternity,* and the *Conferences* with the Daughters, reveal the practical wisdom and humanity of St. Vincent in providing a service to as many people as possible, with a minimum of duplication. They show his knowledge of many matters related to the care of the sick and of human nature, and indicate his common sense in organizing the nursing service for the community in hospital and home.

The effect of this pioneer work was felt not only in France in the time of St. Vincent but also in other countries, as is shown by developments in succeeding centuries. In the early part of the nineteenth century, reforms began to be more marked. The public, the recipients of nursing care, expressed in the press the concern felt over the quality of the care, and medical practitioners, who desired more adequate care for their patients, proposed reforms. The first half of the century saw the establishment of new groups to nurse the sick, first in Germany, and then in England. These set the stage for the more revolutionary reforms instituted by Miss Nightingale in the latter half of the same century.

Some sources illustrating these beginnings in Germany and England will be presented in the next chapter.

Chapter 5

Some References to Nursing Reforms in Europe in the First Half of the Nineteenth Century

INTRODUCTION

ALTHOUGH some changes in the care of the sick took place before the nineteenth century, real and marked reforms came slowly. Even before the establishment by Florence Nightingale of a new kind of nursing service and nursing education in St. Thomas's Hospital in 1860, however, disquietude began to be expressed concerning the nursing of the sick in the hospitals and in the homes. Indeed, the success of Miss Nightingale's plan was in some measure the result of the fact that many people were cognizant of, and agitated about, the lack of adequate care. Public interest in improvement in the first half of the nineteenth century is shown among various groups. Doctors, clergymen, and philanthropic citizens wrote in favor of the establishment of nursing systems of a different character than those then in vogue. Some favored a system under religious auspices, while others advocated a secular nursing plan to be brought about chiefly by utilizing paid nurses rather than the "pauper nurses" who were then employed in many institutions. There was a tendency to increase the numbers of secular nurses in hospitals and also toward organizing new groups under religious auspices.

As a result of the concern of the public, various beginnings were made, some in Germany, and others in England. The first changes came in Germany, mainly through the work of Pastor Fliedner of Kaiserswerth. In England, at this time, the movement took place chiefly under the sponsorship of the Established Church. At the same time efforts were made to improve the care in the large infirmaries through the utilization of paid nurses.

The literature expressing these developments includes materials from

148

the public press, medical writings, pamphlets and books, letters, biographies, prose, and poetry.

Early statements of interest from the public press and a pamphlet are presented in this chapter: a letter to the editor of the *London Times,* dated April 15, 1857 (140); a refutation of the points in this article by Dr. John Flint South, in *Facts Relating to Hospital Nurses* (141); an article by Frances Power Cobbe, in *Macmillan's Magazine,* in the year 1861, entitled "Workhouse Sketches" (142); and one by Ernest Hart, in the *Fortnightly Review* for April, 1866 (143).

The conditions in the homes in the British Isles are pictured by many writers. The classic instance of home nursing is Charles Dickens' description of the fictitious characters Sairey Gamp and Betsy Prig, found in *Martin Chuzzlewit* (144). Nursing in the homes under admittedly unusual conditions is exemplified by that done during cholera epidemics, such as those of Oxford and London. Three references to this phase are: Sir Henry Wentworth Acland's *Memoir of the Cholera at Oxford in the Year 1854* (145); the biography of Felicia Skene by E. C. Rickards, narrating Miss Skene's work in the same epidemic, entitled *Felicia Skene of Oxford A Memoir* (146); and Margaret Goodman's book relating the *Experiences of an English Sister of Mercy* (147), which includes her nursing in a cholera epidemic in London.

Descriptions of hospital nursing at this time are fairly numerous. Among those quoted in this chapter are: Sir James Paget's portrayal of the nursing in St. Bartholomew's Hospital about 1835, given in a speech before the Abernethian Society (148); Pastor Muhlenberg's reference in a letter to nursing in the same hospital in 1855 (149); three descriptions of the "old time nurse"; in particular, Mrs. Porter, at the Royal Infirmary at Edinburgh; one by Lord Lister, told in Sir Rickman Godlee's *Life of Lord Lister* (150); another given by Dr. John Beddoe in his *Memories of Eighty Years* (151); and the third, the well-known poem by Ernest Henley, "Staff Nurse; Old Style," to be found in his volume *In Hospital; Rhymes and Rhythms* (152).[1] A brief reference to nursing in a cholera epidemic in Hamburg is found in letters written by Amelia Sieveking to her mother (153).

Nursing in the hospitals is also described by individuals and groups making investigations into hospital conditions. Among these delineations are the report of the extensive investigation made by *The Lancet Sanitary Commission for Investigating the State of the Infirmaries of Workhouses,* published in *The Lancet* in 1865 (154); and that of Louisa Twining, Guardian of the Poor in Kensington, published as *Workhouses and Pauperism and Women's Work in the Administration of the Poor Law* (155).

As has been stated, suggested remedies to the conditions in nursing in England at this time were mainly two: first, that nursing be conducted under religious auspices; and second, that lay nurses be paid in order to do away with the so-called "pauper nurses." The development of these ideas took place concurrently with the beginning of Florence Nightingale's great reforms. There were advocates of both proposals, and the concern felt by various groups and individuals resulted in progress along both lines. This situation is reflected in many writings, from which selections have been made as follows: the writings of Dr. Robert Gooch, in *Blackwood's Edinburgh Magazine,* July-December, 1825, and the *London Medical Gazette* for 1827 (156, 157); those of Robert Southey in *Sir Thomas More; or Colloquies on the Progress and Prospects of Society* and in *The Life and Correspondence of the Late Robert Southey* (158, 159); [2] a letter written to Rev. [W. F.] Hook by Edward Pusey, Canon of Christ Church, Oxford (160); a paper by Sir Edward Parry, R.N., Superintendent of Haslar Hospital, advocating the training of women as nurses on the Kaiserswerth plan (161); articles which appeared in the *Saturday Review* and the *Pall Mall Gazette* in 1866 (162); a letter written by the Bishop of London on December 27, 1865, expressing his disapproval of vows in the sisterhoods and alluding to the work of St. John's House, St. Peter's House, Deaconess House, and All Saints Sisterhood in London (163); and an article by Dr. John Ogle, "Nurses for the Sick Poor," which appeared in the *Medical Times and Gazette,* April 11, 1874, and which reported the interest of the Epidemiological Society in the matter (164).

As has been indicated, the organization of efforts to improve conditions in nursing was first initiated in Germany. A small beginning was made in this by Amelia Sieveking in 1832, in the founding of a Protestant sisterhood (165). The revival of the work of the Christian deaconesses. which became very widespread in Protestant countries, came through the efforts of Pastor Theodor Fliedner of Kaiserswerth (166–174). As has been seen, [3] the Christian deaconesses had not entirely disappeared in the preceding centuries, although their work had assumed less importance in the Church as the effects of the monastic system became more widespread.

In England the deaconess system was initiated in the Established Church. There the groups did not always assume the title of "deaconess" but rather came to be known as "sisters," the organizations being called "sisterhoods." Their characteristics in England differed in some respects also from those in Germany.

Reference will be made in this chapter to a few additional writings on this subject: a letter of J. J. Ellacombe, touching on the Park Village

Community (175); an allusion by Dr. Lionel S. Beale in the *Medical Times and Gazette* for December 6, 1873, to St. John's House (176); correspondence, journal, and diary of Elizabeth Fry on the Institution of Nursing Sisters (or Protestant Sisters of Charity, as they were sometimes called) (177–179); the *Memoirs of the Life of Elizabeth Fry,* edited by her daughters (180); a letter written by William Makepeace Thackeray to the Nursing Sisters (181); a small extract from the "Minutes of the London Hospital," dated September 2, 1840, alluding to the Nursing Sisters (182); an excerpt from the first printed "Report of the [Mildmay] Deaconesses on East End of London," describing their nursing in the cholera epidemic (183); and the letters written by Sister Dora and others, giving details of the work of Sister Dora in Walsall, a market town of England (184, 185).

Brief reference to the purposes of the Protestant Sisters of Charity of France, found in the "Statutes" of the Order (186), and a statement of the objects of the Roman Catholic order of the Irish Sisters of Charity (187) are included also.

THE SOURCES

140. *London Times,* April 15, 1857

[The writer is a physician expressing his ideas on the uses to be made of the Nightingale Fund. As is seen, while coming to the defense of the "untrained" nurse, whose characteristics he describes, he recognizes the need for training of nurses.]

Letter to the Editor of the *London Times,* dated April 14, 1857.

(Signed) One Who Has Walked a Good Many Hospitals.

Hospital nurses have for the last year or two been the victims of much unmerited abuse. They have their faults, but most of these may be laid to the want of proper treatment. Lectured by committees, preached at by chaplains, scowled on by treasurers and stewards, scolded by Matrons, sworn at by surgeons, bullied by dressers, grumbled at and abused by patients; insulted, if old and ill-favoured; talked flippantly to, if middle-aged and good humoured; tempted and seduced, if young and well-looking,—they are just what any woman might be, exposed to the same influences,—meek, pious, saucy, careless, drunken, or unchaste, according to circumstances or temperament; but mostly attentive, and rarely unkind. . . .

Who . . . that has been inside an hospital, has not constantly seen how urgently a training institution was needed? A poor woman is left a widow with two or three children,—of course, quite unprovided for. What is she to do? She would starve on needlework. She is unfit for domestic service, which besides is too poorly paid to enable her to maintain her children—she knows nobody to give her charring, and has no money to buy a mangle, of which there are already three in the court. So she thinks of an hospital as a natural refuge, as nursing is her natural employment—gets a recommendation from a clergyman to a matron, is engaged, and turned into a ward to pick up a knowledge of her business as she best can; and her first experiences are usually sufficiently disgusting when she encounters an irritable surgeon, who expects to have everything ready to hand from a wretched woman in the last stage of anxiety and nervousness, whom no one has taken the trouble to teach even the names of things she is expected to be ready with.

141. J. F. South. *Facts Relating to Hospital Nurses*

[John Flint South (1797–1882), surgeon, was educated in medicine at St. Thomas's Hospital, where he later became lecturer in anatomy and senior surgeon. He was twice President of the Royal College of Surgeons, in 1851 and in 1860. He is described as a man of varied attainments and many interests outside his profession. As a small boy he began to keep a diary, and continued it during his entire life.[4] The article from which the following extract is taken begins by refuting the statements concerning hospital nurses, which were made in the short letter appearing in the *London Times* on April 15, 1857, signed "One Who Has Walked a Good Many Hospitals." * Dr. South then describes, in some detail, the nursing at St. Thomas's Hospital, which he considers a typical London hospital. His descriptions of the Institute of Nursing Sisters and the Community of St. John's House are apparently based on information which he secured for the purpose. He disagrees with many of the statements made by Miss Nightingale in her book on the Kaiserswerth Institution, which was published anonymously in 1851.[5]]

Having thus reviewed, and I hope refuted, to the satisfaction of the reader, the untrue assertions of the "One Who has Walked a good many Hospitals," I will now state the *facts,* which can be easily verified by any one who may choose to inquire, in reference to the nursing establishment of St. Thomas's Hospital, which may be taken as a fair example of the usage throughout all the "large London Hospitals."

For the ordinary service of each ward, the nurses are of three kinds: two, or it may be three according to the size of the ward, of these are day-nurses, and the third is the night-nurse. The day-nurses are of two and very different grades and qualifications—the head nurse, or "sister," as she is called in three of the "large London Hospitals," and the nurse, as she is there called, or "ward-maid," as she is more properly designated in the Dublin hospitals. Each of the three has her distinct duty; but the control and responsible charge of the ward rests with the "sister," or head nurse, and the nurse, or "ward-maid," has the menial offices to perform.

* See Reading No. 140.

The sister has much the same duty imposed on her as has a good private nurse. She receives the directions of the physician or surgeon to whose ward she is attached as to the administration of medicine, diet, and other matters requiring attention; and she reports to the apothecary or house-surgeon, any circumstances which call for immediate attention; or if not requiring special report, she gives, when the physician or surgeon makes his visit, an account of the condition of the patient since the previous visit. She takes care that the nurse, or ward-maid, does her duty, and that the patients do not infringe the regulations of the hospital. In severe cases she pays more especial attention to the patients; and this is particularly seen in the surgical wards, as regards serious accidents and operations; under which circumstances she is as constantly with the patient, day and night—often for many together—as is the dresser, whose duty is to be on watch at the bedside so long as the surgeon thinks needful. Not infrequently this duty becomes very heavy; but she cheerfully discharges it, in hope of being rewarded by the recovery of the patient and the approbation of her surgical superior, who is almost invariably anxious to encourage her in the laborious discharge of her duty, and to award her just share of praise in assisting him, with God's blessing, to the successful conduct of important cases to their conclusion, which, but for her unremitting care and womanly aid, would not have attained a successful issue, however great and eminent the medical and surgical talents and attainments of the surgeon. Only those who have operated much know how greatly the success of operations depends on good nursing; and it may be taken as an undoubted fact, that in those hospitals where operations and bad accidents do best, there are the sisters, or head nurses, most attentive and intelligent. Each sister is provided with a bed-room and sitting-room adjoining the ward, and one or both opening into it; but the greater part of her day is spent in the ward; and although she is presumed to go to bed regularly each night at a reasonable time, yet, as has been already mentioned, if she have any serious case on hand she is more frequently up night after night. She receives a salary paid quarterly, but has not any perquisites or rations, except beer.

The day-nurse, or ward-maid, performs for the ward the usual duties of a housemaid, as to cleaning and bed-making. She also makes and applies poultices and the like, in less important cases; attends to the wants of the patients confined to their beds or requiring such assistance as she can render; and washes such children as may chance to be in the ward. She comes on duty at six o'clock in the morning, and remains till eight o'clock in the evening, after which she retires to sup and sleep among her fellows in a spacious dormitory specially allotted to them. But though these are her regular hours, she, as well as the sister, is liable to be kept up all night. She is under the immediate superintendence and control of the sister, who reports her to the steward or matron if negligent. She receives wages, which are paid weekly, but she has not any rations except beer.

The night-nurse comes on duty at eight o'clock in the evening, and remains on watch, moving continually about the ward, till six o'clock of the following morning, when the day-nurse arrives. She gives such medicines as may be due during her watch, renders any assistance which the patients require, and informs the sister of any change in the patients' condition which requires her attention. Her watch over, she remains till eleven o'clock assisting to clean up and put the ward to rights, after which she retires to the dormitory, has her dinner, and goes to bed from two till eight o'clock, when she gets up and prepares to go on duty in the ward to which she is attached. She receives weekly wages, but has not any rations except beer.

It would naturally be presumed that the women filling the offices of sisters, and of nurses or ward servants, are not all of the same class. The sisters are selected from among intelligent and active persons in the prime of life—usually about thirty years of age—who are generally ascertained to be quick, and capable of understanding and attaining a knowledge of the duties required of them. They are not thrust at once into the wards, ignorant and unfitted for the responsibilities they assume, "to pick up a knowledge of their business as they best can." They are at first taken as supernumeraries, or unattached, into the matron's office, where, by their frequent errands into the wards, and communication with the attached sisters, they gradually attain an insight into the duties they will have to undertake; and after a while are sent for short periods into a ward, the sister of which is either ill and unable to attend to her duty, or is enjoying her annual short holiday. Her length of probation varies partly on the readiness with which she acquires a knowledge of the ward duties, and in part on the vacancies which occur by the retirement or discharge of sisters . . .

As regards the nurses, or ward-maids, these, as I have said, are much in the condition of housemaids, and require little teaching beyond that of poultice-making, which is easily acquired, and the enforcement of cleanliness, and attention to the patients' wants. They need not be of the class of persons required for sisters, not having such responsibilities.

For the information of the public it is right to state that there have been in London for many years *two training institutions* for nurses, namely, the Institution of Nursing Sisters founded in 1840 by the exertions of the late Mrs. Fry, and the Training Institution for Nurses founded in 1848, principally, I believe, by the exertions of the Rev. E. H. Plumtre and Mr. Bowman.

The Institution of Nursing Sisters proposes only to prepare and provide nurses. They live at the institution house during their instruction at the hospitals, and, when considered capable, remain in the house in readiness for engagement by persons of every station from the highest to the lowest, subject to the control and disposal of the lady superintendent, who appoints them to such cases as she thinks they are best suited to tend. She receives all the applications for sisters, and conducts the correspondence of the institution, being herself subject to the direction of the committee of ladies who manage the establishment without any male assistance. The women who purpose to become *nursing sisters* are examined as to their general qualifications, and the lady committee having been satisfied therewith they are sent, if not previously nurses, to a large hospital, where they remain in the wards for sufficient length of time to attain a knowledge of their required duty by attentively watching the proceedings of the sister of the ward, attending the visits of the medical officers; being present at the performance of operations, and rendering such assistance as they by degrees become competent to afford. They return to their meals and to sleep at the institution house, or some convenient place in the immediate neighbourhood of the hospital, except when prevented by the hospital arrangements. The nursing sisters under instruction have enjoyed the large opportunity for acquiring practical knowledge afforded by Guy's Hospital from the first foundation of the institution in 1840; and within the last five or six years they have been also received at St. Thomas's, where they have constantly two or three of them . . .

When considered qualified they return to the institution house, where they continue under the control of the lady superintendent, who, as sisters are required and applied for, appoints them to such service as they are best fitted for, for a period of six weeks. . . . They receive fixed wages, and wear a modest dark-coloured dress and plain cap, neither of which, however, in its peculiar form or cut, attracts particular attention.

The other institution, the St. John's House *Training Institution for Nurses,* designs "to improve the qualifications and to raise the character of nurses for the sick by providing for them professional training, together with moral and religious discipline, under the care of a clergyman, aided by the influence and example of a lady superintendent and other resident sisters." The officers consist of "a master, lady superintendent, and two physicians;" but "no person who is not a member of the United Church of England and Ireland, as by law established, is competent to act on the council or to fill any office in the institution." . . . . The inmates consist of three classes:—1. *Sisters.* Ladies who are willing to devote themselves to the work of attending the sick and poor and of educating others for those duties. 2. *Probationers.* Women under training in this establishment and in the public hospitals of the metropolis, under the direction of the officers of the institution. 3. *Nurses.* Women who have passed satisfactorily their period of probation. It is further stated that "the probationers will receive instruction from the master and lady superintendent, and be properly trained and exercised in the particular duties of nurses," and "the period of probation will be determined according to their several capacity by the authorities of the hospitals and the officers of the institution." From 1848, at which time the institution was founded, the probationers were received at St. George's and at the Westminster and Middlesex Hospitals; but since Lady-day, 1856, at King's College Hospital. After being admitted nurses, their duties are "to attend the sick, both rich and poor, at hospitals or private houses, as the lady superintendent shall appoint, and when at home in the institution, to perform such domestic duties as shall be assigned to them . . ."

The principal feature in the St. John's House institution is the class of sisters, whose duties are "to assist the master and lady superintendent in the instruction and general training of the probationers and in the domestic management; also, with the sanction of the parochial clergy, to visit such sick and aged poor as may be approved by the master and lady superintendent." [6]

142. Frances Power Cobbe, "Workhouse Sketches," *Macmillan's Magazine,* Vol. III (November, 1860–April, 1861), pp. 448–461

[Frances Power Cobbe (1822–1904) was one of the early women journalists of England. She was the founder and for eighteen years the Honorable Secretary of the Victoria Street Society for Protection of Animals from Vivisection, as well as President of the British Union for Abolition of Vivisection. She published hundreds of articles on the English Poor Laws.[7]]

But even the unfitness of the wards and their furniture is second to the question of medical aid and nursing . . .

Besides the anomalous arrangements of wards and medical attendance in workhouses, which are actually hospitals without proper Hospital Supervision, there remains a third source of misery to the inmates—the *Nurses.* It is easy to understand that the difficulty of obtaining good nurses in ordinary hospitals is doubled here. Indeed it is rarely grappled with at all; for women hired by the Board are so invariably brought into collision with the master and matron, that even the kindest of such officials say (and probably say truly), that it is best to be content with the pauper nurses, over whom at least they can exercise some control. The result is that, in an immensely large proportion of houses, the sick are attended by male and female paupers who are placed in such office without having had the smallest preparatory instruction or experience, and who often have the reverse of kindly feelings towards their helpless patients. As *payments,* they usually receive allowances of beer or gin, which aid their too common propensity to intoxication.

. . . .

3d. It is hoped that it may be possible to reach the monster-evil of unqualified nurses, and to pay from voluntary contributions the salaries of good ones who should be subordinated so completely to the matron as to obviate the existing prejudices and difficulties. Finally, as it is at all times exceedingly difficult to obtain the services of well qualified nurses, it is hoped that it may prove practicable to train the workhouse girls in the "Homes" for such service by attaching to the establishments wards for incurable patients who are in need of careful attendance though able to defray the cost of their own support. Such a class is not rarely to be met, and would be as much benefited as the girls, who (on showing fitness for the task) would receive instruction qualifying them to earn a comfortable livelihood, and to be of essential service to the community.

143. Ernest Hart, in *Fortnightly Review*, April, 1866

[Ernest Abraham Hart (1835–1898) was an English medical journalist, eye specialist, and member of the Royal College of Surgeons. It was as editor of the *British Medical Journal* that he did his best-known work in reform of the care of the sick in workhouse infirmaries and throughout England as a whole.[8]]

In many provincial infirmaries the "straw sack" was found to be still in use, the "assistant nurse" was still receiving her £12 per annum, and night nurses were few and far between. The unpaid pauper had charge of the nursing in many an infirmary, and for the infirm, the sick, and the helpless imbeciles to be mixed up together was the rule rather than the exception.... [At Bath] ... the day nursing was done by one nurse with three untrained assistants. Night nursing there was none, nor even a bell by which assistance could be summoned. At Bristol there were two paid nurses to 132 patients; at Bedminster, two to 128; at Truro, one to 783, and at Falmouth, none at all. At Sedgefield, among other scandals, confinement took place in a corner of the general ward.[9]

144. Charles Dickens. *Martin Chuzzlewit*

[The life and works of Charles Dickens (1812–1870), English novelist, are well known to the world. His works have sometimes been said to be autobiographical. Not himself a professional reformer, he nevertheless brought about, indirectly, many reforms in the social life of his day. In the preface to *Martin Chuzzlewit* (written 1843–1844), Dickens states that "Mrs. Sarah Gamp is a representation of the hired attendant on the poor in sickness.... Mrs. Betsy Prig is a fair specimen of a Hospital Nurse..." Forster, his friend and biographer, adds that "the rich ... [were] no better off, for Mrs. Gamp's original was in reality a person hired by a most distinguished friend of his [Dickens'] own, a lady, to take charge of an invalid very dear to her..." [10] There are two narratives in the book about Mrs. Gamp's and Mrs. Prig's care of patients. That chosen for inclusion here is from Chapter XXIX and is probably the less familiar one; the other will be found in Chapter XXV.]

This lady [Mrs. Gamp] lodged at a bird-fancier's, next door but one to the celebrated mutton-pie shop, and directly opposite to the original cat's-meat warehouse, the renown of which establishments was duly heralded on their respective fronts. It was a little house, and this was the more convenient; for Mrs. Gamp being, in her highest walk of art, a monthly nurse, or, as her signboard boldly had it, "Midwife," and lodging in the first-floor front, was easily assailable at night by pebbles, walking-sticks, and fragments of tobacco-pipe—all much more efficacious than the street-door knocker, which was so constructed as to wake the street with ease, and even spread alarms of fire in Holborn, without making the smallest impression on the premises to which it was addressed.

．　　　．　　　　．　　　　．　　　．

Arriving at the tavern, Mrs. Gamp (who was full-dressed for the journey [to Hartfordshire with a patient], in her latest suit of mourning) left her friends to entertain themselves in the yard, while she ascended to the sick-room, where her fellow-labourer, Mrs. Prig, was dressing the invalid.

He was so wasted, that it seemed as if his bones would rattle when they moved him. His cheeks were sunken, and his eyes unnaturally large. He lay back in the easy-chair like one more dead than living; and rolled his languid eyes towards the door when Mrs. Gamp appeared, as painfully as if their weight alone were burdensome to move.

"And how are we by this time?" Mrs. Gamp observed. "We looks charming."

"We looks a deal charminger than we are then," returned Mrs. Prig, a little chafed in her temper. "We got out of bed back'ards, I think, for we're as cross as two sticks. I never see sich a man. He wouldn't have been washed, if he'd had his own way."

"She put the soap in my mouth," said the unfortunate patient feebly.

"Couldn't you keep it shut then?" retorted Mrs. Prig, "Who do you think's to wash one feater, and miss another, and wear one's eyes out with all manner of fine-work of that description, for half a crown a day? If you wants to be tittivated, you must pay accordin'."

"Oh dear me!" cried the patient, "oh dear, dear!"

"There!" said Mrs. Prig, "That's the way he's been a-conducting of himself, Sarah, ever since I got him out of bed, if you'll believe it."

"Instead of being grateful," Mrs. Gamp observed, "for all our little ways. Oh, fie for shame, sir, fie for shame!"

Here Mrs. Prig seized the patient by the chin, and began to rasp his unhappy head with a hair-brush.

"I suppose you don't like that neither!" she observed, stopping to look at him.

It was just possible that he didn't, for the brush was a specimen of the hardest kind of instrument producible by modern art, and his eyelids were red with the friction. Mrs. Prig was gratified to observe the correctness of her supposition, and said triumphantly, "she know'd as much."

When his hair was smoothed down comfortably into his eyes, Mrs. Prig and Mrs. Gamp put on his neckerchief, adjusting his shirt-collar with great nicety, so that the starched points should also invade those organs, and afflict them with an artificial ophthalmia. His waistcoat and coat were next arranged; and as every button was wrenched into a wrong buttonhole, and the order of his boots was reversed, he presented on the whole rather a melancholy appearance.

"I don't think it's right," said the poor weak invalid. "I feel as if I was in somebody else's clothes. I'm all on one side, and you've made one of my legs shorter than the other. There's a bottle in my pocket too. What do you make me sit upon a bottle for?"

"Deuce take the man!" cried Mrs. Gamp, drawing it forth. "If he an't been and got my night-bottle here. I made a little cupboard of his coat when it hung behind the door, and quite forgot it, Betsy. You'll find a ingun or two, and a little tea and sugar, in his t'other pocket, my dear, if you'll jest be good enough to take 'em out."

Betsy produced the property in question, together with some other articles of general chandlery; and Mrs. Gamp transferred them to her own pocket, which was a species of nankeen pannier. Refreshment then arrived in the form of chops and strong ale for the ladies, and a basin of beef-tea for the patient; which refection was barely at an end when John Westlock appeared.

"Up and dressed!" cried John, sitting down beside him. "That's brave. How do you feel?"

"Much better; but very weak."

"No wonder. You have had a hard bout of it. But country air, and change of scene," said John, "will make another man of you! Why, Mrs. Gamp," he added, laughing, as he kindly arranged the sick man's garments, "you have odd notions of a gentleman's dress!"

"Mr. Lewsome an't a easy gent to get into his clothes, sir," Mrs. Gamp replied with dignity, "as me and Betsy Prig can certify afore the Lord Mayor and Uncommon Counsellors, if needful!"

John was at that moment standing close in front of the sick man, in the act of releasing him from the torture of the collars before mentioned, when he said in a whisper,—

"Mr. Westlock! I don't wish to be overheard. I have something very particular and strange to say to you—something that has been a dreadful weight on my mind through this long illness."

Quick in all his motions, John was turning round to desire the women to leave the room, when the sick man held him by the sleeve.

"Not now. I've not the strength; I've not the courage. May I tell it when I have? May I write it, if I find that easier and better?"

"May you!" cried John. "Why, Lewsome, what is this?"

"Don't ask me what it is. It's unnatural and cruel. Frightful to think of—frightful to tell—frightful to know—frightful to have helped in. Let me kiss your hand for all your goodness to me. Be kinder still, and don't ask me what it is!"

At first John gazed at him in great surprise, but remembering how very much reduced he was, and how recently his brain had been on fire with fever, believed that he was labouring under some imaginary horror or despondent fancy. For further information on this point, he took an opportunity of drawing Mrs. Gamp aside, while Betsy Prig was wrapping him in cloaks and shawls, and asked her whether he was quite collected in his mind.

"Oh, bless you, no!" said Mrs. Gamp. "He hates his nusses to this hour. They always does it, sir. It's a certain sign. If you could have heerd the poor dear soul a-findin' fault with me and Betsy Prig, not half an hour ago, you would have wondered how it is we don't get fretted to the tomb."

This almost confirmed John in his suspicion; so not taking what had passed into any serious account, he resumed his former cheerful manner, and assisted by Mrs. Gamp and Betsy Prig, conducted Lewsome downstairs to the coach, just then upon the point of starting . . .

It was a troublesome matter to adjust Mrs. Gamp's luggage to her satisfaction; for every package belonging to that lady had the inconvenient property of requiring to be put in a boot by itself, and to have no other luggage near it, on pain of actions at law for heavy damages against the proprietors of the coach. The umbrella with the circular patch was particularly hard to be got rid of, and several times thrust out its battered brass nozzle from improper crevices and chinks, to the great terror of the other passengers. Indeed, in her intense anxiety to find a haven of refuge for this chattel, Mrs. Gamp so often moved it, in the course of five minutes, that it seemed not one umbrella but fifty. At length it was lost, or said to be, and for the next five minutes she was face to face with the coachman, go wherever he might, protesting that it should be "made good" though she took the question to the House of Commons.

At last her bundle, and her pattens, and her basket, and everything else being disposed of, she took a friendly leave of Poll and Mr. Bailey, dropped a curtsy to John Westlock, and parted as from a cherished member of the sisterhood with Betsy Prig.

"Wishin' you lots of sickness, my darling creetur," Mrs. Gamp observed, "and good places. It won't be long, I hope, afore we works together, off and on, again, Betsy; and may our next meetin' be at a large family's where they all takes it reg'lar, one from another, turn and turn about, and has it business-like."

"I don't care how soon it is," said Mrs. Prig, "nor how many weeks it lasts." [11]

145. Sir Henry Wentworth Acland. *Memoir of the Cholera at Oxford in the Year 1854*

[Sir Henry Wentworth Acland (1815–1900) was an English physician of note and a man of learning. He studied medicine in London and Edinburgh, and later took an active part in the revival of the Oxford medical school. He also promoted the study of natural science, art, and archeology in the university. As a physician interested in public health and sanitation, he served on the royal commission on sanitary laws in England and Wales in 1869.[12] His study of the outbreak of cholera at

Oxford in 1854 contains an outline of the nursing arrangements during the epidemic, and a suggestion for the future.]

Arrangements Made in Oxford during the Epidemic.

The Nurses

Sect. 6. One consequence of the decision that medical attendance shall be provided at the houses of the poor is, that Nurses must be engaged, and that they should be accessible as readily as the Medical Staff.

This was done as follows:

In the Police Office, which is near the Town Hall and in the most central locality, a list was kept of all the respectable women who were willing and able to nurse in Cholera houses. Their names had been furnished mainly through the local knowledge of the Parochial Clergy. The list was arranged thus:

Name	Address	Gone out	Returned home	Qualifications and Remarks
Anne Walker	19, Osney Lane	To Mrs. W. 84, Speedwell St.		An excellent nurse. A. B. Surgeon

There was no lack of Nurses but on one day. The wages were 1s. 6d. daily, or 10s. 6d. weekly. After they had nursed three nights, they were allowed a day's rest, or the option of going out again to nurse. Rations were given to them every day. A cook was kept at the Town Hall to prepare them. The allowance was,

1 lb. of Cooked Meat.	1 lb. of Bread.	1 Bottle of Ale
2 ounces of Butter.	1 ounce of Sugar.	Half an ounce of Tea.

Except by Medical order, no brandy was allowed.

When a new Case of Cholera was announced, in the house of any poor person, a Messenger from the Police Office proceeded to the house of a Nurse "returned home," and sent her to the place at which her help was required. It was then the business of an Inspector, Condé, an old Waterloo soldier, to go there, to ascertain whether the interior economy of the house was such that the order of the Medical Attendant could be followed. If not, his duty was to forward from the Police Office the deficiency: food, bedding, blankets, hot bottles, &c. And lastly, because the most important, a lady (who desires her name to be withheld,) [13] visited daily every house (within a certain area) to instruct the Nurses, to comfort the sick, to cheer the disconsolate; and, where need was, herself to supply a sudden emergency, or to relieve a wearied attendant. By day and by night she plied this task, and when she rested, or where,—as long at least as she knew of a house where disease had entered,—is known to herself alone.

Over the whole of these arrangements Mr Cartwright, Deputy Chairman of the Board of Guardians, presided; he received the Reports of the Inspector, who gave a list of the daily state of affected houses; he paid the wages, engaged or dismissed the Nurses, and shewed in all his transactions the power of blending acute business habits with a most benevolent humanity.

Chapter IV.   On Certain Points Affecting Voluntary Institutions for giving Medical Aid.

On the necessity of providing Nurses for the Poor.

Far more important than a revolution in Hospital Nurses appears to me the obtaining Nurses trained and qualified to attend the poor at their own homes. There is no object more requiring the energy of the benevolent; none more certain to repay their exertions; none more easy of execution. A very moderate Subscription, the cooperation of Guardians, the consent of the Governors of Hospitals, with the aid of the Parochial Clergy, might at once obtain for every town a corps of Nurses, such as we had at Oxford at the time of the Cholera. A lady, resident here, is willing to undertake the organization and superintend such arrangements for Oxford. A body of more or less competent women would then be ready at all times to wait on the sick poor. They might at once effect good in various ways. Their knowledge of cooking alone would be a positive boon, supposing always they had been properly instructed, as has been proposed, at the Hospital. The more able of them would in time become trained Nurses for all classes; they would be known and certified. This would probably have been attempted here had not the cholera Nurses, for the most part, gone out to the Crimea, and had not other circumstances delayed the public proposal of this plan. What can be effected in Oxford, can be effected elsewhere. Persons might come hither for instruction from parishes in Oxfordshire and the adjoining counties. In connection with every Hospital, through the kingdom, such an institution might soon exist, to the great advantage of every class of society, and to the maintenance of many respectable women, and especially of widows.

The benefit of such an organization is so apparent, that I need not say more on the subject, but only to suggest to the reader, the boon that it would be during the prevalence of Epidemics of whatever kind.[14]

146. E. C. Rickards. *Felicia Skene of Oxford A Memoir*

[Felicia Skene (1821–1899) was born in Aix in Provence, one of a large family. Her father, James Skene, was a lifelong friend of Sir Walter Scott. Their friendship is described in the "Introduction" to the fourth canto of *Marmion*. One brother, James Henry Skene, served in the Crimean War,[15] while another, William Forbes Skene, was a famous historian and antiquarian. Felicia's girlhood was spent in Edinburgh and Athens. One of her most intimate friends was Frances Power Cobbe,[16] whose efforts in antivivisection she eagerly joined. The family later moved to Oxford where Felicia lived for fifty years, becoming active in church work and prison visiting, and writing articles on the latter activity. A friend of Sir Henry Wentworth Acland,[17] she assisted in the nursing of the victims of the cholera epidemic in Oxford in 1854. In the following year she greatly desired to take a group of nurses to the Crimea, but being unable to obtain her parents' permission, she lent her services in the recruiting of suitable nurses for Miss Nightingale's group.[18]]

In 1854 a fresh claim came upon her energies. Oxford was once more attacked by cholera and smallpox. It was the worst visitation of cholera there had been, numbering more victims than either of the two previous ones.

Already in 1849, Felicia had given her services to the sufferers, so that she had had some experience of the terrible disease ...

A noble corps of workers among the doctors, the clergy, and others banded themselves to cope with the scourge. . . . The kind of cases with which Felicia and her fellow-labourers had to deal are painful even to read about ...

The plan of campaign adopted was a double one. Nursing must be carried on in some building in an airy spot apart from the town, for the reception of those patients who could be removed to it; and those who could not must be nursed in their own houses.

For the first a field was found on which three old cattle-sheds were adapted for the use of patients, one for smallpox, two for cholera. Sleeping shelters were provided for members of families of the sufferers; tents were erected for meals and for the reception of children coming from infected houses. There they could be carefully watched to see if symptoms of disease appeared, and removed to the temporary hospital if necessary ...

The nursing itself was carried on under the direction of Felicia's friend Miss Hughes (Sister Marion) ...[19]

The other department of the nursing, that in which Felicia took the leading part, had to be carried on in the homes of the sick ...

At first Felicia tried to carry on her labours among them singlehanded, but it soon became necessary to enlist other helpers. Mr. Cartwright, Deputy Chairman of the Board of Guardians, was made responsible for engaging and dismissing a band of respectable women as nurses, and Felicia was to superintend and instruct them in their duties.

She had undertaken no light task, for if on the whole they did their work satisfactorily, many were ignorant and needed training. How well she acquitted herself Sir Henry Acland shall testify.[20]

At all hours Felicia might have been seen going about the lowest streets, carrying hot water bottles or other comfort for the sufferers. If she were not sitting up at night with one of them, she was willing to be sent for at any moment. The front door of her house was kept on the latch with a policeman walking up and down to guard it, to make her summons easy. The cholera cases were often awfully rapid. The patient would be suddenly seized with violent pains, and in a couple of hours all would be over . . .

Neither had she that special taste and talent for nursing that makes it quite apart from duty, a real pleasure to many women; though she had the moral qualities required, which have led to the saying, that it takes a good woman to be a good nurse. In that, as in so many branches of work, love helps to find out the way. Her quick sympathy gave her insight into the patients' needs. Her tenderness invited confidence, so that they could pour out the anxieties which weighed on their minds and retarded their recovery. Her courage and cheerfulness braced them to make an effort to get well. Her strong will ensured obedience to her orders. Her very presence with its vigorous vitality seemed to inspire them with hope and strength . . .[21]

147. Margaret Goodman. *Experiences of an English Sister of Mercy*

[Margaret Goodman was a member for six years of Miss Sellon's Sisterhood, the Devonport Sisters, founded by Miss Sellon in 1848. During an epidemic of cholera in London, she nursed the victims as a Sister of Mercy. Later, during the Crimean War, she became a member of Miss Nightingale's group of nurses going to Scutari.[22]]

While in the midst of occupations such as these [teaching, etc.] the lady, who, on account of Miss Sellon's illness, had chief charge of the sisterhood, came to me one afternoon to inquire if I had any objection to go into the homes of the Irish in Stoneham Lane; many of whom were dying untended of cholera. We went together to a house in which, after a short stay, she left me for the night at my request, but said I must leave the next morning at five o'clock, when she would ask another sister to take my place; she also expressed her intention of sending one of the old sailor men, who found a home in the sisters' houses, with my tea, and to see if all were right. On this afternoon began my experience of nursing in the cholera, and it appeared to me so awful a pestilence, and caused me to witness such fearful privations, that every minute incident in the scenes of the next few weeks is so graven on my memory, that I believe they will never be effaced until the whole tablet is blotted.

The room in which I found myself, contained a large bedstead, but positively no other article of furniture; not even a cup or spoon. A girl of about seventeen, sister of the sick woman on the bedstead, was sitting on the floor in front of the empty grate, with her knees drawn up to her chin, rocking herself to and fro and moaning piteously. My first care was to quiet her, the noise was so extremely distracting; she was suffering from want, fatigue, and grief, and when she understood that I would take charge of her sister, she was persuaded to lie down in a corner of the room, and, drawing her thin shawl over her head, soon fell asleep. The sick woman was lying on the planks of the bedstead without a vestige of bed to save her from them; the floor would have been less uncomfortable . . .[23]

148. Sir James Paget on the Nursing at St. Bartholomew's Hospital about 1835

[Sir James Paget (1814–1899) taught and practiced medicine at St. Bartholomew's Hospital. He was a skilled diagnostician and an eminent authority on diseases of the bones and joints. His brother, Sir George Paget was also a physician. Sir James is said to have been a delightful speaker.[24] The following description is from his speech entitled "St. Bartholomew's Hospital and School Fifty Years Ago," before the Abernethian Society in 1885.]

1. In the department of nursing, there is the greatest and happiest contrast of all. It is true that even fifty years ago there were some excellent nurses, especially among the sisters in the medical wards, where everything was more gentle and orderly than in the surgical. There was an admirable Sister Hope, who had had her leg amputated in the hospital, and then spent her life giving others the most kindly watchful care. A Sister Mary, a near relative of hers, was as constant to her charge; and there were some good surgical sisters too. They had none of the modern art; they could not have kept a chart or skilfully taken a temperature, but they had an admirable sagacity and a sort of rough practical knowledge which were nearly as good as any acquired skill. An old Sister Rahere was the chief among them, stout, ruddy, positive, very watchful.... And there was her neighbor, Sister Colston, rough-tongued, scolding, not seldom rather tipsy; and yet very watchful and really very helpful, especially in what she felt to be good cases. On the whole, indeed, it may fairly be said that the Sisters were among the very best nurses of the time. The ordinary nurses were not so; the greater part of them were rough, dull, unobservant and untaught women; of the best it could only be said that they were kindly, and careful and attentive in doing what they were told to do.[25]

149. Pastor Muhlenberg on the Nursing at St. Bartholomew's Hospital in 1855

[William Augustus Muhlenberg (1796–1877) was a philanthropist and Protestant Episcopal clergyman. A graduate of the University of Pennsylvania, he became interested in public education, and, largely through his efforts, the Lancaster, Pennsylvania, public-school district became the second to be established in the state. His interest in education also led to the founding of what was probably the first Episcopal "church school" in the United States, at Flushing, Long Island.[26] In New York, in 1846, he instituted the first American order of the Protestant Episcopal deaconesses, the Sisterhood of the Church of the Holy Communion, which led to the establishment of St. Luke's Hospital, the cornerstone of which was laid in 1854.[27] In the interest of nursing in the latter hospital, he visited St. Bartholomew's Hospital in 1855.]

I spent several hours in St. Bartholomew's Hospital. One of the chaplains, a most excellent and earnest man, accompanied me through every part of it. . . . All the Sisters but one are communicants of the Church, and those I spoke to seemed to be good women. . . . The most ample space is allowed for the beds; there not being more than twenty-two or twenty-four in each ward, which is divided into two compartments, leaving to each ten or twelve patients, in a room some forty feet long by twenty-five in width. Each ward has the service of four nurses including the Sister. The atmosphere was as fresh as in our little Infirmary, and the cleanliness everywhere is beautiful. If the other hospitals of London are in like condition, and I am told they are, London has more to boast of than I imagined.[28]

150. Sir Rickman John Godlee. *Life of Lord Lister*

[Lord Lister (1827–1912) brought to surgical practice the principles of antisepsis, and is known as the Father of Antiseptic Surgery.[29] Much of his practice at one period was carried on at the Royal Infirmary at Edinburgh. The nurses were "untrained," not yet having been affected by Florence Nightingale's ideas on nursing. Lister came in contact with good and poor types of these nurses, both of which are described in the following extract from the life of Lister by his nephew. In the preface of this biography, Sir Rickman states that he lived for many years in close personal contact with his uncle. He also had access to his notebooks, many pages of which he wrote at Lister's dictation.[30]]

[Nursing at the Royal Infirmary, Edinburgh, 1870.]

The nurses were probably at least as good as in most hospitals that had not come under the direct influence of Florence Nightingale or her pupils. Educated women had hardly begun to diffuse their leaven in the nursing profession. The fully trained nurse was hardly known and some of the old "Sairey Gamp" type were still to be met with. Lister used to tell of one of these who took advantage of an empty bed to sleep off her potations. Instead of being instantly dismissed, as would be the case now, it was suggested that the effect of a serious reprimand from her surgeon should be tried. Accordingly, he put on his gravest expression—and he could be very grave at times—and asked her whether she never thought of her responsibility for all the poor sufferers under her charge. "Oh, I nae minds o' them," was her unexpected reply, which with its cheery indifference, nearly upset his gravity.

But there was one amongst them, Mrs. Porter, a great character, who might almost be called an institution. She was head nurse in his wards, as she had been under Syme's regime. Edinburgh students of those days remember her well. She kept them all in order, and, it was said, her chiefs also. She acted as if all the responsibility rested on her shoulders, and was in fact an important and efficient personage, whom everyone treated with deference.[31]

151. John Beddoe. *Memories of Eighty Years*

[Dr. John Beddoe (1826–1911) was a fellow student of Lister in London and his colleague at Edinburgh. He was an anthropologist of note, and published several writings on the subject. During the Crimean War he was on the staff of a Civil Hospital.[32] The following is a brief account of an attempt at cliff climbing, which pictures the concern of Mrs. Porter over Lister's bruises, the result of a fall on that occasion, ending with a brief allusion to another nurse of the infirmary staff.]

So we went thither one day to attempt it [the climbing of Cat's Nick]. Lister had been overworking himself, and before I, who was leading, had accomplished more than half the ascent, he said to me—

"Beddoe, I feel giddy; would it not be foolish in me to persevere today?"

"Certainly!" I replied. "Let us postpone it till you are in good condition," and I began to descend.

I suppose much experience of the place had made me careless. A large fragment came away in my hands and the stone and I both fell upon Lister . . .

Lister was badly bruised, but no bone was broken. I went off at once to the Infirmary and procured a litter and four men, wherewith I returned to Lister. As our melancholy procession entered the courtyard of the surgical hospital, there met us Mrs. Porter, the head nurse then and for many years after. She wept and wrung her hands, for Lister was a universal favourite.

"Eh, Doketur Bedie! Doketur Bedie! A kent weel hoo it wad be. Ye Englishmen are aye sae fülish, gaeing aboot fustlin [whistling] upo' Sawbath."

I do not suppose Lister ever whistled on Sunday. I am certain I did not, for I never could whistle in all my life; but we had suffered for the national offence. We were both in bed for a fortnight, at the end of which time, on a Saturday afternoon, up came one of my nurses.

"Eh, Doketur, can ye no coom 'doon? Here's Maggie Dixon's taen a appleplectic fit, and there's naebody in the hoose tae bleed her." [33]

152. Ernest Henley. *In Hospital; Rhymes and Rhythms*

[William Ernest Henley (1849–1903) was an English poet, critic, and editor. Crippled by tuberculosis of the bone, he became the model for Long John Silver in Stevenson's *Treasure Island*. Henley collaborated with Stevenson in four plays.[34] In 1873 he was a patient in Sir Joseph Lister's wards in Edinburgh, and while there wrote some short verses under the title of *In Hospital; Rhymes and Rhythms*. The one called "Staff Nurse: Old Style" is said by Lister's nephew to be a faithful portrayal of Mrs. Porter.[35]]

Staff Nurse: Old Style

The greater masters of the commonplace,
REMBRANDT and good SIR WALTER—only these
Could paint her all to you: experienced ease
And antique liveliness and ponderous grace;
The sweet old roses of her sunken face;
The depth and malice of her sly, grey eyes;
The broad Scots tongue that flatters, scolds, defies;
The thick Scots wit that fells you like a mace.
These thirty years has she been nursing here,
Some of them under SYME, her hero still.
Much is she worth, and even more is made of her.
Patients and students hold her very dear.
The doctors love her, tease her, use her skill.
They say "The Chief" himself is half-afraid of her.[36]

153. Amelia Sieveking's Description of Nursing during the Cholera Epidemic, Hamburg, 1831

[The Sieveking family held an eminent position in Hamburg in commerce and municipal affairs. One branch of the family moved to London in 1809, where Amelia's nephew, later Sir Edward Henry Sieveking (1816–1904),[37] became a physician, a staunch supporter of the British Medical Association, and a Fellow of the Royal College of Physicians. He took an active interest in better nursing for the underprivileged, writing a pamphlet on the subject.[38] Amelia Wilhelmina Sieveking (1794–1859) was one of five children. Her father was a merchant and, subsequently, a senator of the city of Hamburg. Her mother was a highly educated woman. After the death of the latter, Amelia lived with Madame Brunnemann, a wealthy widow whom she calls "Mother" in some of her letters. For many years Amelia was active in improving nursing, in 1832 establishing the first group in Germany organized for nursing service in the homes, the Protestant Sisters of Mercy.[39] The letters from the Cholera Hospital suggest the conditions during the epidemic in Hamburg in 1831.]

Letters from Cholera Hospital of St. Eric on the Hollandisch Brook

October 14, 1831.

My dear and beloved Mother,—The first moment of leisure that I find here—it is now 10 A.M.—my heart impels me to send you word how I am getting on. The house-steward and the other officials show me every attention that I could possibly look for, and in the housekeeper I have unexpectedly found an old acquaintance. . . . Two female patients are all that are under my charge at present, yet I and another nurse have been fully occupied hitherto. In the men's ward there are so far more attendants than patients, and I hear that the physician declares that each sick person properly ought to have two. My patients are both elderly women. . . . Nor is my under-nurse amiss, but she seems to me to need supervision.

.   .   .   .

Sunday morning.

Before the new nurse arrived a female patient was brought in, and soon afterwards another; both, however, were so ill, that they could not be saved. With one of them, a native of Vierlanden, her sufferings, which lasted the whole night, reached a point that I had never seen yet.

My new nurse is a very stupid woman, but as soon as a second is required Dr. Siemers has promised to send me R., who I have been told by one of the best attendants in the men's ward wishes for the post . . .

.   .   .   .

[Monday evening] 11 P.M.

I share the night-watching with the two nurses, and find very little inconvenience from it. When I feel fatigued I lie down for an hour in the day-time, which is better than taking a whole night to myself, for as superintendent to the men's ward I have to make my rounds there every few hours by night as well as by day.

.   .   .   .

Tuesday.

In the morning, I have to see that, before the physician's visit, all the wards are cleaned, the beds made, and that everything is in proper order. Three times a day, morning, afternoon, and evening, I visit the sick-beds in company with the physician, the surgeon, and the apothecary, when Dr. Siemssen gives to each the directions belonging to our respective departments.

In the women's ward, of course, I have to pay particular attention to all the medical orders, as I am responsible there for their exact fulfilment.

In the men's wards my special duty is only to observe that diet is prescribed, according to which I draw up the daily bill of fare for the housekeeper. Not infrequently, too, I have to send the necessary notice of his admission to the relatives of the sick man, as the patients are often brought in unknown to their family. The linen of the wards is also under my charge. At present I also occasionally take part, when I see any need for it, in the actual nursing of the men, but if the number of our patients should greatly increase, I should be obliged to do less of this even in the women's ward, as the general superintendence would be of more importance, and would give me full occupation; but it would then be of great use to me that I have thus acquired experience in the treatment of the patients.

169

November 5th, evening.

I have been obliged to dismiss one of my nurses. I was very sorry, for the woman had been taken on my recommendation. She was very willing, and was not indifferent to me for the sake of old recollections. It was Mrs. H.—, who for several years used to take care of my father's house in the summer, and nursed him in his last illness. It is to be hoped she was then younger, quicker, and at least somewhat fitter for a nurse than she is now. Thus, for instance, she cannot read the labels on the medicine bottles; if a draught is to be given every two or three hours, she cannot calculate the time, and if she is told the hour she cannot remember it.[40]

154. *The Lancet Sanitary Commission for Investigating the State of the Infirmaries of Workhouses*

[*The Lancet,* a weekly medical journal, was founded in 1823.[41] Through the years it interested itself not only in the medical profession and medical practice but also in health questions in general. Its commissions, from time to time, investigated conditions in the health field and made recommendations for improvement. The findings of the Lancet Commission for investigating the care of the sick in the workhouse infirmaries presented, among other matters, observations of the conditions in nursing, and suggested appropriate remedies.]

We have no wish to make "sensation" statements against the pauper nurses. But, in the first place, it is notorious that the majority of them are aged and feeble and past work, or have strong tendencies to drink, and in many cases have otherwise led vicious lives. Even those workhouse officials who on principle oppose the employment of paid nurses, allow that, as a rule, there is no managing pauper nurses, except by confining them strictly to the house— a regime which must undermine their health and unfit them for their work. Secondly, their inefficiency is borne out by the character of their ward work as to the details of cleanliness, etc., which we have mentioned, and also by the united testimony of those benevolent persons who have visited the workhouses in a philanthropic spirit, and have been taken into the confidence of the patients; which testimony asserts that, in the great majority of cases, pauper nurses can only manage their patients by inspiring fear, and that their conduct is consequently often brutal.

There *is* a solution of the difficulty which, however distant, lies plainly before us. . . . In the district suburban schools, to which the workhouse children are now almost universally drafted off at an early age, there are immense numbers of girls daily growing up to a healthy womanhood under good physical and moral influences. What worthier means of completing their emancipation from the inherited curse of pauperism could be devised than the training of them to the respectable and truly dignified calling of skilled nurses? Surely, by means of the teaching of some of the nursing institutions these girls might (save for the one pecuniary difficulty of maintaining them during the probation) be readily converted into first-rate nurses upon condition of their agreeing to serve the infirmaries of the workhouses for a moderate, but sufficient stipend.

There is one aspect of nursing which bears so powerfully on the question of paid versus pauper nurses, that we must dwell on it for a moment: we refer to the duty of night-nursing. It is well known by all hospital physicians and surgeons that it is most difficult to secure the efficient performance of this work, and that nurses of a low *morale* are totally unfit to be trusted with it. At present mode of its performance, or non-performance, in our workhouse infirmaries is one of the greatest scandals attaching to these institutions. In our investigations we have almost uniformly failed to obtain any satisfactory account of the behavior of paupers as night-nurses, while we have received a great deal of positive evidence of their frequent gross neglect of that sort of duty.

St. Giles and St. George, Bloomsbury Infirmary

Disorder and neglect appeared to be in authority as a direct consequence of the so-called system of nursing which obtains here, directed by an aged female, 63 years old, with a salary of £20 per annum. Under her supervision there are fourteen pauper assistants or helpers, with two night-nurses, selected from those who perform the day-nursing, none of whom receive remuneration for their labours.

St. Leonard's, Shoreditch

To make matters as bad as possible, the nurses, with one exception, are pauper nurses, having improved rations and different dress, but no pecuniary encouragements. They are mostly a very inferior set of women; and the males, who are "nursed" by male paupers, are yet worse off. The nursing organization at this establishment is as bad as can be. The male nurses especially struck us as a peculiarly rough, ignorant, and uncouth set. There are no night-nurses ...

A poor fellow lying very dangerously ill with gangrene of the leg had had no medicine for three days, because, as the male "nurse" said, his mouth had been too sore.... A female, also very ill, had not had her medicine for two days, because the very infirm old lady in the next bed, who it seemed was appointed by the nurse to fulfil this duty, had been too completely bedridden for the last few days to rise and give it to her.... The nurses generally had the most imperfect idea of their duties in this respect. One nurse plainly avowed that she gave medicines three times a day to those who were very ill, and twice or once a day as they improved. The medicines were given all

171

down a ward in a cup; elsewhere in a gallipot. The nurse said she "poured out the medicine, and judged according." In other respects the nursing was equally deficient. The dressings were roughly and badly applied. Lotion and water-dressings were applied in rags, which were allowed to dry and stick. In fact, this was the rule. Bandages seemed to be unknown. But the general character of the nursing will be appreciated by the detail of the one fact, that we found in one ward two paralytic patients with frightful sloughs of the back: they were both dirty, *and lying on hard straw-mattresses;* the one dressed only with a rag steeped in chloride of lime solution, the other with a rag thickly covered with ointment. This latter was a fearful and very extensive sore, in a state of absolute putridity; the buttocks of the patient were covered with filth and excoriated, and the stench was masked by strewing dry chloride of lime on the floor under the bed. A spectacle more saddening or more discreditable cannot be imagined. Both these patients have since died: no inquest has been held on either.

A severe commentary on the nursing staff is supplied by the information given to us by the master, that the average age of the nurses is sixty, and their average duration in office from six to nine months.

The Islington Workhouse.

The infirmary accommodates 150 patients. Mr. Ede, the medical officer visits daily; there is a resident dispenser, and the guardians find the drugs. Thus there are the best elements of successful medical care. . . . The wards, low, small and ill-lighted as they were, have yet an aspect of cheerfulness and comfort. . . . Every ward had a full supply of bed-rests for bed-ridden patients. . . . At the end of each ward was its clean and shining array of stomach and feet warmers for three or four aged and sick persons. Each ward had its proportion of shawls for the use of the sick in cold weather. . . . In every case they had had their medicines regularly. The dressings were well applied. Sore backs were unknown . . .

The nurses are chosen from amongst the paupers; they are, however, paid from 1s. to 1s 6d. a week, and are well dressed. One sees here certainly the best side of parish nursing. Most of them have been in office for long terms of years; and they seem on the whole well-conducted, zealous, and well-managed, conscious that they are thoroughly looked after, and anxious to deserve good opinion . . .

The midwifery ward is the only ward which calls for animadversion . . . the women were very unkempt; the bed-linen was unclean, and their personal linen in some instances filthy. . . . It is managed by a midwife and nurse, . . . this ward is something of a reproach.

The Strand Infirmary.

In this great workhouse hospital we find that there are, for all purposes of superintendence, a master and matron, who do indeed happen to be unusually intelligent, active, and humane, but who are seconded by *no paid nurses*

172

whatever! There are twenty-two pauper nurses, and twenty-two pauper helpers. Of the former, very few can be considered fitted for their work as far as regards knowledge, and many are plainly incompetent from age or physical feebleness. The helpers are, of course, mere ignorant drudges. And yet this nursing staff has to minister to the wants of a sick population ... [of] nearly 200 sick, besides 260 infirm or insane.

Greenwich Infirmary.

[In] the infirmary ... there are eight wards for men, containing eighty-one beds. ... There are ten female wards, which contain 107 beds. ... The nursing arrangements are very improper, their being no paid nurse, except for the insane, throughout the whole establishment, although there are 198 beds in the infirmary and over 200 other cases under medical treatment. There are twenty-six pauper nurses, of ages varying from thirty to seventy-six; they are distinguished by a special dress, and have allowances of tea, sugar, meat, and beer daily; and occasionally gin, but get no money payment. Sixteen of these do the whole duty of the infirmary *by day and night,* sleeping in the wards to which they are attached. Thus there is no night-nursing properly so-called. It is right to say that as much care as is possible seems to be taken in selecting the fittest of the pauper inmates for the duties of nursing.

Bermondsey Infirmary.

[In the lying-in ward] the Nurse, an aged woman of seventy-four, is far too old and feeble for her onerous duties.

.   .   .   .

Bethnal Green.

The responsible work of nursing the sick, 550 to 600 in number, is committed to the care of two paid nurses, who receive £30 and £24, a year respectively, and about forty pauper nurses and helpers. Neither of these paid officials have been trained, but both displayed considerable aptitude for their duties. On being questioned as to the amount of work, both said they had more to do than they could get through, independently of the difficulty of managing the forty pauper nurses, whose tendencies to drink cannot be controlled.

.   .   .   .

Association for the Improvement of the Infirmaries of Workhouses.

Having been requested to express an opinion of the principles which should guide any efforts to improve the State treatment of the Sick Poor in Workhouse Infirmaries, we beg to state that any scheme, in order to be satisfactory, should, in our judgment, be based upon the following principles:—

1. The Sick Poor should be separated from the ablebodied paupers, and their treatment should be placed under a distinct management.

2. In lieu of Sick Wards annexed to each Workhouse, consolidated Infirmaries should be provided, where the following rules of Hospital

Management should be adopted under skilled supervision. They are those generally accepted in this and other European countries ...

3. The nursing should be conducted entirely by a paid staff, and there should be not less than one day nurse, one night nurse, and one assistant nurse for each fifty patients ...

(Signed.) Thomas Watson, M.D.,
President of the College of Physicians.

George Burrows, M.D.,
President of the General Medical Council.

James Clark, M.D.
William Jenner, M.D.
Edward Sieveking, M.D.
William Fergusson.
James Paget.[42]

155. Louisa Twining. *Workhouses and Pauperism and Women's Work in the Administration of the Poor Law*

[Louisa Twining (b. 1820) was the daughter of a well-known merchant in the Strand, London. At one time she gave serious consideration to becoming a nurse.[43] She was twice Guardian of the Poor, in Kensington from 1884 to 1890, and in Tonbridge Union from 1893 to 1896.[44] She wrote many papers on the management of workhouses, referring repeatedly to the nursing arrangements in them. Her diary and reports tell of visits to various workhouses, and her impressions of the conditions found.]

From Louisa Twining's Diary.
[1853] June 26th.—I went with Mrs. Jameson to see the St. Pancras workhouse with Mrs. Tomlinson, who had been mentioned to me as being one of the committee forming for visiting the workhouse. We heard much of the new arrangements, and of the miserable old state of things. One poor woman said their sheets had not been changed formerly for months. The matron of the infirmary seemed a good woman, and paid nurses were just being tried ...
[1853] June 27th.—I went with Mrs. Goodfellow to see the Holborn Workhouse; she and one other lady take a ward there. The matron, as usual, looked old and dirty; ... the matron owned she had great difficulty in finding proper persons among the paupers to be nurses.
[1858] February 28th.—In the sick ward I visit at the West London, there is a poor girl of sixteen, a cripple, always sitting in a low chair by the fire; she was sometimes doing needlework. I asked her why she did not read, and found that she could not; so I took her a little book, and the nurse promised to teach her: she knew her letters.
Notes of Six Years' Work as Guardian of the Poor 1884–1890.
[Lunatic Asylum at Barming] In conversation with the nurses in the

Infirmary . . . I found that none had any training in Hospitals, such as is now beginning to be thought necessary, one only having learnt a little from a matron in an institution, during a few months.

.   .   .   .   .   .

[In one large country infirmary] It was surprising to find that in so extensive and complete a workhouse no Entrance Lodge had been provided, the gates being far away below the House, so that any or every body could come and go as he liked, without coming near the porter and his vigilant eye; it can of course only be surmised what may have left the House or been brought in by inmates. One instance of the latter practice was discovered within a fortnight of the arrival of the new master and matron, in consequence of which a nurse of long standing was dismissed. One old member of the Board was so tender-hearted as to stand up for her, and lamented the disappearance of "a well-known old face!" but as may be supposed, he was in a minority. Other dismissals have taken place, all more or less, through faults of character and drink, five, besides nurses.

.   .   .   .

[Barming Lunatic Asylum] . . . a Report was read by the Medical Officer on the "Nursing System" of the Infirmary, or, as it was expressed by one Guardian, the "No System." During my whole tenure of office this had been my chief trouble and anxiety, seeing that though a fine building had been erected with good arrangements, no trained Nurses had been substituted for those who had been thought sufficient during all the previous years in the "Old Hospital." I therefore was ever looking for an opening and opportunity to introduce the subject, although the difficulty of realising any distinction between "trained" and "untrained" women seemed to be almost hopeless,— one idea about the former being that "they would not do anything," though I could not ascertain that those who expressed this opinion had any experience of Trained Nurses.

.   .   .   .

The workhouse has a modern, well-appointed infirmary, while the infirm male patients are in the old hospital, distinct from the quarters of the able-bodied. Except in some minor details . . . the structure and arrangements are those of a general hospital. But what would be said of a hospital of 230 beds which was entirely nursed by untrained persons assisted by paupers? Yet this is the state of the case in the Tonbridge Union. The only trained nurse is the temporary night nurse, and she has no assistant, so that, since her charges are in three distinct buildings, her nursing must be merely nominal. This is an anomalous state of things, and one which surely cannot be long maintained by a Board of Guardians who have shown themselves anxious to provide for the comfort of the sick in so many other ways. No merits of structure can ever compensate for the lack of nursing, and much

175

complex machinery is simply thrown away without the skilled management of those who understand it.

.   .   .   .

During five weeks we inserted advertisements in the best papers, and out of the large number of applications received, four only were found to be available, all others being thoroughly unsatisfactory, although in many instances holding *good testimonials*. . . . One might have hoped and expected that the nurse "Gamp" of the past, with her love for the bottle, was long since extinct, but alas! experience shows she is not, and intemperance continues to rank as one of the chief causes of failure in those who apply, especially for posts in a workhouse, where it is hoped so high a standard as in other institutions is hardly expected.

In descending to the lowest class of all in the Poor Law service, we come to the Pauper helps, who, if no longer called by the dignified title of "Nurse," still exercise a considerable amount of control in Workhouses throughout the country. . . . When it is considered that a certain number of these so-called "able-bodied" inmates are of the semi-imbecile, or, at least, feeble-minded class, both men and women, the latter too often of immoral character, it is easy to suppose what the result must be during the long hours when, in the nurses' absence, the sick are left to their control. . . . The fact that these persons have been, to a great extent, employed as sole attendants on the sick at night (night nurses being, till quite recently, the exception, even when trained women were employed by day) makes the evil only more obvious and censurable.[45]

156. Dr. Robert Gooch, "Protestant Sisters of Charity," *Blackwood's Edinburgh Magazine*, July–December, 1825, pp. 732–735

[Dr. Robert Gooch (1784–1830) was the son of Robert Gooch of Yarmouth, a sea captain. Graduating in medicine from the University of Edinburgh in 1807, he was elected lecturer on midwifery at St. Bartholomew's Hospital.[46] His interest in improved care of mothers and babies, particularly in the rural areas, is expressed in his periodical articles.[47] In the excerpts given here and in Reading No. 157, his insight into the relation of nursing to other problems is apparent.]

Let the Church, or if not, let that class of Christians, in whom, above all others, religion is not a mere Sunday ceremony, but the daily and hourly principle of their thoughts and actions . . . let all serious Christians, I say, join, and found an order of women like the Sisters of Charity in Catholic countries, let them be selected for good plain sense, kindness of disposition, indefatigable industry, and deep piety; let them receive not a technical and scientific, but a practical medical education; for this purpose, let them be placed both as nurses and pupils in the hospitals of Edinburgh or London, or in the county hospitals; let their attention be pointed by the attending physician to the particular symptoms by which he distinguishes the disease; let them be made as familiar with the best remedies, which are always few, as they are with barley-water, gruel and beeftea. Let them learn the rules by which these remedies are to be employed; let them be examined frequently on these subjects, in order to see that they carry these rules clearly in their heads; let books be framed for them containing the essential rules of practice; briefly, clearly, and untechnically written; let such women, thus educated, be distributed among the country parishes of the kingdom, and be maintained by the parish allowance, which now goes to the parish surgeon; let him be resorted to only in difficult cases; let them be examined every half year by competent physicians about the state of their medical knowledge; let this be done, and I fearlessly predict that my friend [a country clergyman], and all those who are similarly situated, and zealous with himself, will no longer complain that their sick flocks suffer from medical neglect.

It may be objected, that women with such an education would form a bad substitute for a scientific medical attendant. Be it remembered, however, that the choice is not between such women and a profound and perfect physician, or surgeon, but between such women and the ordinary run of country apothecaries; the latter labouring under the additional disadvantage of wanting time for the application of what skill they have ...

London, 1st Nov. 1825.

157. Dr. Robert Gooch in *The London Medical Gazette*, 1827, pp. 55–58

Those who live in the country, at a distance from towns and cities, especially parish priests, charitable ladies, and that hard working and useful class of medical men, who, in a worldly point of view, may be said to have the misfortune to have settled in these thinly-populated districts, well know the deplorable medical attendance which the poor receive in sickness. . . .

To supply the poor with medical attendance more adequate to their wants; to relieve more speedily their sufferings, shorten their illnesses, and, in some instances, save their lives, two plans have been proposed which I shall proceed to describe. In the year 1823, some opulent and benevolent persons held a meeting at Southam, a small country town of Warwickshire, near Stratford-upon-Avon, where Mr. Smith, a surgeon of the town, proposed the establishment of a Dispensary for the sick poor of that neighborhood ...

The Southam Dispensary has now been in operation four years, and the results appear to be highly satisfactory to the members.

The other plan proposed for supplying the sick poor in the country with medical attendance more adequate to their wants, is to form an order of women similar to the Beguines of Flanders, and the Soeurs de la Charité of France, to instruct them in medicine, as far as can be done as a practical art; and to station them in the country parishes of England. What I know about these singular and admirable orders of women, and how they might be adopted, and adapted to the station for which they are proposed, I will relate in a subsequent letter.

> I am, Sir,
> Your obedient humble servant,
> A Country Surgeon.

· · · · · · · ·

I concluded my former letter by remarking that another plan for supplying the sick poor in the country with better medical attendance than that they now receive was to form an order of women similar to the Beguines of Flanders, and the Soeurs de la Charité of France; to give them such practical instructions in medicine as would enable them to detect and relieve the common forms of disease, and to station them in the country parishes of England. This plan was first proposed two years ago by an anonymous writer in *Blackwood's Magazine,* in a paper entitled "Protestant Sisters of Charity."

The proposal was soon followed by a pamphlet under the same title, addressed to the Bishop of London, and signed "A Country Clergyman," in which the proposal of the anonymous writer was adopted and enforced. Some efforts were made to induce the established church to put the plan to the test of experiment, both without success.

If an attempt should be made to introduce Sisters of Charity into England, I would advise the experiment to be made at first on a small scale. They should be not mere nurses, and religious instructors, but a set of religious female physicians. . . . There are only two classes of people whom I have any hope of influencing in favour of this plan—one are the Church Methodists, the other the Society of Friends. . . . Could not Mrs. Fry divert a little of her zeal from the female convicts in Newgate to the sick poor of the country? or could not her friend, Mrs. Opie, the daughter of a physician, and, if her writings are to be trusted, a tender-hearted woman, become the Mademoiselle le Gras to an order of female religious physicians, by which they might bless their country and immortalize their names?

158. Robert Southey. *Sir Thomas More; or Colloquies on the Progress and Prospects of Society*

[Robert Southey (1774–1843), English man of letters, was much agitated about the state of the care of the sick of his day. His interest in reform led him to advocate, in his writings and in his correspondence, the establishment of Sisters of Charity in the English Church for the improvement of the care in hospitals and homes.[48]]

Piety has found its way into your prisons; your hospitals are imploring it in vain; nothing is wanting in them but religious charity; and oh! what a want is that! and how different would be the moral effect which those medical schools produce upon the pupils educated there, if this lamentable deficiency were supplied. I know not whether they or the patients suffer most from its absence. Many are the lives which might be saved by it; many are the death-beds to which it would administer a consolation that is now too often wanted. . . . England is grievously in need of its Sisters of Charity.[49]

159. *The Life and Correspondence of the Late Robert Southey*

[The editor of this work was the poet's son, Charles Cuthbert Southey, Curate of Plumbland, Cumberland.]

To Sharon Turner, Esq. Keswick, April 2, 1816.
I wish we had reformed the monastic institutions instead of overthrowing them. Mischievous as they are in Catholic countries, they have got this good about them, that they hold up something besides worldly distinction to the respect and admiration of the people and fix the standard of virtue higher than we do in Protestant countries. Would that we had an order of Beguines in England.

To John Rickman, Esq. March 1, 1820.
I like your Beguinage scheme in all its parts. Endowments (analogous to college fellowships) would grow out of it in due course of time. And great part of the business of female education would be transferred to these institutions to the advantage of all parties.

To Dr. [Robert] Gooch. Keswick, Dec. 18, 1825.
My dear Gooch,
I cannot refer you to any other account of the Sisters of Charity than is to be found in Helyot's Histoire des Ordres Monastiques, a very meagre but useful book;—compared to what a history ought to be, it is somewhat like what a skeleton is to the body. When I was first in the Low Countries, I endeavoured to collect what information I could concerning the Beguines, and got into their principal establishment at Ghent. Their history is curiously uncertain which I found not only from themselves but from pursuing the subject in books; and as I have those books at hand, I can at any time tell you what is not known about them, for to that the information which they contain amounts. The Beguines are much esteemed in the Low Countries as the Soeurs de la Charité in France, but I have incidentally learnt from books that scandal used to be busy with them. A profession of religion naturally affords cover for hypocrisy, and it is therefore to be expected that scandal should sometimes arise, and more frequently be imputed; but the general utility of the institution is unquestionable; and I do not know that there is anything to be set against it, for they are bound by no vows, nor to any of those observances which are at once absurd and onerous. I will have the notes which I made concerning them at Ghent transcribed for you. As your

adventures were in Flanders, not in France, have you not mistaken the Beguines for the Sisters of Charity?

.   .   .   .   .   .

> Yours affectionately,
> R. Southey.

.   .   .   .   .   .

To the Rev. Nicholas Lightfoot. Keswick, July 12, 1829.

Among the letters pertinent and impertinent which have reached me . . . [is one which] relates to the scheme for directing the personal charity of females to hospitals rather than prisons; to the sick, rather than to the profligate. This is from Mr. [J. J.] Hornby, the Rector of Winwick, who had before hinted at such a thing in a sermon preached upon the opening of the Liverpool Infirmary, and who now offers his purse and his personal exertions to promote it. You will readily suppose that I am gratified by this.

[Remarks by the Editor]

. . . several letters . . . passed between my father and Mr. Hornby, chiefly upon the plan of educating a better order of persons as nurses for the poor; and through the exertions of the latter, a beginning was made, which unfortunately was prevented by untoward circumstances from producing any permanent results.

It appears that Mr. Hornby, in contact with Adam Hodgson, Esq. of Liverpool, undertook to set on foot an institution for this purpose as an experiment, and to maintain it for two years. They hired a house, engaged a matron, received a number of inmates, and had educated and sent out some few as nurses. Other individuals now became anxious to join them in the responsibility and superintendence, and there not being sufficient unity of purpose among all the managers, the scheme, which was prospering, fell to the ground. As soon as it appeared that they were educating a valuable class of persons, it was sought to make them available to the upper classes as monthly nurses; and this being an entire perversion of the original plan, Mr. Hornby and Mr. Hodgson withdrew at the end of two years, and the whole scheme quickly fell to the ground.[50]

160. Letter of Edward Pusey to Rev. Dr. [Walter Farquhar] Hook

[Edward Bouverie Pusey (1800–1882), English divine and Canon of Christ Church, Oxford, for fifty-four years, was eminent chiefly for his leadership of the High Church movement in England. One of the phases of his leadership was the fostering of sisterhoods in the Church of England, the first attempt to establish them being made at Park Village West, Regents' Park, on March 26, 1845.[51] Dr. Hook (1798–1875) was eventually Dean of Chichester. The following letter, dated six years before the founding of Park Village Community, advocates such sister-hoods.]

Christ Church, Dec. 1839.

I want very much to have one or more societies of 'Soeur de la Charite' formed: I think them desirable (1) in themselves as belonging to and foster-ing a high tone in the Church, (2) as giving a holy employment to many who yearn for something, (3) as directing zeal which will otherwise often go off in some irregular way, or go over to Rome. . . . It seemed best that at first they should . . . be employed in hospitals, lunatic asylums, prisons, among the females. Do you know of any who would engage in it in a small scale, quietly, or one who would be a Mother Superior, i. e. one fitted to guide it? . . .

Ever your very affectionate friend,
E. B. Pusey [52]

161. Sir Edward Parry, R.N., on Nursing

[Sir Edward Parry was Superintendent of Haslar Hospital at Gosport, in the early nineteenth century. The following paper was written in June, 1847, and advocated the training of nurses on the Kaiserswerth plan for the naval hospitals of England.[53]]

It would be scarcely possible to overrate the importance, both to the souls and bodies of men, of employing in public hospitals, nurses possessing not merely the requisite mechanical skill, but likewise a high tone of religious and moral principle. Considering the circumstances under which they exert an influence, for good or for evil, there are perhaps few situations in life in which a discharge of duty *upon truly Christian principles,*—"doing it heartily as to the Lord and not to men,"—may be productive of more beneficial consequences.

The locality of the noble institution which I have the honour to superin-tend, renders it extremely difficult,—I may say impossible upon the present system,—to secure the services of a sufficient number of nurses of even tolerably fair character; and as the patients must have a certain number in constant attendance, it unavoidably follows that a considerable proportion of those who are thus employed, are such as nothing but necessity would justify admitting into the establishment.

The same difficulty, though perhaps never in the same degree as in *Naval* Hospitals, has been experienced in other establishments for the reception of the sick in this as well as in foreign countries; and many attempts have been made to remedy the evil. The most successful of these, because it was founded on the right principle, has been made at Kaiserswerth, near Dussel-dorf, in Prussia, where an institution for the training of nurses (among other benevolent objects) was established about ten years ago by the Rev. Th. Fliedner. Mr. Fliedner's plan consists in the training of a number of Protestant Deaconesses, or Nursing Sisters, who, from the pure motives of

181

Christian charity, are willing to enter upon this service, without taking any vows, but agreeing to serve for at least five years, and expecting no salary or other recompense beyond a decent and comfortable maintenance.

With these facts before our eyes, showing with what complete success the efforts of the Pastor Fliedner have been attended, and the extensive benefits likely to follow them, it is the earnest wish of the principal medical officers of Haslar Hospital, no less than my own, to avail ourselves of similar nurses for improving the class of nurses in this institution. As we cannot for a moment admit a doubt of being able to find, among our own countrywomen, individuals as willing to devote themselves to this "work and labour of love" upon the highest principles of Christian philanthropy, as those who have entered upon the same field of benevolence in foreign countries, we are desirous of proposing to our friends to assist us in this undertaking.

The plan we contemplate is as follows:

1. To endeavour to engage, *in the first instance,* the services of three or four Christian women, between the ages of thirty and fifty, who upon the principles and conditions adopted at Kaiserswerth, are willing to devote themselves to this work at Haslar Hospital.

2. These persons, when engaged, to be placed for about six months at the German Hospital at Dalston, by permission of the authorities of that institution, for the purpose of receiving the necessary instruction in the duties of nursing, and to be trained according to the system pursued at Kaiserswerth—or, if circumstances permit, to be placed *at* Kaiserswerth for this purpose.

3. Their training being completed, the nurses to be admitted into Haslar Hospital, when, although they will receive no pecuniary remuneration, a comfortable home, with a certain allowance for neat and respectable clothing, and a sufficient maintenance, will be provided for them. In the discharge of their arduous and self-denying duties, in which they must expect to meet with much to exercise their Christian patience and forbearance, they may depend on receiving from the Captain-superintendent, and other principal officers of the establishment, the most cordial encouragement and friendly support.

Having thus explained the plan we propose to pursue, we would now very earnestly solicit the help of our Christian friends, in seeking out from the circle of their *personal* acquaintances such individuals as they *confidently* believe to possess the character and qualifications requisite for this arduous but honourable office.

Although it is fully expected that the nurses, when once they have entered on their duties at Haslar, will be adequately maintained on the present Government allowance, yet it is obvious that some extra expense must be at first incurred by the proposed system of previous training. For this purpose we do not hesitate to ask the contribution of those who are willing to assist us in making this experiment, which, if successful (and we see no reason to doubt it), will not only materially improve the comfort and promote the welfare of the patients in this Hospital, but may lead to the introduction of a similar system of nursing throughout the hospitals of this kingdom.

William Edward Parry
Captain-Superintendent.

Haslar Hospital, Gosport, June, 1847.

We cordially concur in the sentiments expressed in the foregoing statement, and earnestly desire to try the plan therein proposed, in the several departments of Haslar Hospital respectively under our charge.

John Richardson, M.D., *Medical Inspector.*
James Anderson, M.D., *Medical Inspector.*
James Allan, M.D., *Deputy Medical Inspector.*
Alexander M'Kechnie, M.D., *Surgeon and Medical Storekeeper.*
Alexander Stuart, *Assisting Surgeon.*[54]

162. Articles from *Saturday Review* and *Pall Mall Gazette*

[In 1865 and 1866 in England, considerable interest was expressed by the public in the betterment of nursing in workhouse infirmaries and hospitals. Not all institutions came immediately under the influence of Miss Nightingale's new system. Various groups advocated varying solutions to the problem. In the following articles from the *Saturday Review,* and the pamphlet, *Sisterhoods; Schools for Nurses,* which combined certain articles from the *Saturday Review* and the *Pall Mall Gazette,* two main solutions were offered, namely, the creation of additional sisterhoods and the improvement of economic conditions in nursing.]

"The Sick in the Workhouse," *Saturday Review,* March 10, 1866

Even such deficiencies as these might be in a measure supplemented by good nursing; but imperfect as the workhouse system appears on every other point, it is indisputably weakest upon this one. The nurses are usually paupers, generally unpaid, or only rewarded by a somewhat superior scale of dietary. They are utterly without any training for their office, besides being old, infirm, and occasionally almost bed-ridden. The men are frequently nursed by men who are even more uncouth and ignorant than the women, and in most of the London workhouses whatever nursing there is is altogether suspended at night.

"Sick Wards in Workhouses," *Saturday Review,* June 30, 1866

The last case that has become public is that of Paddington Workhouse. It is only fair to say that it favourably differs in some respects from the others which have been exposed. . . . Still, at this admirable institution persons suffering from all sorts of complaints were crowded together; three or four patients were sometimes put in one bed; the screams of wretched lunatics were allowed to disturb the sick-ward day and night; the paid nurse had more work to do than she could possibly manage; the pauper nurses who worked under her were almost all incompetent; they took bribes, got drunk, and were occasionally cruel; the lady visitors, who complained of these nurses, were assured that no better substitutes could be got in their place; and it was asserted that the master of the workhouse had behaved very harshly to the patients in the infirmary.

"Sisterhoods in England," *Saturday Review,* August 25, 1866

Not long ago we drew public attention to the opposition offered by a majority of the Governors of St. George's Hospital to a proposal that the nursing department should be entrusted to St. Peter's Sisterhood, Brompton Square.... It is generally admitted that the nursing department of St. George's Hospital requires material improvement and would be considerably the better for the introduction of a few first-class nurses ...

All England is just now cordially agreed that our system of nursing in workhouses, hospitals, and public institutions calls for a radical reform, and by many it is thought that even for the ordinary purposes of private life, for every-day medical work, a sufficient supply of good nurses is not at present to be procured for money or love. On the other hand, there is scarcely less unanimity as to the character of Sisterhoods viewed merely as schools for training nurses. Religious considerations apart, the stoutest Protestant will admit that they are of the highest value. They not only supply nurses of the very best kind, ladies well-educated and high principled, but they present the additional, and perhaps still more important, advantages of strict organization. A striking proof of their superiority has just been furnished during the distress occasioned by the cholera. Notwithstanding the urgent need felt for nurses, it has been thought advisable to decline desultory and individual offers of assistance from charitable ladies where the organized efforts of trained Sisters have been gratefully welcomed ...

Pall Mall Gazette, 1866

Our readers will no doubt have observed some able letters by Mr. Capes, lately published in these columns on the subject of nursing and the establishment of sisterhoods. His arguments on these topics may be stated in a few words. He begins by showing that the existing arrangements at hospitals for the supply of nurses are altogether inefficient. This want, he adds, cannot be supplied by mere hired servants. On the other hand, there are a large number of ladies who are much in want of some occupation and who are very unwilling to marry. They are the natural persons to undertake the duties in question, but they will not do so unless they are combined into sisterhoods. ... This is Mr. Capes' argument ...

As to the matter of fact that the present system of nursing in our hospitals is unsatisfactory, and that it would be much improved if ladies undertook the superintendence of the hospital servants, we need raise no question; and the establishment of a great number of what are called sisterhoods might have, or at least might contribute to, this effect . . .

Why should not there be well paid and well lodged superintendents of hospital nurses just as there are well paid and well lodged governors of gaols? For £150 a year and comfortable rooms, ladies might be got to look after the nurses of a hospital who would stand in need of no religious dresses or names . . .

Every one must admit that the position of women of the middle class who are compelled by circumstances to earn their own livelihood is a peculiarly hard one. They are as honourably and justly reluctant as men to sink below the social rank in which they were born; or to adopt occupations inconsistent with its supposed dignity; and they have the utmost difficulty in finding employment which society will not pronounce degrading to a lady, or which will not force upon them unsuitable companionship and disagreeable associations. Professions for women are few, and terribly overcrowded. . . . For ladies, or those who call themselves such—for women who have been well brought up, and enjoyed some sort of education—there is a deplorable dearth of fitting occupation. And yet the most important of feminine professions, eminently suited to and requiring a higher class of workers is almost entirely monopolized by the lower; and while thousands of women pine or starve for want of work, one of the most essential of women's duties is left undone, or done very badly, for want of proper candidates for employment therein.[55]

163. Letter from the Bishop of London

[The sisterhood movement became an inherent part of the High Church revival in England. The Archbishop of Canterbury, at that time the Rev. Archibald Campbell Tait (1811–1882), approved of the establishment of women's orders for the care of the sick but did not look with favor on the taking of perpetual vows. With his wife, he did much to help with the organization of the sisterhoods.[56]]

The Bishop of London to Mr. ———— ————.

Fulham Palace, London, S. W.,
Dec. 27, 1865.

Dear Sir—

There is no warrant for supposing that I in any way approve of Sisterhoods in which perpetual vows are administered. . . . I do fully approve of ladies who have no home duties, and who think they are fitted for such work, associating themselves together for the care of the poor and the sick. Such an institution, under my presidency, is St. John's House of Nurses in Northumberland St., Strand, and St. Peter's House, Brompton Square, and the Deaconesses' Home in Burton Crescent,—in all three of which institutions arrangements are made whereby, I believe, anything I objected to as to dress, mode of life, or any other point, would at once be altered. There is also the All Saints Home, Margaret Street, with which I am connected as diocesan. Over this institution I have not the same direct control, but I cannot but admire the self-denying spirit in which Miss Byron and her ladies have undertaken their difficult work in the hospitals and among the destitute . . .

A. C. London.[57]

164. John W. Ogle, "Nurses for the Sick Poor," *Medical Times and Gazette*, April 11, 1874, pp. 395–396

[John William Ogle (1824–1905) received his education at Trinity College, Oxford, and at the medical school attached to St. George's Hospital. He became a Fellow of the Royal College of Physicians in 1855. His main interest was in the treatment of nervous diseases. He was very active in the field of medical literature.[58]]

. . . in May, 1854, the Epidemiological Society, under the presidency of the late Dr. Babington, appointed a committee to take into consideration the question of supplying the labouring classes throughout the country with nurses in epidemic and other diseases, and during the period of childbirth. The Committee eventually was a large one, and consisted chiefly of members of the medical and clerical professions, but contained also no less than five masters of metropolitan workhouses. It assumed not only that such nurses were required for the speedy recovery of the sick, but also that it was the duty and interest of society to acknowledge and provide for this want, inasmuch as sickness, which in many ways presses more on the needy than the affluent, ruins and degrades the families of the poor, throws them as a burden on parish relief, and tends to decrease the wealth of the country by the loss of life which it occasions. Considering that the providing of nurses, easily available throughout the country, would diminish disease, and consequently mortality and pauperism, among the poor, arrest contagion, and lessen poor and county rates, they concluded that the workhouses present the training schools wherein these nurses may be trained, the 553 unions of England containing (in 1854) 20,000 able-bodied women, at present a source of unproductive expense to the country. They proposed that by an order of the Poor-Law Board "it be made imperative upon the master and matron of each workhouse to put the able-bodied females through a systematic training in the kitchen and infirmary; that when found sufficiently qualified to act as nurses, they shall receive a certificate of fitness, signed by the medical officer and master; and that a register of all such qualified nurses, whether residing in or out of the workhouse, be kept at the workhouse, and be open to the public as a means of obtaining nurses" . . . . In the meantime the Poor-Law Board sent word to the Nursing Committee that their proposal appeared to involve great difficulties of a legal and practical nature. . . . No result . . . of an immediate character came of this and not long afterwards, owing to a variety of circumstances interest began to lag, and the Committee ceased to sit.

165. Emma Pöel. *Life of Amelia Wilhelmina Sieveking*

[The idea in Miss Sieveking's mind, of a Protestant Sisterhood in Germany, took shape in 1832. The founding of the group antedated that of Kaiserswerth, of which Miss Sieveking was to be asked in 1837 by Pastor Fliedner to become the head.[59] It has been said of Miss Sieveking that she had thorough simplicity of mind and an entire unconsciousness of the fact that she was doing a great and good work.[60] Catherine Winkworth, the translator of the *Life,* said in a letter to Richard Massie, dated February 25, 1864, "Many of those who make so much noise about 'women's work' nowadays might learn too, from her how much work may be accomplished by *quietly* embracing any opportunity of usefulness opened to the mind, and making no unnecessary stir about it." [61]]

[Letter to Minna Hosch, March, 1852.]

. . . that confidence is reposed in me . . . is especially important for the carrying out of a new plan, which has occupied me very seriously since I have been in the hospital—namely, the foundation of an association for the care of the sick and poor. The object of it is, more frequent and regular visiting of the sick poor in their own dwellings, and a closer supervision of them than is possible for the General Poor's Board, with care to promote order and cleanliness, and whatever else may be helpful to them either in body or in soul. The project was put on paper by me during one of the last days of my residence in the hospital, and submitted to Dr. Siemssen and Dr. Siemers, who gave it their approbation, and promised me their support as far as I might need it. Similar assurances have been sent to me by other friends, and especially by several gentlemen who are thoroughly acquainted with our system of out-door relief, its advantages and deficiencies, and are themselves actively at work in the matter.

The principal difficulty lies in finding the needful number of helpers to carry out the plan, and here I find more obstacles in fact than I had anticipated.

[The beginning of the association, as described by Miss Sieveking to her pupils.]

I had entered the hospital with the thought that my services there would become the commencement of a new kind of labour for the good of the poor, and it had in fact brought me into much closer contact with the lower class; what they lacked, and how much consequently might be done for them, had become clearer to me, and all this experience was not to pass by unused.

On the last Sunday of my residence there, I wrote down the scheme of an Association for the care of the sick and poor, founded on the principle of a Sisterhood of Mercy, and certainly very different from that which was ultimately carried out. For instance, I had chiefly in view, the cooperation of women of the lower middle class, because, repelled by the disapprobation I had met with among the higher classes, I did not venture to approach them. I also thought that this class of persons were nearer to the poor, and could better judge of their necessities. Originally I had several of these in the Association; yet there is much to be said against such a plan, because as a rule higher cultivation creates a sounder judgment, which is often wanting in this middle-class. . . . My scheme at that time required of the members of the Association that they should take part with their own hands in cleaning and setting in order the dwellings of the poor, when it should seem desirable; that they should undertake to watch by the sick, &c, &c. In practice these things took another shape. The first principles of the plan however remained the same; personal intercourse with the poor, and the exhibition of a love towards them manifested by action and rooted in faith; nor do I believe that a work founded on any other principles could endure.

My plan being complete, I left the hospital and sought to win some to take part in the undertaking. Among many refusals, I met with a cheerful response from several, and so on the 23rd of May, 1832, thirteen of us met for the first time in my mother's house.

The first difficulty was in our position with regard to the medical men. I had learnt to know them well while in the hospital, and now it was proposed that they should recommend their poor patients to us. Several made me a friendly promise to do so. Dr. M———, however, decidedly refused, on the ground that in his opinion our labours would destroy the one good and admirable thing which he still found among the poor, namely, their readiness to help each other . . .[62]

166. Theodor Fliedner. *Kurzer Abriss seines Lebens*

[Theodore Fliedner (1800–1864), German Protestant minister and philanthropist, was appointed pastor of the small Protestant congregation in Kaiserswerth in 1822. The bankruptcy of the manufacturing firm upon which almost the entire congregation depended caused him to go to England to obtain funds. There he met Mrs. Elizabeth Fry, and became interested in prison work. When he returned he founded, in 1826, the first prison society of Germany, the Rhenish-Westphalian Prison Association. From this beginning, the sympathies of Pastor Fliedner and his wife Friederike turned to the sick.[63] In 1836 he established the Kaiserswerth Deaconess Institution.[64] It is evident from his description of the beginning of these efforts that Pastor Fliedner thought of his

instituting of the deaconess movement in Germany as a restoration of the
system which had existed in the early Christian church for the care of
the sick and unfortunate.]

The state of the sick poor had long weighed heavily on our hearts. How
often had I seen them fading away like autumn leaves, in their unhealthy
rooms, lonely and ill cared for, physically and spiritually neglected! And
where hospitals existed—I had seen many in my travels through Holland,
Brabant, England, and Scotland,—I had not infrequently found the gates
adorned with marbles, when the nursing within was bad. The medical staff
complained bitterly of the hireling attendants, of their carelessness by day
and by night, of their drunkenness and other immoralities. And what should
I say of the spiritual attendance. Little thought was given to that. Hospital
chaplains were unknown in many cases, hospital chapels in still more. . . .
Did not such abuses cry to heaven against us? Did not that terrible saying of
our Lord apply to us, "I was sick, and ye visited me not"?

Or shall we deem our evangelical Christian women incapable or unwilling
to undertake the task of Christian nursing? Had not numbers of them done
wonders of self-sacrificing love in the military hospitals during the war of
liberation in 1813–15? If again, the Church of apostolic days made use of
their powers for relief of its suffering members, and organised them into a
recognised body, under the title of deaconesses, and if for many centuries
the Church had continued to appoint such deaconesses, why should we
longer delay the revival of such an order of handmaids devoted to the
service of their Lord? . . .

These reflections left me no peace, and my wife [Fredericke] was of the
same mind with myself, and of greater courage . . .

We now quietly looked around for a house for the hospital. Suddenly the
largest and finest house in Kaiserswerth came into the market. . . . We commended our cause to the Lord, and behold ere long He sent us some bright
gleams through our many clouds . . .

As we say, the ground was burning hot under our feet, until the hospital
opened. Then the Lord sent it into the heart of a Christian maiden in Düssel-
dorf, Albertina P., to help us for some months in the housekeeping, though
she did not wish to become a deaconess, while our children's nurse, Catherine
B., offered to act as temporary nurse to the sick people. Thus the Deaconess
House began without any deaconesses. On October 13, the two young women
entered the house, and arranged the ground floor for themselves and a few
sick persons, very scantily; one table, some chairs, with half-broken arms, a
few worn knives, forks with only two prongs, wormeaten bedsteads, and
other similar furniture which had been given to us. . . . Our first deaconess,
Sister Gertrude [Reichardt] duly appeared on October 20 [1836], and she
was soon followed by other aspirants to the office.[65]

167. Fredericke Fliedner on the Deaconesses

[Fredericke Münster (1806–1842) became Theodor Fliedner's first wife and first "Mother" of the Deaconess Order. Before her death she made notes on her interpretation of the rules of the order.[66] These are revealing particularly in their emphasis on discipline. The following statement, taken from the notes, was given by her granddaughter at the 1934 meeting of the International Council of Nurses.]

On Rules.

No institution can exist without man-made rules; but they should not be so framed as to neglect the essential godliness (1. Tim. 4, 8.).

Deaconesses should submit for the Lord's sake to the will of their superiors in all things, even in man-made rules. But their superiors should be on their guard lest the rules exceed God's commandment. For it may be that a nurse is offended by the rules; but let it not be imputed to her for a sin. It may be that she is perfect in the rules; but let it not be ascribed to her for a virtue. For the Lord seeth the heart. I hate monastic rules. I must obey the apostolic admonition for the Lord's sake (1 Peter, 3, 3.). Not the clothing is essential, but the quiet spirit. The uniform may be a yoke to a nurse; then must she be lovingly helped to bear it, and led by a loving spirit into the right path, and hearts must not be closed against her because of something that is of no account in the Lord's eyes. If my opinion is a wrong one, teach me to think otherwise, O true and loving Lord!

Remarks Based on Experience as Mother Superior of the Deaconesses, 1836–1842.

Definitive Admission to the Deaconess' Office.

We read in 1 Tim. 5, 22, "Lay hands suddenly on no man, neither be partakers of other men's sins: Keep thyself pure."

Since there is so great a lack of enlightened women: since the need is so pressing; since the Deaconesses Association is trying to do many things at once; therefore it happens that persons are admitted simply because there is no one else suitable. When accepting a person, the Board must see that that person is pious and experienced in God, truthful and domesticated. Those who, though they possess other good qualities, are vain and desirous of admiration, must not be accepted, for they are unsuitable to be sent out; in the House, too, they do harm, and their reading and praying will have no influence upon an unconverted heart. Nor have they any true love in their hearts for the sick, for they love themselves too much for that. The Board (the Director) should ask the Superior about this point, for she, as a woman, will see more clearly. For just as a woman cannot properly judge of a man in his mentality and his motives, so cannot a man judge of a woman, since her inner motives also are hidden from him.

A woman's capacity is cured by a heavy fall. That is not the position of a servant of Christ. Any fall of hers is not a fall that the world sees. Moreover, the Lord protects those whom he loves. He can do it in whatever way he will. Those whom the Lord chooses as overseers must take good heed of this.

Concerning the ordinary common people who seek to become deaconesses, I cannot refrain myself from this thought: that, just as clergy, schoolmasters, and vergers are necessary to the service of the church, yet it would be to the detriment of the congregation if the schoolmaster and verger were also the clergyman; so does the deaconess's office come to harm through unsuitable persons. On the other hand, there is no harm to the congregation if the clergyman performs the duties of schoolmaster and verger. So likewise I believe that these ordinary people must be useful, if they have a seed of God's word in them, but not under the name of deaconess. For a deaconess cannot be an ordinary person, else is a lie told to the world. Let all the spiritual content be taken from her service, and let her be made into a nurse for the physically sick, just as the verger's service of the church has no spiritual content.

The Attitude To Be Adopted by the Superior to a Sister Who Has Special Gifts.

First and foremost, she should use these gifts to the advantage of the community. Then she should also bring them to the attention of the Director. She should rejoice at the gifts, and seek to develop them; but she should be very cautious in so doing. Her position allows of no sharing of authority, and the sister must be subordinate to her. She must avoid any false humility, even though she should be thought arrogant. If she cares for the peace of the institution, and for the Director's peace and her own, she must remain firm.

Since her office is no honorary office, but one of labour and suffering, let her rejoice when she perceives such splendid gifts as can endure more than she can endure. Let her be the first to be humble with gladness. But not in false humility; let her only be humble when her sister has attained a maturity greater than her own. Let no soul venture itself to measure the degrees of humility. Let her entrust her desire to the Lord, who will grant it at the right time. Let her put her case before the Director in clear, plain words ...

How the Young Sisters Can Best Learn the Bodily Care of the Sick.

In my opinion (I know not whether it be the true one), it is fitting that the young sisters should learn all that they have to learn of the bodily service of the sick on the persons of women. None should perform any duty in the men's ward unless she is specially ordered thereto by the Director. This applies likewise to all other cases, such as autopsies and operations. The Director must carefully weigh the temperamental conditions of the nurse. If there seems any remnant of lightmindedness or pride, *let none sacrifice the soul for the sake of art.* Any appointment to the men's ward calls for great consciousness and a careful enquiry into the nurse's temperament. A nurse may have many good qualities, and may even be sound at heart; but if nature has made her at all indolent or excitable, she must not be put to the test during her probation. Even after appointment as ward-sister, that will call for much consideration. Therefore the Director must take care to place the members so that they become a complete whole; and every member must make her own feeble contribution to that end. And may the good God help the work.[67]

168. [Florence Nightingale.] *The Institution of Kaiserswerth on the Rhine, for the Practical Training of Deaconesses*

[The first edition of the earliest published work of Florence Nightingale was issued anonymously in London in 1851 and printed by the inmates of the London Ragged Colonial Training School, Westminster. Another edition was printed for the Invalid Gentlewomen's Establishment, 1 Upper Harley Street.[68]]

But how has Pastor Fliedner secured such a class of women, as he finds himself able to trust with spiritual influence in this Kaiserswerth Hospital? First, by his own self-denial. An institution will never succeed, which is intended to be worked mainly by the middle and lower classes, if left to occasional inspection. The middle class cannot be expected to give up the idea of saving money, the "cynosure" of English eyes, as long as they say, "The directors might, if they pleased, out of their easy chairs and good dinners, give me as high a salary as my services are worth." In Kaiserswerth there are, for all, the same privations, the same self-denial, the same object —one spirit, one love, one Lord.

Another secret of Pastor Fliedner's education is, that he really, not nominally, delegates his authority. Every master and parent knows how difficult this is. He does not like to see another do ill what he can do well. He doubts how far it is right to allow it, and much as he feels the importance of forming his monitors or children, he ends by waiting till they are fit for their office, like the man who waited to go into the water till he had learnt to swim. Pastor Fliedner, from the unexampled plainness of his instructions to his nurses, and from the constant vigilance with which he follows them up, guards both them and the patients from danger. Every week he gives a lecture to the nurses; before which each has to report to him all that she has read to her patients at morning and evening prayers during the week, and generally what has passed in her ward, and to receive his advice as to how she should proceed. He then places before them particular cases which are likely to occur, *e. g.* where the patient is distressed in mind, where he is self-righteous, etc., and questions them what, in such cases, they would do, attentively listening to, and correcting their answers. His instructions are never in the shape of a formal lecture, but of question and answer. He shows them how they are to approach the hearts of the patients, without assuming the tone of a father confessor, how they are to act in cases of emergency, and at all times they have access to him to ask his advice . . .

One great reason which deters women of education from this work of love is, that, having seen the unutterable dulness of a common hospital, they say to themselves, "If I am to have no moral or spiritual work to do, if I am only to sweep, and comb out dirty heads, and dress loathsome wounds, as I have no idea of buying heaven by such works, I may as well leave them to those who must earn their livelihood, and not take away their trade." Let such as feel this go to Kaiserswerth, and see the delicacy, the cheerfulness, the grace of Christian kindness, the moral atmosphere, in short, which may be diffused through a hospital, by making it one of God's schools, where both patients and nurses come to learn of Him.

We are aware of the difficulty and the disgust, which would attend a woman who wished to learn in a hospital, as commonly conducted. None such need deter her from visiting Kaiserswerth. First, the kindness of the sisters in imparting their own knowledge is as remarkable, when contrasted with the jealousy of nurses and surgeons, in general, as the refinement with which it is done. The Pastor's spirit seems to pervade the whole sisterhood.

The hospital contains above one hundred beds, and is divided into four departments—for men, for women, for boys, and for children, which last includes girls under seventeen and boys under six years of age.

The wards are all small. This gives, it is true, more trouble, but also far more decency and comfort. None of the female wards have more than four beds. When an examination takes place, or when a particular case requires it, the patient can thus easily have a ward to herself. In no private house is decorum more observed than in this hospital, and the influence this continues to exercise upon the patients after their return home can well be believed.

The male wards are served by men-nurses, of whom there are five, who have been educated in the hospital, and are under the authority of the Sisters. After eight P.M. no Sister goes into the men's wards; the men-nurses sleep in the wards, and sit up in case of need. Even in the boys' ward the Sister does not sleep. No Sister is called upon to do anything for a male patient but that which, in a private house, a lady would perform for a brother. Everything else is done by the men-nurses, who, brought up in this atmosphere, have always been found faithful and careful. The most fastidious could find nothing to object to in the intercourse which takes place between patient, surgeon, and Sisters.

No medical man resides in the hospital. Why should he? In a private family, a patient only receives a visit once or perhaps twice a day from the physician. Why he should *not* reside in the house is sufficiently obvious. He is then master. Whereas, at Kaiserswerth, the clergyman is master. The Sisters are, however, bound, of course, punctually to obey the directions of the medical man, and they are too well trained not to do so, with far more correctness than is found in other hospitals.

The superintending Sister of every ward is always present during the daily visits of the medical man. The apothecary is a Sister, and she also goes the round of the patients with him, noting down all his prescriptions and directions, which she afterwards transcribes into a book. By the presence of this

Sister and the head Sister of the ward, all giggling, all familiarity, everything but the strictest propriety is prevented. The Sisters are perfectly well bred.

Every head Sister has family prayers, morning and evening, in her ward. She generally sings a hymn with the patients, reads a very short portion of the Bible, or of some other book chosen by the Pastor, and prays. All the male patients, who are able to leave the wards, assemble in a schoolroom for prayer, which is conducted by one of the Sisters, whose practical remarks on the Bible are listened to by the patients with eager interest ...

The night-watching seems remarkably well managed. ... The nurse is made to feel the night-watch more a blessing than a burden. She never sits up more than three hours and a half, and the whole establishment takes it in turn, so that it comes once a week at most to each Sister. The Sisters go to bed at ten and rise at five. One Sister sleeps in every ward; but the watcher is for the whole house; at half-past one, A.M. she is relieved by another. Every hour she makes the round of all the wards, goes softly into each room, excepting those of the male patients; and thus a double advantage is secured; the watcher is not likely to fall asleep, and she can minister to the little wants of the patients not dangerously ill, without waking the ward Sister. In cases of severe illness, and in surgical cases, the Sister of the ward is, of course, obliged to sit up. The station of the watcher is in the children's room, where her attention is most frequently wanted, as infants are received at any age ...

But we are not describing the Hospital as a hospital, but as a Training School for the Deaconesses. *Probation* is its grand principle—one which we are familiar with in all God's dealings with us; one which St. Paul speaks of, when he says, "And let these also first be proved, then let them use the office of a deacon, being found blameless."

A period of from one to three years is allowed for probation. As nothing is offered to the Sisters, neither the prospect of saving money, nor reputation, nothing but the opportunity of working in the cause for which Christ worked and still works; so if this does not appear to be their ruling principle, they are dismissed, however painful to the Pastor. They are also at liberty to leave any day. The probationary Sister receives nothing for six months but food and lodging; after that a small salary. The Deaconesses,—that is, those who, after their probation, have received a solemn blessing in the church, are paid, but only sufficient to keep them in clothes. Board, lodging, and the Deaconess's upper dress are given to them. There is therefore no pecuniary inducement to come to this work; but a provision is secured for those who have become ill or infirm in the service, to whom the *Mother-house* always opens her arms. "You have been wounded with honour in the field," as the Pastor said one day to a Deaconess, about to undergo a painful operation.

No establishment can subsist which does not offer this prospect to those who have disinterestedly spent the best years of life in its service; and it is beautiful to see the attachment which the Deaconesses of Kaiserswerth feel to their *"Mother-House."*

The Christian liberty of the Deaconess is carefully preserved. Even during the five years, for which a Deaconess engages herself after her solemn consecration in the Church, should marriage, or her parents, or any important duty claim her, she is free, she is never held fast to conclude the term of years . . .

The Institution stands in the place of a parent to the Deaconesses, who have been sent out to other establishments, such as Hospitals, Poorhouses, &c. It has the right of recalling them, without giving any reason to the directors who have, on the other hand, the right of dismissing sisters and of asking for others. The Institutions of Paris, Strasburg, Echallens, and Utrecht, have reserved to themselves the same right as that of Kaiserswerth. Even Deaconesses may sometimes disagree among themselves, and a timely exchange may save much evil. This provision is necessary, if the Institution is to remain a "Mother-house" to the Deaconesses, to afford them protection from the demands (often exorbitant) of the other institution which they serve, and to continue their home for times of sickness and old age. The Deaconess has a vote on the reception of a new sister into the Institution, and in the choice of a superintendent.[69]

169. Letters of Florence Nightingale Relating to Kaiserswerth

[Florence Nightingale planned, in 1848, to visit Kaiserswerth. This visit did not materialize. A brief sojourn of two weeks took place in 1850. At this time she wrote a short account of *The Institution of Kaiserswerth on the Rhine,* the first edition of which was published anonymously in 1851.[70] It is to this pamphlet that the first letter below refers. In this letter Miss Nightingale speaks of two visits to Pastor Fliedner's institution, the second of which, of three months' duration, was in 1851.[71] She alludes here also to the spirit which pervaded the place fifteen years after its founding, and during the lifetime of its founder. Her manner of life in her longer sojourn is told in the letters to her mother.]

Letter to the British Museum.

September 24, 1897,
10, South Street, Park Lane.

Messrs Duban—

A gentleman called here yesterday from you, asking for a copy of my Kaiserswerth for I believe, the British Museum.

Since yesterday, a search has been instituted—but only two copies have been found, and one of these is torn and dirty. I send you the least bad-looking. You will see the date is 1851, and after the copies then printed were given away, I don't think I have ever thought of it.

I was twice in training there myself. Of course, since then hospital and district nursing have made great strides. Indeed, district nursing has been **invented.**

195

But never have I met with a higher love, a purer devotion than there. There was no neglect.

It was the more remarkable because many of the deaconesses had been only peasants—(none were gentlewomen when I was there). The food was poor—no coffee but bean coffee—no luxury but cleanliness.

Florence Nightingale.[72]

Letters to Frances Nightingale [1851].

On Sunday I took the sick boys a long walk along the Rhine; two Sisters were with me to help me to keep order. They were all in ecstasies with the beauty of the scenery, and really I thought it very fine too in its way—the broad mass of waters flowing ever on slowly and calmly to their destination, and all that unvarying horizon—so like the slow, calm, earnest, meditative German character.

The world here fills my life with interest, and strengthens me in body and mind. I succeeded directly to an office, and am now in another, so that until yesterday I never had time even to send my things to the wash. We have ten minutes for each of our meals, of which we have four. We get up at 5; breakfast ¼ before 6. The patients dine at 11; the Sisters at 12. We drink tea (i. e. a drink made of ground rye) between 2 and 3, and sup at 7. We have two ryes and two broths—ryes at 6 and 3, broths at 12 and 7; bread at the two former, vegetables at 12. Several evenings in the week we collect in the Great Hall for a Bible lesson. The Pastor sent for me once to give me some of his unexampled instructions; the man's wisdom and knowledge of human nature is wonderful; he has an instinctive acquaintance with every character in his place. Except that once I have only seen him in his rounds.

The operation to which Mrs. Bracebridge alludes was an amputation at which I was present, but which I did not mention to ———, knowing that she would see no more in my interest in it than the pleasure dirty boys have in playing in the puddles about a butcher's shop. I find the deepest interest in everything here, and am so well in body and mind. This is life. Now I know what it is to live and to love life, and really I should be very sorry now to leave life. I know you will be glad to hear this, dearest Mum. God has indeed made life rich in interests and blessings, and I wish for no other earth, no other world but this.[73]

170. Two Letters of Agnes Elizabeth Jones

[Agnes Elizabeth Jones was of Irish Protestant ancestry, the daughter of Colonel Jones of Fahan, Londonderry, and niece of Sir John Lawrence, Viceroy of India from 1863 to 1869. She is described as beautiful and intensely religious. She had admired Miss Nightingale's work in the Crimea, and spent eight months at Kaiserswerth before entering St. Thomas's Hospital as a Nightingale probationer. She was the pioneer of improved nursing in workhouses at the Liverpool Workhouse where she

196

died in 1868.[74] The following quotations from Miss Jones' letters and journal, describe her impressions of Kaiserswerth.]

[July, 1853]

My darling J.,—. . . .

This is a very busy day, and we have seen neither Louisa Fliedner [the pastor's daughter] nor my dear friend Hedwig, who are generally much with us. . . . They both speak English very well, especially the latter. Yesterday I had such a pleasant talk with her; she believes that I shall come back here; I am sure I shall if it be for my good. . . . She belongs to one of the very highest families in Germany; now she is principally engaged in teaching in the seminarist's house, but even the pastor himself was astonished at the cheerfulness with which, as "probe Schwester," she did any menial work. Each person here is, as far as possible, assigned to the work for which they are best fitted. There is much freedom in every way. Each ward has its deaconess, who has many "probe Schwestern" under her, all responsibility devolves on the Sister, and one evening every week each Sister comes to consult with the mother (Madame Fliedner) and tells her difficulties and trials. The mother is indeed a mother, overseeing all, helping and advising all. . . . There is such love between all, and everyone is so free, no one would think it a convent. Love seems indeed, as far as human nature permits, to pervade every action . . .

[1860]

My darling Mother,—This has been such a day of visiting and variety. . . . I must tell you of my day; as usual, up at 5; hospital for half an hour; at 6.15, breakfast and prayers; at 7, hospital again until 10.30, when I was called to the head sister's room to Pastor Fliedner. Now I must tell you that I fancied he had forgotten me, except the dinner on Sunday, at which he scarcely spoke, I have not seen him. With all his bad health, however (consumption), it is wonderful how he is yet the head and mainspring of this great establishment; and how training others for usefulness is understood by him, and by those who are heads of the different divisions. Now there is Sister Sophie, the hospital superintendent, no matter at what hour I go to visit her, some one comes in at every moment for directions, or to tell how such-and-such a thing is going on; yet every little detail I am to see and know, everything I should be present at, a message comes to me,—nothing ever seems forgotten. But to return to the pastor; though he is not very formidable, a little quaking one came in to him. He had a book of his printed directions for parish visiting to give me, and then asked me to take a walk with him in the garden. I was soon quite at my ease, and we were talking busily. He spoke most strongly to me of what he himself has quite acted up to—of our not only seeking to be ourselves useful, but to be the preparers of others to take our place: and *that,* if nothing else, is the art here.[75]

197

171. Agnes Elizabeth Jones' Journal [1861]

October 3rd.— . . . at 7, to the men's hospital. Sister M., to my great delight, put me at once to work, first washing the glasses, etc., used by the sick during the night, then dusting and washing furniture in the bedrooms, seeing the dressing of the wounds, etc., washing up of breakfast things, and then I was sent to sit in the room with a dying man. . . . After dinner, returned to my post. At 2, Pastor S.'s class; then my English lesson, and then to men's hospital again till 7; after tea, a visit to Sister G., and then to the female wards to say good-night to my friends.

My routine is now: up at 5, dress, make bed, sweep room, and read till 6.15, breakfast and prayers, go to hospital at 7, give children cod-liver oil and other medicines, then begins the washing and dressing till 8.30, children's luncheon, then there are several who must be fed, mending to be done, etc., 10 to 11, English class, 11 children's dinner, and after it is over, and faces and hands washed, our own dinner comes; then I take the children a walk till 2, children's coffee etc., 3.30 to 4 the "stille stunde" in the church, 4 medicines given, 5 undressing and washing of children for bed, 7 supper; some evenings I have the charge of the hospital till 9.30. This is the daily routine.

April 10th.—I am now at home in my new station. I have the entire care of four women, also of the medicines of the twenty-four in the ward. My own special charge have sore legs, which must be hourly attended to, beds made twice a day, rooms cleaned, etc., then, as far as I can, I help with the other patients. I have such delight in the women, reading to them is like reading to my poor at home.[76]

172. Mme Elizabeth S. (Gurney) De Bunsen. *Elizabeth Fry's Journeys on the Continent, 1840–1841*

[Mme Elizabeth De Bunsen was the niece of Elizabeth Fry, the great Quaker prison reformer. While on a journey to Holland, Belgium, and Germany in 1840 and 1841, in company with Mrs. Fry and others, she kept a diary. The following excerpt from it gives her impressions of Kaiserswerth four years after its founding.]

Dusseldorf, May 6, 1840.

One morning we drove over to Kaiserswerth an old town on the Rhine and the residence of Pastor Fliedner. An eminently good man. He has established a small hospital close to his own house which is evidently beautifully arranged. He has also instituted Protestant Sisters of Charity whom he terms Deaconesses. These are all dressed alike in blue print gowns and neat white caps. They wait entirely on the patients, go out to visit the poor and are sent to any parts of the Kingdom where real good Christian Nurses are required. They appeared a capital set of women and were pleased when they saw our great interest in them. Our Aunt had them assembled after dinner at the Pastor's house and he interpreted to them her beautiful address giving them excellent hints on nursing the sick and the necessity of true quiet, Christian Manners of Gentleness and Eveness of temper to form a real Nurse. This had been *her* experience and she felt sure from their looks and manners it had been theirs also. A refuge for discharged prisoners and a bright little Infant School are both under his immediate care. Whilst our Aunt rested the Pastor took us a walk to the old Castle, long the residence of the German Emperors as the name of the town implies. We had passed many of these old ruins whilst coming up the Rhine, but this was the first of them that we had visited. We admired the Rhine (unpicturesque as it is here) and the distant country thro' the broken arches and Windows.[77]

173. Pastor Fliedner's Letter Describing Mrs. Fry's Visit to Kaiserswerth

[This letter, written in 1848, not only expresses Pastor Fliedner's recollections of Mrs. Fry's visit to Kaiserswerth in 1840 but also reviews his founding of the institution in 1836.]

The 8th of May, 1840, was a great holiday to us; Elizabeth Fry of London visited our institution. Of all my contemporaries none has exercised a like influence on my heart and life: truly her friendship was one of the "all things," which God, in sovereign mercy, has worked for my good. In January, 1824, I had had the privilege of witnessing the effects of Mrs. Fry's wonder-working visits among the miserable prisoners of Newgate. On my return to my father-land, my object was to found a society entitled the "Rhenish West-phalian Prison Association," having ramifications in all the provinces of Germany. In this I was greatly assisted by the advice and experience afforded me by this eminent servant of God. During my second stay in England, in 1834, I had the happiness, in common with Dr. Steinkopff, of spending a day with Mrs. Fry, at her own home, and also of accompanying her in one of her visits of mercy to Newgate. By this means, I was enabled to see and admire her, in her domestic, as well as public character. Thus may my happiness be estimated, when in 1840, Mrs. Fry, accompanied by her brother, her young niece, William Allen and Lucy Bradshaw, came in person to see and rejoice over the growing establishment of Kaiserswerth. She saw the whole house, going into every room, and minutely examining each detail, and then delivered to the inmates a deeply interesting discourse. Many were the tears shed, and I have a bright hope, not in vain.

To the "helping sisters" of the institution she gave much motherly advice, and told the results of her own labours, showing that truly she estimated the great difficulties in educating those aright who are hereafter to have the care of the sick and suffering. It was a particular matter of rejoicing to that dear mother in Christ that so many of those trained at Kaiserswerth were earnestly desirous of filling places of trust in other institutions of a similar nature. She examined thoroughly the "Mutter Haus," and the wards for the sick, which contained at that time between forty and fifty, and was much interested in the infant school connected with the institution: she assembled the twenty working deaconesses, and those who were undergoing their time of probation also. . . . Truly God was in the midst of us, and the remembrance of that spirit of active, self-denying love, is one of the sweetest consolations which I possess, amid the trials and difficulties which every such institution must afford.

Thomas Fliedner.

May 26, 1848.[78]

174. Kaiserswerth as Seen by Pastor Passavant

[William Alfred Passavant (1821–1894), Lutheran pastor of Pittsburgh, visited Kaiserswerth in 1846, ten years after the founding of the deaconess institution there. At that time, he made arrangements for the coming to America of four deaconesses for work in a proposed deaconess institution in Pittsburgh. In 1849 Pastor Fliedner himself accompanied the deaconesses to Pittsburgh.[79] The following letter describes Pastor Passavant's impressions of his visit.]

Letter of Pastor Passavant to his wife (date not given).

Again I am on the mystic Rhine at Kaiserswerth, an obscure village of two thousand inhabitants but celebrated all over Europe for the interesting institution of Protestant deaconesses which Pastor Fliedner, an unobtrusive Lutheran minister, has established there. As I had letters from Bremen and from the Sisters in the hospital in Frankfurt and London, Fliedner at once made me welcome and we were soon seated around a frugal but comfortable repast to which my long walk enabled me to do ample justice. During the afternoon, we went over the whole institution which, from nothing but a believing heart, has gradually increased to an ample establishment, consisting of a hospital, an orphan home, an infant school, a day school, an asylum for released female prisoners, an institution for the training of Evangelical teachers, and a mother house for deaconesses! Building after building goes up and, with nothing but faith for a capital, the necessary means are always at hand. Though the institution is only a few years old, it has already sent forth two hundred and sixty female teachers and a large number of nursing Sisters who are scattered over Europe in hospitals, from St. Petersburg to Rome! . . .

Among the deaconesses were several ladies of the nobility, one of whom came from Sweden with the purpose of remaining a year and then founding a similar institution in her own land . . .[80]

200

175. Letter Describing the Work of the Sisters of Park Village Community

[The following brief fragment from a letter giving the merest suggestion of the work of the sisters of the Park Village Community was written by Jane Ellacombe, or Sister Anne, as she came to be known. Sister Anne was the daughter of Rev. H. T. Ellacombe, rector of Clyst St. George, a leading authority on church bells, and an intimate friend of Newman. Sister Anne was one of the first two to enter Park Village Community on March 26, 1845, when it was founded.[81]]

> 17 Park Village, West,
> April 11, 1845.

The people are all very glad and thankful at our coming to them—and we have not met with anything like a word of rudeness. We go to them to relieve their bodily wants, but principally our office lies in religious instruction and guidance as far as God gives us help. . . . We are out from 9 till 1, and again after dinner from a little after 3 till 5. The recreation hours are from a quarter to 2 till 3, and from 7 till 8 . . .

> Believe me to remain,
> Your very thankful and affectionate child,
> J. J. Ellacombe.[82]

176. Lionel S. Beale, "Nursing the Sick in Hospitals, Private Families, and Among the Poor," *Medical Times and Gazette*, December 6, 1873, pp. 630–632

[In 1873 Dr. Lionel S. Beale, Fellow of the Royal Society of Physicians and physician in Kings College Hospital, wrote a series of articles on nursing for the *Medical Times and Gazette*. The following brief statement is taken from the fourth in the series. In earlier articles Dr. Beale had expressed his conviction that nursing was and must be a special calling, or profession, and that if the nurse were educated as a professional person she would desire to devote her entire energies to nursing the patient rather than dividing herself between nursing and domestic matters in the household.[83]]

About seventeen years ago, then, the responsibility of nursing our hospital was transferred from hospital servants to the sisters and nurses of St. John's House. No hospital could be better nursed than ours has been during these seventeen years . . .

St. John's House is a comfortable *home* as well as a nursing institution, and when our nurses become old and can no longer work they receive a pension, which though not so large as we desire it should be, nevertheless represents an amount of capital which very few people in the enjoyment of an income far higher than that of a nurse can manage to save. Our nurses belong to a sisterhood—a religious sisterhood. . . . Our workers take no vows —they can come and go as they think right. They freely give their services . . .

177. Correspondence of Elizabeth Fry Regarding the Nursing Sisters

[Elizabeth Gurney Fry (1780–1845) was an eminent Quaker prison reformer and philanthropist in England. For many years she worked tirelessly in the interest of the women prisoners at Newgate Prison, and is best known for that work. Pastor Fliedner twice visited her in England, and in 1840 she visited Kaiserswerth.[84] Her habitual acquaintance with sickness prompted her to establish the Institution of Nursing Sisters in 1840, the actual plan being carried out by her sister, Mrs. Samuel Gurney, with the assistance of her daughters and some friends.[85] In addition to these letters, extracts from her journal and diary are given in Readings Nos. 178 to 180.]

Elizabeth Fry to the Bishop of London

Upton, 5th Month, 1841.

Elizabeth Fry presents her respects to the Bishop of London [Dr. Blomfield] and if convenient to the Bishop to receive her she proposes calling upon him in St James's Sq^{re} about twelve o'clock this morning as the Queen Dowager wished the Bishop of London would inform Elizth Fry his views respecting the new institution for the Protestant Sisters of Charity. Elizth Fry would have written before had not the illness of her daughter made it very uncertain whether she could attend to any engagement for a future day.

To the Bishop of London

.   .   .   .

Earl Howe to Elizabeth Fry

Bushey House,
July 8, 1841.

My dear Mrs. Fry,

Queen Adelaide commands me to state with what sincere pleasure she will place her name in your Society of Sisters of Charity. Her Majesty adds that you may call upon her as an extra nurse if *shorthanded*.

Seriously, it is satisfactory to find any little objection the Archbishop has felt now removed, and Her Majesty will gladly become an annual subscriber to your excellent and, I am satisfied, most useful institution.

Believe me, with greatest respect,

Very truly and faithfully,
Howe.[86]

178. Journal of Elizabeth Fry

Twelfth Month, 31st, 1840.

I deeply feel coming to the close of this year, rather unusually so: it finds me in a rather low estate, and from circumstances my spirit is rather overwhelmed although I am sensible that blessings abound, through unmerited mercy. I think the prison cause, at home and abroad, much prospering, many happy results from our foreign expedition, and much doing at home. Among other things the establishment of a Patronage Society for prisoners, by which many poor wanderers appear to be helped and protected, and a Society for the Sisters of Charity to visit and attend the sick.[87]

179. Diary of Elizabeth Fry

June 28th, 1841.

My sister Gurney [Mrs. Samuel Gurney] and my dear friend Charlotte Upcler, went with me to the Bishop of London on Sixth Day, on the subject of the Sisters of Charity. It has been a great pleasure to me, the Queen Dowager giving her name as patroness.[88]

180. *Memoirs of the Life of Elizabeth Fry*

[The *Memoirs,* containing extracts from Elizabeth Fry's journal and letters, were edited in 1848 by Mrs. Fry's daughters, Katharine Fry and Rachel Elizabeth Cresswell. Because of the ill health of Mrs. Fry, the actual founding of the Nursing Sisters was entrusted to Mrs. Fry's sister.[89] The following quotation gives briefly the outline of the plan for instituting the Nursing Sisters.]

The plan of proceeding is this: suitable women are selected with great care, and their characters minutely inquired into. They are regularly trained for a certain time in one of the public hospitals, in order to prepare them for their important duties. At the expiration of this period of probation, if their conduct and qualifications be found satisfactory, they are received as sisters. They are allowed an annual stipend of £20, (which is raised to £23 after three years' service,) supplied with an appropriate dress, and maintained in a home provided for them during the intervals of their engagements.

There is . . . a small distinct fund under the name of the "Superannuated Fund," for the assistance of such of the sisters as may after long and faithful service be disqualified for labour.

By the rules of the institution, Christian women of various denominations are admitted to join its ranks. No direct system of religious instruction is pursued, although the Sisters are required to attend family and public worship when in the house. They are encouraged to read the Scriptures to their patients; and to endeavour to promote their spiritual welfare, as well as to labour for their bodily comfort. . . . Whilst at the Home the sisters visit and nurse the sick poor in its neighbourhood. But there is another class of persons to whom their services are invaluable, persons of comparative refinement, but who are in circumstances of great limitation, perhaps wholly dependent on their own exertions for support. To such as these the boon is great indeed, of a careful, experienced, conscientious nurse: not one who squanders the little substance of the sufferer, not one who watches harpylike for perquisites and profit, nor "snores the sick man dead," but carefully and with fidelity discharges her onerous duties. In cases of this kind a large proportion of their time is occupied, often entirely gratuitously, at other times, on terms proportioned to the means of the patient, but which are very far from repaying the institution. The lowest sum which is considered to cover its current expenses is £1, 1s. a-week, but when circumstances claim a pecuniary sacrifice, the Committee on their part are ready to make arrangements accordingly, as well as to render assistance entirely gratuitous, in cases of great necessity.

The sisters are not permitted to receive mourning or presents directly or indirectly, from the patients or the families on whom they attend. The funds of the Society depend partly upon subscriptions, and partly upon the liberality of those who have benefited from the institution. The help of the nursing Sisters has been sought and greatly valued, by persons of all classes, from royalty to the poorest and most destitute.[90]

181. Letter of William Makepeace Thackeray to Mrs. Robinson

[William Makepeace Thackeray (1811–1863), English novelist, having had occasion to employ a nurse from the Institution of Nursing Sisters, sent payment and a contribution to Mrs. Robinson, the head of the organization.]

36, Ouslow Square,
January 17, 1860.

Dear Madam,
I have the pleasure of sending you ten guineas, for the five weeks' service of the excellent nurse I had from your institution, and beg it to accept the other five pounds.
With the thanks and good wishes of your obliged serv[t].

W. M. Thackeray.

To Mrs. Robinson,
Lady Superintendent.[91]

182. Minutes of the London Hospital, September 2, 1840

[The voluntary hospital movement of the eighteenth century in England began in a small way when the Royal College of Physicians encouraged its members to give, when desired, "gratuitous advice to the sick poor in their localities in London and seven miles around." This made the voluntary hospital a possibility. The second hospital of this character to be founded in London was the London Hospital, in 1740. The physician, surgeon, and apothecary were to attend for a few hours a day, and a man and his wife were engaged to carry out all other duties.

Nurses began to be employed at a later date. The beginnings of a medical school followed.[92]]

The Committee met on special summons to consider a communication from a deputation of the Provisional Board of Management of a projected Society for the establishment of Protestant Sisters of Charity, especially with the view to improve the class of women employed in nursing the sick, requesting the Committee to admit two or three respectable women to be trained under the superintendence of the matron. Resolved that the application be complied with, under definite understanding that it shall in no manner be permitted to interfere with the discipline or arrangements of the hospital.[93]

183. Report of the Deaconesses of East End of London

[This group, known as the Mildmay Deaconesses, was so named from the Mildmay estate in the locality, rather than from any contribution of the Mildmay family to its work. It was founded by the Reverend William Pennefather, clergyman of the Church of England and for twelve years Vicar of Christ Church, Barnet. He later removed to London where the deaconess group was established.[94]]

The summer of 1866, with its terrible visitation of the fatal disease of cholera, is still fresh in all our memories and it seems scarcely necessary even to remind our readers of the many hundreds who, day after day, were swept into eternity in the sorrowful and benighted East End of our vast metropolis. Great and dire distress was the lot of thousands, while the work that fell upon the ministers of these densely peopled districts was altogether overwhelming. In this extremity the Rev. J. Trevitt, Vicar of St. Philip's, Bethnal Green, accepted the offer of the Rev. W. Pennefather to assist him by means of his trained deaconesses; and allotted to them a district for visitation containing some 5700 souls.[95]

184. The Letters of Sister Dora

[Sister Dora (Dorothy Wyndlow) Pattison (1832–1878) was a member of the Sisterhood of the Good Samaritans.[96] She was the tenth and youngest sister of Mark Pattison, English author and rector of Lincoln College, Oxford. Her work was carried out mainly in the hospital in Walsall, a market town of Staffordshire, where she greatly endeared herself to those with whom she worked.[97]]

> The Hospital North Ormsby,
> Jan. 5th, 1865.

My dear Miss F———, . . .

I have been ordered off the hospital to-day, and am sitting up to-night with a poor man who is suffering from concussion of the brain; and he alarms me by getting up and trying to get away, and he is insensible (*i. e.*

not himself), so that it is useless speaking to him. It is so cold at night that, though sitting over the fire, I am shivering. I have put a blister on my patient. I hope, when it takes effect, there will be an improvement.

I remain, yours sincerely,
Dora Pattison

.   .   .   .   .   .

[Epidemic Hospital]
February 28th [1875].

My dear Sister

I have been wondering how you are getting on. . . . The old Irishwoman, sixty-seven! who shouts at the patients, and is a regular old Sarah Gamp and Grimes, who cannot crawl, and is so dirty. If only S——— would have come, I should have done. My room is between the wards, with little windows as you have, peeping into both. My bed in one corner, chest of drawers, and slip for my basin. The doctor said it "smelt of pox" this morning; and no wonder—they were airing all the sheets by my fire when I came in. I think the most infectious thing I have to do is to nurse the babies, taking them streaming out of their mothers' arms. One has the pox on its arms and chest very slightly. Our worst case is a lad of eighteen. He vomits everything; and is so delirious; he got out of his bed this morning, and I thought he had escaped into the town, but I found him in an empty ward . . .

One of the police came to see me to-day, and he said they declared in the town they should not mind having the small-pox with "Sister" to nurse them. I declare I taste it in my tea. I have made my room look as respectable as I can. . . . Is not this a glorious retreat for me in Lent? I can have no idle chatter.

With love,
Sister Dora.

.   .   .   .   .   .

The Epidemic Hospital,
Walsall, March 1, 1875,

My dear———

I do not know what my darling will say to me when she hears where I am. I came and opened the small-pox hospital on Saturday. It was spreading in the town, and no one could be found to come; also, the people could not be persuaded to come until they heard I was here. So I came on Saturday, and had not been here half an hour before seven arrived; so I have my hands full, for I cannot get a decent woman to come and help, though we pay well. I have got two "critters" from the workhouse; one is so helpless, I have to do her work for her, and the other sits up at nights; so can do no more. One man is so delirious I cannot keep my eye off him, or else he is out of bed. Then I have a baby a *year* old, and another youngster, and they are so cross; they keep up their music night and day. They are all so pleased to have me here. I had such a nice Sunday. God's blessing seemed very much on the place. I spoke to them. . . . O that I had Mr. Twigg's power to help souls! I know you will all pray for me, that, living or dying, I may glorify Him. You must not fret for me. A kiss to all my beloved children . . .

Your faithful friend,
Sister Dora.[98]

185. Letter of a Visitor to Walsall Hospital

[This letter was written in 1872 by a lady who was staying in the neighborhood of the Walsall Hospital and, having heard of the excellence of Sister Dora's nursing, went to see it for herself.[99]]

We have been to see the celebrated Sister Dora, and I must tell you about her at once. "Cottage Hospital" is hardly a name for it, for Walsall is an enormous place; and there are something like a score of beds, with only Sister and one paid nurse (Mrs. H.———), and two or three scrubber folk to look after them. I wish you had been with us. She is a tall, black-haired, handsome woman, brimming over with fun and energy. I think the most striking part of her is the way she picks out the humorous side of everything she tells one, and laughs over it heartily, that the first moment I thought her unfeeling. But then the next minute she had brought tears into my eyes, and I saw that her sense of humor must be the greatest blessing and help to her in the midst of such melancholy scenes. . . . On Saturday, at midnight, a man was brought in with his throat cut, dead to all appearance. He had cut his sweetheart's throat first, and all the doctors were with her, for he had rushed away into the fields, and had not been found for some time. So Sister Dora sewed up his wounds as he lay in the hall, thinking that, if he were not dead, he would be in a few minutes, and it was not worth moving him. But as she finished, he began to breathe again with a gasp, and now he is likely to get well . . .

She has not slept out of the hospital since November twelvemonth! but she looks anything rather than ill. She has been nursing eleven years. I can fancy that she would not make as good a second in command as she does chief, being human, and taking an evident pride in her own good management, which she is much too transparent and openhearted to hide. But she is certainly as fascinating a woman as I ever came across, to use only mild language. You might as well keep this letter, please; I should like to be reminded of our visit to Sister Dora some time hence, when the impression is faded.[100]

186. Article I of the Statutes of the Protestant Sisters of Charity in France

[The French order of the deaconesses in the Protestant Church was established in 1841.[101] The following, from the first article of the statutes, is cited by James Meeker Ludlow, American Presbyterian clergyman, in his book on the deaconesses. It states the objectives of the group.]

The Institute of Deaconesses is a free association having for its object the instructing and directing, in the practice of active charity, of such Protestant women as shall devote themselves within its bosom to the relief of bodily and spiritual misery, and particularly to the care of the sick, the young, and the poor.[102]

187. Two Documents Relating to the Irish Sisters of Charity

[The Roman Catholic Order of the Irish Sisters of Charity was founded in 1816 by Mother Mary Aikenhead (1787–1858). The religious community selected by the Archbishop for Mary to enter was the Convent of the Institute of the Blessed Virgin Mary at Micklegate Bar, York, because the nuns there took no vows of enclosure and went out to visit the sick.[103] The letter below, addressed to Mother de Chantal, describes the work of the hospital of the Sisters in Dublin. The statement of the purposes of the order was in answer to a query by a commission set up to inquire into the state of the poor in Ireland.]

To Mother de Chantal [Dublin, c. Aug. 21, 1833].

Here we are going on with cholera still, Sister M. Jerome and Francis Teresa spending all their time at the poor little hospital. We hear that the great physicians say that this disease is no longer prevalent—God help them if they should be taught to their cost. However, it is the fashion to make light of it, and no hospitals are opened except this poor thing of twelve beds for the parish. Certainly it is not so bad as last year, but it is bad enough, and the poor sufferers are without relief.

.   .   .   .   .   .

Convent of the Sisters of Charity,
Sandymount,
30th December, 1833.

My Lords and Gentlemen,

A copy of the "Queries for Parishes in Large Towns" has been sent to me, requesting that I will favour "The Commissioners of Inquiry into the State of the Irish Poor," with an early reply to such of them as may come within my cognisance.

There are many of the queries which I cannot be expected to reply to; therefore I have preferred furnishing the Commissioners with such information on the state of the poor, in the district in which our convent is situated, as I have been able to collect in the discharge of the duties of a Sister of Charity.

Our convent has been established at Sandy-mount, Parish of St. Mary, Donnybrook, City of Dublin, about three years. The object of our Institute is to attend to the comforts of the poor, both spiritual and temporal; to visit them at their dwellings and in hospitals, to attend them in sickness, to administer consolation in their afflictions, and to reconcile them to the dispensations of an all-wise Providence in the many trials to which they are subject . . .

I have the honour to be my Lords and Gentlemen,

Your obedient servant,

Mary Aikenhead.[104]

CONCLUDING STATEMENT

The work of St. Vincent de Paul in France, in the seventeenth century, illustrated in the preceding chapter, served to improve the nursing care of the sick wherever the Sisters of Charity were engaged in this activity in hospital and home. It was a beginning in meeting the vast need in one country.

In the nineteenth century in England, the concern felt over conditions in the nursing care of the sick was expressed in the writings of physicians, philanthropists, and novelists such as Charles Dickens. The nurse, as described in the writings quoted in this chapter, was often uneducated, sometimes drunken and immoral, occasionally kindly, and rarely skillful. She was usually a "pauper nurse," or poorly paid, and, perhaps understandably, was mainly interested in her own welfare rather than that of her patients. Exceptions were found in the nurses described by Sir James Paget, Dr. John Flint South, Dr. John Beddoe, and others.

The nursing in the infirmaries of workhouses as investigated by the *Lancet* Commission, and by Louisa Twining in connection with the administration of the Poor Law, was generally done by unpaid nurses and was, more often than not, unsatisfactory in character.

Into this picture is projected a different kind of nurse, the volunteer nurse in epidemics—a nurse such as Felicia Skene, whose contribution to the welfare of the sick was temporary and atypical, and another, like Sister Dora, who for a number of years devoted herself to hospital nursing.

Many of the writers suggested remedies which fall into two main categories, namely: (1) payment of the nurses; and (2) establishment of nursing under religious auspices. Physicians such as Dr. Robert Gooch advocated nursing by an order of women in the Church of England, resembling the Sisters of Charity in Catholic countries, or the Beguines of Flanders. Robert Southey also favored this method. Others, writing in the *Saturday Review* and the *Pall Mall Gazette,* advocated this or the alternative method of improving the economic status of nursing.

Actual beginnings in establishing nursing under religious auspices were made first in Germany by Amelia Sieveking, and, through the revival of the Christian deaconess system, by Pastor Fliedner of Kaiserswerth and his wife, Fredericke. In England several attempts succeeded in the form of orders in the Established Church, such as the Park Village Community, the Community of St. John's House, and the Institution of Nursing Sisters.

In the present chapter the founding and characteristics of the Kaiserswerth Institution are outlined by Pastor and Fredericke Fliedner, Florence Nightingale, Agnes Elizabeth Jones, Mrs. Elizabeth Fry, and Pastor Passavant. These descriptions illustrate two chief characteristics of the deaconess group—their religious devotion to the sick and their attention to discipline. The institutions in England are described by various writers who were instrumental in their founding, were participants in their nursing, or utilized their services. Religious fervor plays a part here also, coupled with practical application to the needs of the patients being cared for by the sisters.

These beginnings of better nursing in Germany and in England form the background for the founding of a new system of nursing by Florence Nightingale, whose reforms revolutionized the care of the sick in hospitals and homes throughout the world. These changes, beneficial as they proved to be when adopted, did not occur all at once, as will be seen by the descriptions of conditions which lingered long past the time of the founding of the Nightingale School in 1860. Miss Nightingale's life and work are the subject of the next two chapters. The chapter immediately following this one draws upon the sources for her early life and preparation for the founding of the new system, while the following one deals with the latter development and its widespread influence.

PART II

*The Origins of Professional Nursing
as Shown in Selected Manuscripts*

Chapter 6

Some References to the Life of
Florence Nightingale Before 1860

INTRODUCTION

FLORENCE NIGHTINGALE is the acknowledged founder of modern professional nursing. Her accomplishments in the reform of nursing, particularly in the Crimean War, are familiar in some degree to large numbers of the English-speaking world as well as to those of other countries. The events of her youth, and her efforts to find satisfactory means for a life of service before the time of her departure for the war are, however, less well known, although now becoming more a part of common knowledge. The fact that Miss Nightingale, a member of a well-to-do family with high social status in English society, lived at a time when nursing was at a very low ebb gave to her desire to become a nurse and to her accomplishments in the struggle to reform hospitals and to improve nursing education a highly dramatic quality. The importance of her contributions to society was equaled by that of few women of her day—or, indeed, of any day.

The details of Miss Nightingale's life at home, her education, her friends, and her many activities have been told countless times. Repetition of these, which would necessarily be brief and therefore incomplete, has not been attempted for the purposes of this book. It has been deemed more desirable to let the sources which it has been practicable to include speak for themselves.

The familiarity of large numbers of people with the life of Florence Nightingale is in some measure the result of the biographies, among which is the indispensable two-volume work by Sir Edward Cook, *The Life of Florence Nightingale,* published in 1913, and more recently made available in one volume. The new biography by Cecil Woodham-Smith, *Florence Nightingale,* documented with new as well as with the more familiar sources, is valuable as well as scholarly. A less well-known, undated biography by Annie Matheson, evidently published, or at least written before Cook's work, makes use of primary and secondary sources, and contains much interesting and valuable material.

These writings present all aspects of Miss Nightingale's life and work: her early life and interest in nursing; her preparation for nursing, at Kaiserswerth, and in other experiences; the story of the Crimean War reforms which affected the nursing in army hospitals in England and elsewhere; the establishment of an improved system of nursing service and nursing education at St. Thomas's Hospital, London, which left its imprint on nursing and nursing education everywhere; Miss Nightingale's other contributions to social welfare; and finally her writings.

The readings selected for presentation in this chapter have been chosen to throw light on Miss Nightingale's life before the founding of the school at St. Thomas's Hospital in 1860. It has been deemed advisable to include mainly selections from the sources which are relatively less accessible, rather than from those which are available in Cook's *Life* and in periodical literature, such as the *American Journal of Nursing*. The readings refer to two phases of Miss Nightingale's life: her activities before the Crimean War, and her reforms of military hospital nursing during the Crimean War itself.

In the first category, the following are of interest: Julia Ward Howe's *Reminiscences, 1819–1899,* describing Miss Nightingale's appearance and referring to her desire to become a nurse (188); two letters of Florence Nightingale to Dr. and Mrs. Howe, the first expressing her keen interest in the improvement of nursing in England, and the second briefly alluding to her visit to Kaiserswerth (189); a short excerpt from Elizabeth Blackwell's diary, describing a visit to Embley Park (190); and Elizabeth Gaskell's long letter to Catherine Winkworth eulogizing Miss Nightingale and describing several incidents in her early life (191).

From the large number of references to Miss Nightingale's work in the Scutari hospitals and the Crimea, a few have been selected as best illustrating Miss Nightingale's activities and influence. These include letters, newspaper articles, personal reminiscences, diaries and memoirs, and official records. The following are included: letters from Fanny Allen to her niece Elizabeth Wedgwood and others, describing Florence Nightingale's skill in the hospital (192); a brief description of the asssistance given by Felicia Skene to Miss Nightingale in recruiting nurses for war service, from E. C. Rickards' *Felicia Skene of Oxford A Memoir* (193); letters of Bishop Thomas Grant regarding the Bermondsey nuns who were assigned to Miss Nightingale's contingent of nurses going to the Crimea (194); two articles from the *Illustrated London News* of 1854 and 1855, describing Miss Nightingale's journey to the East and her character and appearance (195); a long article from the *London Times,* October 30, 1854, answering the query, which was prevalent at the time among the English people, as to the identity of Miss Nightingale (196); a letter from Mr. Bracebridge to Mr. Herbert, giving a picture of the Barrack Hospital (197); a letter from Richard Monckton Milnes to his wife, referring to the high regard in which Miss Nightingale was held by the soldiers (198); a letter of Lady Hornby, describing Miss Nightingale's appearance (199); a description of Miss Nightingale and the hospitals at Scutari, by Rev. Sydney Godolphin Osborne in *Scutari and Its Hospitals* (200); that of Peter Pincoffs, in *Experiences of a Civilian in Eastern Military Hospitals* (201); L. Dunne's remarks in *A Trip to Constantinople . . . and Miss Nightingale at Scutari Hospital* (202); a letter of Sir Sidney Herbert to Florence Nightingale, explaining the reasons for the sending of the second group of nurses to the Crimea (203); six letters of Mary Stanley, referring to the work at the Koulali hospital (204); the account of Fanny M. Taylor in *Eastern Hospitals and English Nurses . . . ,* describing her experiences at Koulali and Scutari (205); Sister Mary Aloysius' vivid portrayal of her work at Balaklava and Scutari, in *Memories of the Crimea* (206); Sister Margaret Goodman's account of the journey from London to Scutari and of the nursing in the Eastern hospitals, as given in *Experiences of an English Sister of Mercy* (207).

Several brief quotations referring to events of the war and afterward include: a letter from Mrs. Sidney Herbert to Mrs. S. C. Hall, suggesting the form of the testimonial in Miss Nightingale's honor, which the English people proposed to subscribe (208); a brief extract from the evidence given by the Duke of Newcastle before the Roebuck Committee relative to the employment of nurses in the hospital at Scutari (209); James Henry Skene's description of Miss Nightingale in his book, *With Lord Stratford in the Crimean War* (210); a tribute to Miss Nightingale given by the Rt. Hon. Sir John McNeill, quoted in his *Memoir* (211); and that of Gen. Sir George Higginson in his *Seventy-one Years of a Guardsman's Life* (212).

Included in this chapter also, are two examples of the many tributes in song, prose, and poetry which appeared at the time of Miss Nightingale's dramatic contribution to the betterment of nursing in the hospitals of the Crimea. One is "Santa Filomena" (213), first published in the *Atlantic Monthly;* and the other is from *Punch,* an English periodical, entitled "The Nightingale's Song to the Sick Soldier" (214).

THE SOURCES

188. Julia Ward Howe. *Reminiscences, 1819–1899*

[Julia Ward Howe (1819–1899), American author, lecturer, and social reformer, was the composer of the "Battle Hymn of the Republic," published in the *Atlantic Monthly* in 1862. Her husband, Dr. Samuel Gridley Howe, was the editor of the *Boston Commonwealth,* in which work he was assisted by his wife. Dr. and Mrs. Howe were ardent advocates of Negro emancipation, woman suffrage, and other causes. Mrs. Howe was elected the first woman member of the American Academy of Arts and Letters.[1] The incident described below occurred at the home of Florence Nightingale.]

Florence, the younger sister, was rather elegant than beautiful; she was tall and graceful of figure, her countenance mobile and expressive, her conversation most interesting. Having heard much of Dr. Howe as a philanthropist, she resolved to consult him upon a matter which she already had at heart. She accordingly requested him one day to meet her on the following morning, before the hour for the family breakfast. He did so, and she opened the way to the desired conference by saying, "Dr. Howe, if I should determine to study nursing, and to devote my life to that profession, do you think it would be a dreadful thing?"

"By no means," replied my husband. "I think that it would be a very good thing."

So much and no more of the conversation Dr. Howe repeated to me. We soon learned that Miss Florence was devoting herself to the study of her predilection; and when, years after this time, the Crimean war broke out, we were among the few who were not astonished at the undertaking which made her name world famous.[2]

189. Two Letters of Florence Nightingale to Dr. and Mrs. Howe

[These letters were selected from among several which appeared in the *Yale Review* in the winter of 1935, edited by Laura E. Richards. Mrs. Richards (1850–1943) was the daughter of Dr. and Mrs. Samuel Gridley Howe and was a writer of children's books. She is best known for her book, *Captain January,* and for the "Hildegarde Books" for girls.[3]]

Dec. 26, 1845
Embley Park, Romsey.

[My dear kind Friends]

...I have failed in three beautiful plans this autumn, and generally believe that man counts his years by their failures and not by their months, and that it is of his early miscarriages that are made up his own experience and his neighbor's amusement. Girls seem to me to be the least happy class of the community—and the misery is greatly increased by the feeling that it is a very wicked thing, in such a position, not to be very happy. Their friends always tell them that when they have a vocation, a family dependent upon them, they will find all come right—but I cannot believe that God has created a whole class merely to wait until they are something else. Oh the wasted energies that I see, and the field there is for them—why cannot the two be brought together? Who would fear being an old maid, if she had such a prospect before her, as to be the creature behind whom Providence hides himself—I do not mean only in broth or a load of coals or 2 s. 6 d. I saw a poor woman die before my eyes this summer, whom her well-intentioned nurses had poisoned, as certainly as if they had given her Prussic Acid. She died of ignorant nursing—and such things happen constantly—as well as all sorts (some, from pure ignorance) of misery and profligacy, which good healthful intimacies among the poor people, made by the better educated, under the shelter of a rhubarb powder or a dressed leg, might go far to avert . . .

Oh if we could but live to see Protestant Sisterhoods of Charity without vows, for women of education—but the difficulties of the first step are so great in England—I do not mean the physically-revolting parts of a hospital, but things about the surgeons and the nurses, who are generally most unlike Soeurs, which you may guess. Yet I know a young German Protestant lady, who studied in a hospital—and if women would have a career like this in England, what would become of those much-dreaded, much maligned later years? Would they not be all *verklart,* would not that terror of a life without love, an activity without an aim, be done away with? I am afraid everybody is not so fond of hospitals, but I wish you would tell me, whether in America pupil-nurses could be ever taken there merely to learn . . .

If I could live to see anything in England, "my eyes would indeed have seen His salvation," but now I see nothing but a mist, and only hope, when the mist clears away, to see something else.

· · · · · · ·

Embley, June 20, 1852.

My dear Dr. Howe,

It is so long since we have heard from you or yours that I feel a great desire to renew our intercourse . . .

I went for three months to an Institution of Protestant Deaconesses in Germany last year, at Kaiserswerth—perhaps you may know it. It is first rate, I wish the system could be introduced in England, where thousands of women have nothing to do and where hospitals are ill nursed by a class of women not fit to be household servants . . .[4]

190. From Elizabeth Blackwell's Diary

[Elizabeth Blackwell (1821–1910), graduate in medicine at Geneva Medical College, Geneva, New York, was the first woman to receive a medical degree in the United States. She was the sister-in-law of Lucy Stone, American leader in the struggle for "women's rights." Together with her sister, Dr. Emily Blackwell, she founded the New York Infirmary and College for Women and Children. During the Civil War, Dr. Elizabeth Blackwell was the moving spirit of the Women's Relief Association whose primary purpose was to provide care, including nursing, for wounded Union soldiers.[5]]

April 17 [1851].—Went down with my friend Florence to Embley Park. The laurels were in full bloom. Examined the handsome house and beautiful grounds. Saturday a perfect day. Walked much with Florence in the delicious air, amid a luxury of sights and sounds, conversing on the future. As we walked on the lawn in front of the noble drawing-room she said, "Do you know what I always think when I look at that row of windows? I think how I should turn it into a hospital ward, and just how I should place the beds! She said she should be perfectly happy working with me, and should want no other husband.[6]

191. Letter of Elizabeth Gaskell to Catherine Winkworth

[Elizabeth Cleghorn Gaskell (1810–1865), English novelist and biographer, is best known for her novel, *Cranford,* which was published first in serial form in *Household Words,* in 1851–1855, under the management of Charles Dickens. Mrs. Gaskell also wrote poetry and a life of Charlotte Brontë.[7] Catherine Winkworth (1827–1878) is remembered chiefly for her translations of German hymns and other works, including the *Life of Pastor Fliedner of Kaiserswerth,* and *The Life of Amelia Wilhelmina Sieveking.* She was interested in and helped to promote higher education for women.[8]]

Lea Hurst, near Matlock,
October 20, 1854.

My dearest Kate,

I am going to begin a letter to you, which you must forward to Emily, please. . . . Miss Florence Nightingale went on the 31st of August to take superintendence of the Cholera patients in the Middlesex Hospital (where they were obliged to send out their usual patients in order to take in the patients brought in every half-hour from the Soho district, Broad Street, etc.). She says cholera is not infectious, from person to person. Only two of the nurses had it, one of them died, the other recovered; that one of the porters, etc., had it. She herself was up day and night from Friday afternoon (Sept. 1) to Sunday afternoon, receiving the poor creatures (chiefly fallen women of that neighbourhood, they had it the worst) who were being constantly brought in—undressing them . . . putting on turpentine stupes, etc. herself, to as many as she could manage, never even had a touch of the

the complaint. She says, moreover, that one week the chances of recovery seemed as 1 to 10, but that since then the chances of recovery are as 20 to 1.

Oh! Katie! I wish you could see her—outsidedly only! She is tall, very slight and willowy in figure; thick shortish rich brown hair; very delicate pretty complexion, rather like my Flossy's, only more delicate colouring; grey eyes which are generally pensive and drooping, but when they choose can be the merriest eyes I ever saw; and perfect teeth, making her smile the sweetest I ever saw. Put a long piece of soft net, say 1¼ yards long and half a yard wide, and tie it round this beautifully-shaped head, so as to form a soft white framework for the full oval of her face (for she had the tooth-ache and so wore this little piece of drapery), and dress her up in black silk high up to the long white round throat; and a black shawl on—and you may get *near* an idea of her perfect grace and lovely appearance.

She is so like a saint. Mrs. Nightingale tells me that when a girl of 15 or so she was often nursing in the evening, and Mrs. N. would take a lantern and go up into the village to find her sitting by the bedside of some one who was ill, and saying she could not sit down to a grand 7 o'clock dinner while this was going on, etc. Then Mr. and Mrs. Nightingale took their two daughters to Italy, and they lived there till it was time for them to be presented at Court. In London she was excessively admired and had (this I have heard from other people) no end of offers—but she studied hard with her father, and is a perfect Greek and Latin scholar; so perfect that when they went to travel a few years later with Mr. and Mrs. Bracebridge, and they were in Transylvania, she was always chosen to address the old Abbots, etc., at the convents in Latin, to state their wants. She travelled for a year and a half with them, going to Athens and all sorts of classical Greek places; then up the Nile to the Second Cataract with these Bracebridges. Her mother says that, when she started, they equipped her *en princesse,* and when she came back, she had little besides the clothes she had on; she had given away her linen, etc., right and left to those who wanted it. Then she said that life was too serious a thing to be wasted in pleasure-seeking; and she went to Kaiserswerth, and was there for three months, taking her turn as a Deaconess, scouring rooms and all the other menial work, etc. Then she went to Paris, where she studied nursing in the hospitals, in the dress of a nun or abbess; and besides was for a month serving at a *bureau* in an *arrondissement,* in order to learn from the Sisters of their mode of visiting the poor.

And now she is at the head of the "Establishment for Invalid Gentle-women"; nursing continually, and *present at every operation.* She has a great deal of fun, and is carried along by that, I think. She mimics most capitally; mimics for instance the way of talking of some of the poor Governesses in the Establishment, with their delight at having a man servant, and at having *Lady* Canning and *Lady* Monteagle to do this and that for them. And then at that cholera time she went off, leaving word where she could be sent for, for she considered her "Gentlewomen" to have a prior claim on her services to the Middlesex Hospital, etc. I came in here for the end of her fortnight of holiday in the year. Is it not like St. Elizabeth of Hungary? The efforts of her

family to interest her in other occupations by allowing her to travel, etc.—
but the clinging to one object! Now I must go to dress for dinner. We dine
at 7.

.   .   .   .

[Later]

She must be a creature of another race, so high and mighty and angelic,
doing things by impulse or some divine inspiration—not by effort and
struggle of will. But she seems almost too holy to be talked about as a mere
wonder. Mrs. Nightingale says, with tears in her eyes (alluding to Andersen's
"Fairy Tales"), that they are ducks and have hatched a wild swan. She seems
as completely led by God as Joan of Arc.

I never heard of anyone like her. It makes one feel the livingness of God
more than ever to think how straight He is sending His spirit down into her,
as into the prophets and saints of old. I dare say all this sounds rather like
"bosh"—but indeed if you had heard all about her that I have you would
feel as I do. You must take a good deal upon trust.[9]

192. Letters of Fanny Allen

[Fanny Allen was the youngest of eleven children of John Bartlett
Allen of Cresselly. Her oldest sister Elizabeth married Josiah Wedgwood
of Maer, one of the sons of Josiah Wedgwood of Etruria. There were
nine children of this marriage, the youngest of whom, Emma, married
Charles Darwin. The oldest, Elizabeth, is the niece to whom Fanny
Allen writes in the first letter below.[10]]

Dec. 15th, 1854.

My dear Elizabeth . . .

Yet what a trifling world it was, and what women were his [Sydney Smith's]
fashionable ladies, in comparison with the noble Flo Nightingale and her
companions! Have you heard that she astonishes all the surgeons by her
skill and presence of mind? After amputating a limb, they pass on to another,
leaving her to take up the artery and do all that is necessary. Miss Stanley
is gone out I believe, and the Miss Stewart who so impressed John [Allen]
at the hospital he visits, is the Duchess of Somerset's sister, and is going or
gone out too, I believe.

.   .   .   .   .   .

December 3rd, 1856.

The Nightingale meeting was successful, I think, on the whole. There
did not seem to be much enthusiasm among them, but the time is too far gone
for that, and there is a more enduring stamp on Flo and her work which no
time will change. Sidney Herbert's speech pleased me most. Those three
touching anecdotes of her influence over the minds of the soldiers are beautiful, particularly the one of the soldiers kissing her shadow as it passed over

the beds. What woman ever took so high a position as she does now! I was dreaming of her all last night.

.   .   .   .

April 15th [1857].

I fear from a line in one of the newspapers that Florence Nightingale's life is approaching its end, as Mrs Rich would say. I have been deeply impressed by her life these last few days, which in respect to mine, forms but a fragment in regard to time, and what she has accomplished! I remember her a little girl of 3 or 4 years, then the girl of 16 of high promise when I next met her at Geneva, and which she has most faithfully kept. A high mission has been given her, which has cost her her life to fulfil, and now when I look back on every time I saw her after her sixteenth year, I see that she was ripening constantly for her work, and that her mind was dwelling on the painful difference of man and man in this life, and the trap that a luxurious life laid for the affluent. A conversation on this subject between the father and daughter made me laugh at the time, the contrast was so striking, but now as I remember it, it was the divine spirit breathing in her . . .[11]

193. E. C. Rickards. *Felicia Skene of Oxford A Memoir*

[Felicia Skene (1821–1899) had been active in the cholera epidemic of Oxford in 1854.[12] Thinking that this experience with nurses would be valuable, she offered her services for the recruiting of nurses for Miss Nightingale's group, which was preparing for departure to the Crimea.]

Felicia's work at the time of the cholera was to lead to fresh enterprise on her part, when in the following year the Crimean War began . . .

It struck Felicia that having with great pains trained her corps of nurses for the cholera, they might now be used at Scutari, her great desire being to go out herself at the head of them. Had these events occurred at the present day, when ideas of what ladies, still young, may and may not do in the way of bold enterprise, perhaps she might have obtained her parents' permission to go. As it was, the notion was too new and startling to be taken into consideration; and she had to content herself with doing all she could at home to send out others.

Her zeal was quickened by a letter she received from Lord Stratford de Redcliffe, who had been much struck by her energy and ability, urging her to do all she could in England to send to the rescue. At once she set to work as a pioneer in the undertaking, delighted to encourage her nurses to take their part in the patriotic task.

Meantime Miss Nightingale was hard at work enlisting recruits, thankful to secure Felicia's services as agent in Oxford. She sent her friends Mr and Mrs Bracebridge down there, that they might inspect the volunteers and select the women they thought would be suitable . . .

When the corps was complete, Felicia was requested to escort the party to London, to the house of Lady Canning, where they were to be provided with their outfit and despatched without delay to the seat of war. . . . When Felicia returned to Oxford, a close correspondence was begun between her and Miss Nightingale . . .[13]

194.   Grace Ramsey. *Thomas Grant, First Bishop of Southwark*

[Thomas Grant (1816–1870), first Roman Catholic Bishop of Southwark, a borough of London, was born in France but was driven from his home with his family by a band of incendiaries in one of the fanatical riots between Roman Catholics and Protestants. The family migrated to Ireland, and eventually Thomas entered military service. A pious man, he later entered the priesthood, and in 1844 was named rector of English College in Rome. The Crimean War came when he was Bishop of Southwark. Wishing his diocese to furnish its share of nurses for the troops, he requested a group of Bermondsey nuns, who were under his jurisdiction, to accompany Miss Nightingale to Scutari and the Crimea.[14]]

October 16, 1854.

My dear Daughters in Christ,—In times of real difficulty the children of Mary must be ready to imitate her in her journey with haste into the mountains. Four of your number must start to-morrow for Turkey to nurse the sick.[15] Our Dear Mother will guard those who remain, and as the lot of those who go will be the more difficult; it is necessary for her sake that your Reverend Mother should be one of the four. . . . May our Dear Lord guide and guard you all.

October 19, 1854.

Dear Reverend Mother,—Since you left London on Tuesday, the Government has arranged to have a complete establishment, or staff of nurses for Turkey under the superintendence of the charitable lady who will deliver this paper—Miss Nightingale. The nuns will be all under the care of a religious Superior, as they must be collected from different houses in England and Ireland; but, of course, your nuns will always have the benefit of your advice and direction. The object is that one should act as representing all the nuns as *nuns,* whilst Miss Nightingale will be their superintendent as nurses.

You can explain to the Sisters that you are all to start from Paris and travel with Miss Nightingale, whom you will find very kind and attentive.

When you reach Turkey the chief duty of the Sisters will be to act as hospital nurses, but they will be free to say prayers with all who are Catholics.

It is probable that the religious Superior over all the nuns will be some one accustomed to manage hospitals.

I hope you will have many blessings for your journey, and for your work and duties. Blessings to all.

☩ Thomas Grant.[16]

. . . .

[Agreement for the government drawn up by the bishop, in the name of the Sisters.]

To the Secretary of State.

St. George's: October 20, 1854.

Sir,—Having learned that you are willing to include among the nurses now about to proceed at the expense of Government to the Military Hospitals in the East, a number of Sisters of Mercy, I have offered five under my spiritual care, and I now beg to express my acceptance for their guidance of the conditions which have been laid down as follows.

1. Her Majesty's Government having appointed Miss Nightingale to be Superintendent of the nurses' department, it will belong in her office to regulate all the duties of the nurses in the hospital, their employment, hours, places in the wards, & c., and in general all that falls under the head of hospital regulations. The Sisters of Mercy will therefore place themselves in these respects under her sole direction.

2. Inasmuch as the Sisters of Mercy or others depend on their respective superiors in England and Ireland for direction in the manner of their religious duty, it will be requisite that one of their number be appointed by competent authority in this country, to act as Superior in this respect while they are employed abroad. The Superintendent of the Nurses will communicate with them through their Superior; and in the event of any of them being judged by the Superintendent incompetent to fulfil the duties of nursing, the Superior will at once intimate to her the cessation of her employment in the Hospital.

If the Superior, on her part, should find it necessary that any of their number should return to England, the Superintendent will arrange for her passage home.

3. As no one will be admitted as a nurse in the Hospitals without the sanction of the Government, those who accompany the Superintendent from England, will receive their approval from her; and any Sisters who may hereafter be sent will be approved as nurses by Dr. Andrew Smith, if they are in London; or by a Medical Officer appointed by him in the neighborhood of their residence if they are out of London.

4. The greatest caution being necessary on all hands, in the matter of religion, the Sisters of Mercy will hold themselves free to introduce such subjects only with patients of their own faith.

I have already mentioned that the Sisters now proceeding through France with Miss Nightingale have been taken from the Convent of Mercy under my charge, and as the Sisters of other Houses who may be required will be presented by their respective Superiors, I have endeavoured in this short space of time to communicate with them, and from the answers received, I have every reason to believe that they will fully acquiesce in these conditions.

Signed ✠ Thomas Grant.

. . . .

October 20, 1854.

Dear Reverend Mother,—Since you started things have advanced very rapidly. When the Government saw the zeal of the Sisters, they resolved to encourage the work, and they found at the same time that many nurses would be required for the sick, who are beyond two thousand. For this purpose they selected Miss Nightingale as Superintendent of the nurses and they enquired whether the Sisters would co-operate with her. Knowing that in the work-houses, etc., we are obliged to work under the superintendence of matrons and other officials, I replied, that there would be no difficulty, provided the Sisters were free as nuns to act under their own Superior. Of course as nurses the Sisters have no objection to be distributed by her over the wards (two nuns at least being always together, although not necessarily both of the same Institute, e. g., you might allow one of your Sisters to be with a Sister of Charity). If the Superintendent wishes to communicate with the nuns they are to receive the orders from their Superior. As nuns of various orders will be together, the Archbishop of Westminster will name one of the whole number to act as general Superior, but of course in ordinary matters you will guide your own nuns. I hope you will understand that I give you full power to act for the best, and to dispense them from fastings and abstinence and all other duties you may judge fit till they return home. You will have many opportunities of learning and practising mortification.

Your Sisters must learn to nurse, bandage wounds, dress them, and do all that you are accustomed to do for the poor in sickness. But you will submit to all these trials for the love of Our Dear Lord.

As to money matters, Miss Nightingale will pay all travelling expenses from Paris, and will give you the usual allowance in Turkey,[17] and if any of the Sisters come home before the others, she will find a passage for them.

I wish you to have 50*l.* for any little comforts you may wish to procure for the Sisters after you leave Paris, and whilst you are away. I wish you likewise to charge me, in addition to the 50*l.* with all your expenses for clothing, journey to Paris, and stay there; and when you are leaving and have seen Miss Nightingale (who will call on you perhaps before you receive this letter) you may leave the rest of the money with Mr. Goldsmid. But take as much as you need of it, even beyond the 50*l.* and do not pay any to Mr. Goldsmid until you have ascertained that Miss Nightingale will pay passage, etc. The Government gives her means to do it, and you may take all you can get without scruple.

I hope you will understand this money business. Government has under-taken to pay for you from Paris onwards, and you may talk quite freely to Miss Nightingale about every arrangement, and after you have assured yourself that all your wants will be cared for, keep *at least* 50*l.* for comforts (such as fire in winter, etc.), and keep more if you see you are likely to require it. I wish I could get to Paris before you start, but it is not possible, and therefore I must commend you and your four companions to our dear Mother. You must ask Her to make you good nurses. . . . Tell the Sisters to throw their will into the work, and not be afraid of wounds and death, and to help the sick in every way. You will disarm prejudice by your zeal and charity, and you will help many to die in peace. *Do not introduce religion to any but Catholics,* but if others speak do not be afraid to answer. When you can, suggest an act to the dying of Contrition, Faith, etc. But avoid beginning the subject of controversy to those who are not dying, *unless they are Catholics;* to whom speak quite freely always. The regulations of Miss Nightingale specify that you are not to introduce religion to any but Catholics. Mind, nurse well and efficiently, and encourage one another. Write when you can. God bless you all.

Yours very respectfully,
✠ Thomas Grant.

November 19, 1855.

I cannot express to you, dear Reverend Mother, the gratitude which I and the whole country feel to you for your goodness. You have been one of our chief main-stays, and without you, I do not know what would have become of the work. With love to all my sisters, believe me, dear Reverend Mother,

Ever yours affectionately and gratefully,
Florence Nightingale.[18]

195. Two articles in the *Illustrated London News*

[These articles are but two of the many which appeared in English periodicals and newspapers during Miss Nightingale's period of service in the war hospitals. They describe her activities at that time.]

[*Illustrated London News,* November 4, 1854.]

The Nurses for the East

On Thursday week the Folkstone Steamer carried, amongst other passengers, thirty-seven of the nurses attached to Miss Nightingale's staff. They were accompanied by Mr. and Mrs. Bainbridge [sic], a clergyman, and a courier, who will see them safely landed at Constantinople. The authorities at Boulogne had received orders to pay every attention to them, and the news of their arrival having spread, a crowd had assembled to welcome the self-devoted band, and bid them "God Speed!" on their mission of charity. Mr. Hamilton, the English consul, was in attendance to receive them and conduct them to the Hotel des Bains, where a good dinner had been prepared for them.

On the Friday following Miss Nightingale and the thirty-seven nurses who accompanied her sailed, from Marseilles, in the *Vectis* Steamer, for Constantinople. Throughout the whole of their journey through France they were everywhere received with demonstrations of sympathy and respect. The *Semaphore* of Marseilles, pays them the following compliment:—

Miss Nightingale possesses all that could render existence happy and brilliant. Young, handsome and wealthy, she has chosen a life of abnegation and self denial, and, after having presided over one of those institutions in London of which the idea was suggested by a true spirit of Christianity, her feelings of charity still more excited by the details of the sufferings of the sick and wounded soldiers in the hospital of Scutari, she has chosen a new sphere of action a place where glory is purchased by the severest privations. Nothing could deter her, and at this moment the *Vectis* is conveying her to the East. She and her companions will find there their field of battle in the hospital wards and ambulances, where their sex so well qualifies them to fill a dangerous though heroic position. Captain Powell, the commander of the *Vectis*, received these ladies with perfect courtesy, the officers and crew vied with each other in their attention in conducting them to the places reserved for them with all the respect due to their sex and their affecting mission.

[*Illustrated London News,* February 24, 1855.]

Miss Nightingale

Although the public have been presented with several portrait-sketches of the lady who has so generously left this country to attend to the sufferings of the sick and wounded at Constantinople, we have assurance that these pictures are "singularly and painfully unlike." We have, therefore, taken the most direct means of obtaining a sketch of this excellent lady, in the dress she now wears, in one of "the corridors of the sick," in the Hospital at Scutari. A recent letter in the Times bears the following testimony to the humane services of Miss Nightingale:—

Wherever there is disease in its most dangerous form, and the hand of the spoiler distressingly nigh, there is that incomparable woman sure to be seen; her benignant presence is an influence for good comfort even amid the struggles of expiring nature. She is a "ministering angel" without any exaggeration in these hospitals, and, as her slender form glides quietly along each corridor, every poor fellow's face softens with gratitude at the sight of her. When all the medical officers have retired for the night, and silence and darkness have settled down upon those miles of prostrate sick, she may be observed alone, with a little lamp in her hand, making her solitary rounds. The popular instinct was not mistaken, which, when she set out from England on her mission of mercy, hailed her as a heroine; I trust that she may not earn her title to a higher though sadder appellation. No one who observed her fragile and delicate health can avoid misgivings lest these should fail. With the heart of a true woman, and the manners of a lady, accomplished and refined beyond most of her sex, she combines a surprising calmness of judgment and promptitude and decision of character. I have hesitated to speak of her hitherto as she deserves, because I well know that no praise of mine could do justice to her merits while it might have tended to embarrass the frankness with which she has always accepted the aid furnished her through the Fund. As that source of supply is now nearly exhausted, and my mission approaches its close, I can express myself with more freedom on this subject; and I confidently assert, that but for Miss Nightingale the people of England would scarcely, with all their solicitude, have been spared the additional pang of knowing, which they must have done sooner or later, that their soldiers, even in hospital, had found scanty refuge and relief from the unparalleled miseries with which this war has hitherto been attended.

196. *London Times,* October 30, 1854

[The following article, calling Miss Nightingale "Mrs." Nightingale, is expressed in euphuistic language, as judged by today's standards. It reflects the emotion which was associated with Miss Nightingale's name in England at the time of the Crimean War.]

Who is Mrs. Nightingale?
(From the Examiner.)

Many ask this question, and it has not yet been adequately answered. We reply, then, Mrs. Nightingale is Miss Nightingale, or rather Miss Florence Nightingale, the youngest daughter and presumptive co-heiress of her father, William Shore Nightingale, of Embley-park, Hampshire, and the Lea Hurst, Derbyshire. She is, moreover, a young lady of singular endowments both natural and acquired. In a knowledge of the ancient languages and of the higher branches of mathematics, in general art, science, and literature, her attainments are extraordinary. There is scarcely a modern language which she does not understand, and she speaks French, German, and Italian as fluently as her native English. She has visited and studied the various nations of Europe, and has ascended the Nile to its remotest cataract. Young (about the age of our Queen), graceful, feminine, rich, and popular, she holds a singularly gentle and persuasive influence over all with whom she comes in contact. Her friends and acquaintances are of all classes and persuasions, but her happiest place is at home, in the centre of a very large band of ac-complished relatives, and in simplest obedience to her admiring parents.

Why, then, should a being so highly blessed with all that should render life bright, innocent, and to a considerable extent useful, forego such palpable and heartfelt attractions? Why quit all this to become—a nurse? From her infancy she has had a yearning affection for her kind—a sympathy with the weak, the oppressed, the destitute, the suffering, and the desolate. The schools and the poor around Lea Hurst and Embley first saw and felt her as a visitor, teacher, consoler, expounder. Then she frequented and studied the schools, hospitals, and reformatory institutions of London, Edinburgh, and the continent. Three years ago when all of Europe had a holy day on and after the Great Exhibition, when the highlands of Scotland, the lakes of Switzerland, and all the bright spots of the continent were filled with parties of pleasure, Miss Nightingale was within the walls of one of the German houses or hospitals for the care or the reformation of the lost and infirm. For three long months she was in daily and nightly attendance, accumulating experience in all the duties and labours of female ministration. She then returned to be once more the delight of her own happy home. But the strong tendency of her mind to look beyond its own circle for the relief of those who nominally having all practically have but too frequently none to help them prevailed; and therefore, when the hospital established in London for sick governesses was about to fail for want of proper management she stepped forward and consented to be placed at its head. Derbyshire and Hampshire were exchanged for the narrow, dreary establishment in Harley-street, to which she devoted all her time and fortune, while her friends missed her at assemblies, lectures, concerts, exhibitions, and all the entertainments for taste and intellect with which London in its season abounds, she, whose powers could have best appreciated these, was sitting beside the bed and soothing the last complaints of some poor dying, homeless, querulous governess. The homelessness might not improbably, indeed, result from that very querulousness; but this is too frequently fomented, if not created, by the hard, unreflecting folly which regards fellow-creatures intrusted with forming the minds and dispositions of its children as ingenious, disagreeable machines, needing, like the steam-engine, sustenance and covering, but, like it, quite beyond or beneath all sympathy, passions, or affections. Miss Nightingale thought otherwise, and found pleasure in tending those poor destitute governesses in their infirmities, their sorrows, their deaths, or their recoveries. She was seldom seen out of the walls of the institution, and the few friends whom she admitted found her in the midst of nurses, letters, prescriptions, accounts, and interruptions. Her health sank under the heavy pressure, but a little Hampshire fresh air restored her, and the failing institution was saved.

Meanwhile a cry of distress for additional comforts beyond those of mere hospital treatment came home from the East from our wounded brethren in arms. There instantly arose an enthusiastic desire to answer it. But inexperienced zeal could perform little, and a bevy of ill-organized nurses might do more harm than good. There was a fear lest a noble impulse should fail for the want of a head, a hand, and a heart to direct it. It was then that a field was opened for the wider exercise of Miss Nightingale's sympathies, experience, and powers of command and control. But at what cost? At the risk of her own life—at the pang of separation from all her friends and family, and at the certainty of encountering hardship, dangers, toils, and the constantly renewing scene of human suffering, amid all the worst horrors of war. There are few who would not recoil from such realities, but Miss Nightingale shrank not, and at once accepted the request that was made her to form and control the entire nursing establishment for our sick and wounded soldiers and sailors in the Levant. While we write, this deliberate, sensitive, and highly-endowed young lady is already at her post, rendering the holiest of woman's charities to the sick, the dying, and the convalescent. There is a heroism in dashing up the heights of Alma in defiance of death and all mortal opposition, and let all praise and honour be, as they are, bestowed upon it; but there is a quiet forecasting heroism and largeness of heart in this lady's resolute accumulation of the powers of consolation, and her devoted application of them, which rank as high, and are at least as pure. A safe few will no doubt condemn, sneer at, or pity an enthusiasm which to them seems eccentric or at best misplaced; but to the true heart of the country it will speak home, and be there felt, that there is not one of England's proudest and purest daughters who at this moment stands on so high a pinnacle as Florence Nightingale.

197. Letter of Mr. Bracebridge to Sidney Herbert

[Charles H. Bracebridge (d. 1872) and his wife, Selina Mills Bracebridge (d. 1874), were friends of the Sidney Herberts, and Florence Nightingale made their acquaintance in Rome. They became her devoted friends, and together they explored the beauties of Rome and the antiquities of Egypt. The Bracebridges accompanied Miss Nightingale to the Crimea, and were credited by her with doing much to assist her in her work there.[19] Sidney Herbert (1810–1861), Lord Herbert of Lea, was educated at Harrow and at Oxford. He entered the House of Commons and held minor offices before being appointed Secretary at War in 1845, and again in 1852–1855. He was the leader of the movement for reform of the War Office after the Crimean War.[20] The following letter was written from the scene of the War.]

November 8th [1854].

We have one sitting-room with divans, where I and the courier sleep; a small room for Mrs. B. and Miss N. one room for thirteen nurses, one room for eight sisters, and one room for ten R. C. Sisters . . .

We have been well received by the doctors and Commandant; the orders for us were received by the preceding mail.

The Barrack Hospital is a quadrangle of 500 by 200 paces inside, arcades and corridors all round within, glazed; and rooms behind them to the external walls. A huge kitchen and offices in the centre; the building three stories high in some places, two in others. The General Hospital is on the same plan, but much smaller.

The great corridor, 450 yards long, and four rooms holding 27 each, have been filled with beds and men in double rows, leaving 4 feet to walk in the middle. This was done from 12 o'clock to 6 o'clock today. They were all dressed and fed by 8 o'clock. Miss N. and all her staff assisted. The sisters washed and dressed the wounds . . .

Dr. Cumming has given up his private kitchen to Miss N. for her nurses. She began yesterday, after a day's arrangement with Dr. Cumming,

Menzies, and MacGregor. She went from ward to ward, with nine nurses, and after dressing 62 people after the surgeon, she placed them two and two along wards. To-day a number of bad cases are given to them. In several days they will all be distributed.

Miss N. is decidedly well received . . .

Miss N. is organising a separate kitchen for her people to have charge of, making and giving delicacies, etc. No doubt many have been lost for want of nourishment, not being able to eat the food they get; they tire of boiled food cooked in great coppers, and the officers complain more than the men . . .

The arrival of Miss N. and her staff has put new life in the hospital . . .

In case of sending out other nurses it is easy. Our expenses were by Marseilles £307, not including passages in the *Vectis* . . .

Ever Yours,

C. Bracebridge.[21]

198.   Letter of Richard Monckton Milnes to His Wife

[Richard Monckton Milnes (1809–1885), first Lord Houghton, English writer, philanthropist, and patron of letters, was educated at Trinity College, Cambridge. He was active in politics and counted among his friends Tennyson, Thackeray, Hallam, Swinburne, Carlyle, Charlotte Brontë, Elizabeth Gaskell, Macaulay, the Nightingales, and many other well-known personalities.[22] He wrote the first published life of Keats, reckoned by many to be one of the best. He married the Honorable Annabel Crewe. In his early life he asked Florence Nightingale to become his wife.[23] The following letter, written during one of Lord Houghton's absences from home, begins with a reference to parliamentary affairs and ends with one to the attitude of the soldiers toward Florence Nightingale.]

Upper Brook St., Friday

[January, 1855]

I write this in the morning, and will write to my father from the House if there is anything of interest. Lord John's withdrawal was as much a surprise as a harlequin going through a window. If it means that he wishes to be free at the break-up, and therefore, all ready to head a new Government, I do not think it will succeed. I hope Stafford will speak tonight or Monday; he is only too full of interesting matter. He says Florence in the Hospital quite makes intelligible to him the saints of the Middle Ages. If the soldiers were told that the roof had opened, and she had gone up palpably to heaven, they would not be the least surprised. They quite believe she is in several places at once . . .[24]

199.   Letter of Lady Bithynia Hornby to "Julia"

[Lady Hornby was the wife of Sir Edmund Grimani Hornby, British Commissioner to Turkey during the Crimean War. Sir Edmund was one

of those who worked out the idea of the Hague Tribunal. While judge
of the British Court at Constantinople in 1865, he was appointed the
first judge of the British Supreme Court for China and Japan at Shanghai.[25] The following impression of Miss Nightingale's personal appearance was gained while Lady Hornby was attending a Christmas dinner
at the British Embassy in Constantinople in 1855.]

Orta-Kioy, January 5th, 1856.

My dear Julia . . .

But by-and-by the drawing room doors are thrown open, and the ambas-
sadress enters, smiling a kind and gracious welcome. Behind her are her
daughters; by her side, a tall, fashionable, haughty beauty. I could not help
thinking how beautiful she looked; but the next instant my eyes wandered
from her cold unamiable face to a lady modestly standing on the other side of
Lady Stratford. At first I thought she was a nun, from her black dress and
close cap. She was not introduced, and yet Edmund and I looked at each
other at the same moment to whisper, "It is Miss Nightingale!" Yes, it was
Florence Nightingale, greatest of all now in name and honor among women.
I assure you that I was glad not to be obliged to speak just then, for I felt
quite dumb as I looked at her wasted figure and the short brown hair combed
over her forehead like a child's, cut so when her life was despaired of from
fever but a short time ago. Her dress, as I have said, was black, made high
in the throat, its only ornament being a large enameled broach, which
looked to me like the colors of a regiment surmounted with a wreath of
laurel, no doubt some grateful offering from our men. To hide the close white
cap a little she had tied a white crepe handkerchief over the back of it, only
allowing the border of lace to be seen; and this gave the nunlike appearance
which first struck me on her entering the room, otherwise Miss Nightingale
is by no means striking in appearance. Only her plain black dress, quiet
manner, and great renown, told so powerfully altogether in that assembly of
brilliant dress and uniforms. She is very slight, rather above the middle
height, her face is long and thin, but this may be from recent illness and
great fatigue. She has a very prominent nose, slightly Roman; and small dark
eyes, kind, yet penetrating; but her face does not give you at all the idea of
great talent. She looks a quiet, persevering, orderly, lady-like woman. I have
done my best to give you a true pen-and-ink portrait of this celebrated lady.
I suppose there is a hum all over the world of "What is she like?" [26]

200. Rev. & Hon. Sydney Godolphin Osborne. *Scutari and Its Hospitals*

[Lord Sydney Godolphin Osborne (1808–1899), British philanthropist, was known chiefly in connection with a series of "lay sermons"
which were delivered from the "pulpit" of the *London Times,* under the
signature of "SGO." His philanthropy was of a militant type, inasmuch
as he was always looking for abuses and provoking controversy. He

went to Scutari voluntarily and was publicly thanked by Parliament for his work there.[27] Mr. Osborne championed the cause of Florence Nightingale in her efforts to reform the Scutari hospitals. Portions of the following are quoted in Cook's *The Life of Florence Nightingale*.]

I must now conduct my readers to another part of the Barrack Hospital, and one most interesting. On entering by the gate at the "main guard," turning directly to the left, at a short distance there is a wooden partition across a corridor; passing through the door in this you come to one of the usual lanes hedged in by the beds of the wounded; at its further extremity is the tower, in which the "sisters" have their "quarters." Whatever of neglect may attach elsewhere, none can be imputed here. From this tower flowed that well directed stream of untiring benevolence and charitable exertion, which has been deservedly the theme of so much praise. Here there has been no idleness, no standing still, no waiting for orders from home, no quibbling with any requisition made upon those, who so cheerfully administered the stores at their disposal.

Entering the door leading into the "sisters" tower, you at once found yourself a spectator of a busy and most interesting scene. There is a large room, with two or three doors opening from it on one side; on the other, one door opening into an apartment in which many of the Nurses and Sisters slept, and had I believe their meals. In the centre was a large kitchen table; bustling about this, might be seen the High Priestess of the room Mrs. C———; often as I have had occasion to pass through this room, I do not ever recollect finding her either absent from it, or unoccupied.

At this table she received the various matters from the kitchen and stores of the Sisterhood, which attendant Sisters or Nurses were ever ready to take to the sick in any and every part of these gigantic hospitals. It was a curious scene, and a close study of it affords a practical lesson in the working of true common sense benevolence. There were constant fresh arrivals of various matters ready for immediate distribution, or for preparation for it; there was also as frequent an arrival of requisitions for some of the many good things, over which Mrs. C——— presided with untiring perseverance.

The floor on one side of the room, was loaded with packages of all kinds, stores of things for internal and external consumption of the patients; bales of shirts, socks, slippers, dressing gowns, flannel; heaps of every sort of article, likely to be of use in affording comfort and securing cleanliness. . . . On the right hand side of the room, were doors leading to the private room of Miss Nightingale, and to the dormitories of the Nuns, and their Reverend Mother, a lady of whom all spoke in the highest terms.

In the further corner on the right hand side, was the entrance to the sitting room occupied by Miss Nightingale and her friends the Bracebridges. I shall ever recall with the liveliest satisfaction, the many visits I paid to this apartment. Here were held those councils over which Miss Nightingale so ably presided, at which were discussed the measures necessary to meet the daily varying exigencies of the hospitals. From hence were given the orders which regulated the female staff, working under this most gifted Head. This too was the office from which were sent those many letters to the government, to friends and supporters at home, which told such awful tales of sufferings of the sick and wounded, their utter want of so many necessaries. Here might be seen the "Times" almoner, taking down in his note book from day to day, the list of things he was pressed to obtain, which might all with a little activity have been provided as easily by the authorities of the hospital.

My readers will very naturally expect that I should give them some particulars regarding this lady [Miss Nightingale]. I can only give the result of my own observation and experience; for on such a matter, I should be sorry to draw for my information from other sources. Miss Nightingale in appearance, is just what you would expect in any other well-bred woman, who may have seen perhaps rather more than thirty years of life; her manner and countenance are prepossessing, and this without the possession of positive beauty; it is a face not easily forgotten, pleasing in its smile, with an eye betokening great self-possession, and giving when she wishes, a quiet look of firm determination to every feature. Her general demeanour is quiet and rather reserved; still I am much mistaken if she is not gifted with a very lively sense of the ridiculous. In conversation, she speaks on matters of business with a grave earnestness, one would not expect from her appearance. She has evidently a mind disciplined to restrain under the principles of the action of the moment, every feeling which would interfere with it. She has trained herself to command, and learned the value of conciliation towards others, and constraint over herself. I can conceive her to be a strict disciplinarian; she throws herself into a work—as it's Head—as such she knows well how much success must depend upon literal obedience to her every order. She seems to understand business thoroughly, though to me she had the failure common to many "heads," a too great love of management in the small details which had better perhaps have been left to others. Her nerve is wonderful; I have been with her at very severe operations; she was more than equal to the trial. She has an utter disregard of contagion; I have known her spend hours over men dying of cholera or fever. The more awful to every sense any particular case, especially if it was that of a dying man, her slight form would be seen bending over him, administering to his ease in every way in her power, and seldom quitting his side till death released him.

I have heard and read with indignation, the remarks hazarded upon her religious character. I found her myself to be in her every word and action a Christian; I thought this quite enough. It would have been in my opinion the most cruel impertinence, to scrutinize her words and acts, to discover to which of the many bodies of true Christians she belonged. I have conversed with her several times on the deaths of those, who I had visited ministerially in the hospitals, with whom she had been when they died. I never heard one word from her lips, that would not have been just what I should have expected from the lips of those who I have known to be the most experienced and devout of our common faith. Her work ought to answer for her faith; at least none should dare to call that faith in question, in opposition to such work, on grounds so weak and trivial as those I have seen urged. That she has been equally kind and attentive to men of every creed; that she would smooth the pillow and give water to a dying fellow creature who might own no creed, I have no doubt; all honour to her that she does feel, that her's is the Samaritan's—not the Pharisee's work. If there is blame in looking for a Roman Catholic priest to attend a dying Romanist, let me share it with her— I did it again and again . . .

We all did what we could . . . but this was a hospital, Miss Nightingale and her staff were nurses, cooks, purveyors; they were not, they could not be but in a very minor degree—missionaries . . .

I do not think it is possible to measure the real difficulties of the work Miss Nightingale has done, and is doing, by the mere magnitude of the field, and its peculiarly horrible nature. Every day brought some new complication of misery, to be somehow unravelled by the power ruling in the Sisters' tower. . . . Her's was a post requiring the courage of a Cardigan, the tact and diplomacy of a Palmerston, the endurance of a Howard, the cheerful philanthropy of a Mrs. Fry or a Miss Neave; Miss Nightingale yet fills that post, and in my opinion is the one individual, who in this whole unhappy war, has shown more than any other, what real energy guided by good sense can do, to meet the calls of sudden emergency.

There must have been when I left Scutari little less than four miles of ground occupied in lines of beds; the reader may from this conceive the pressure upon the physical and mental powers of the sisters. That many of them proved unequal to the work was to be expected; the wonder to me is, how any have survived it. Many ought never to have entered upon it . . .

In my own opinion it would be most advisable that the hired professional nurses, should wear some dress distinguishing them from the sisters. There are many offices about the sick and wounded which the surgeons would at once require, and with reason, of a hired hospital nurse, which nothing could induce them to ask of a "sister." I am also quite satisfied that this is no field of usefulness proper for young English women. . . . I have little doubt but the majority would agree with me, that very much of it had been better left, had it been possible, to trained paid nurses; and that there would have still remained a large field of more fitting usefulness for the zeal of unpaid volunteers.

.   .   .   .

They [the sick and wounded officers in the hospital] most of them had their own servants, and the means of procuring any extra comforts of which they stood in need . . .

As nurses to each other, no sister or mother could have been more kind and patient.[28]

201. Peter Pincoffs. *Experiences of a Civilian in Eastern Military Hospitals*

[Peter Pincoffs, M.D., was civil physician to the Scutari hospitals during the Crimean War. He held membership and many honors in the British Medical Association as well as in medical and philosophical societies of other countries.[29]]

And now I must speak of her who was emphatically the providence of this Barrack-Hospital, whose ministry brought comfort to the sick and consolation to the dying, whose energy and self-devotion compassed miracles in times of fearful woe and calamity, as evidenced by the testimony of those who shared her labors at the outset, and whose untiring patience under difficulties of no common order, whose open-handed benevolence, extended alike to all the suffering, without regard either to country or religion, and whose invaluable support to the medical officer in carrying out any plan for the benefit of the patients and the alleviation of their sufferings, it was my own lot to witness during many months subsequent to the eventful period, when she of whom I speak first landed on the Asiatic shore, strong in the holy purpose of fulfilling her vocation.

The great secret of FLORENCE NIGHTINGALE'S success in the noble task she undertook lay in her perfect training for the duties which it entailed. Her enthusiasm for the self-sacrificing calling of a nurse was not the hot-bed production of the harrowing accounts of the "Times' correspondent," the premature birth of the excitement which then prevailed in England, it was the steady growth and full development of years of patient preparatory initiation. She had gone on "from strength to strength," had fed long on "the milk of babes" and was "able to bear the strong meat" which now became her portion. No doubt that many emergencies did occur she never could have calculated upon and that her strong natural intellect and talent for administration carried her through such triumphantly, but the groundwork was there, she had experience of hospitals, was inured to sights and sounds with which most females in her sphere of life are unacquainted, and was practically *au fait* in the art of nursing, and above all, had from early youth had the one object of hospital regeneration ever in view and the whole faculties of a mind of no common order had been brought to bear on this one subject. Her exclusive leaning in this direction was at first discountenanced by her parents, but she was not to be dissuaded from following her vocation, and gently and steadily she pursued the object of which she never lost sight.

．　　．　　．　　．　　．　　．　　．

It was not my privilege to be a witness of Miss Nightingale's personal efforts as a nurse at the time when our hospitals were overcrowded with sick and wounded, but I can from personal experience testify that she never spared herself when unusual pressure did arise. She was in the Crimea at the time of the sudden alarming outbreak of cholera in the Barrack-Hospital in Nov. 1855. Directly the news reached her, she hurried back to Scutari and in those cholera wards resumed her useful labors with her accustomed activity; I believe that there never was a severe case of any kind that escaped her notice, and some times it was wonderful to see her at the bed-side of a patient who had been admitted perhaps but an hour before, and of whose arrival one would hardly have supposed it possible she could already be cognizant.

Her assistance was invaluable to those medical men who desired to procure any extra comfort for their patients; from her kitchen the dainty pudding was never withheld, a warming-bottle, a hip-bath, an air-pillow, an easy chair—freed from the vexatious operation of signed and counter-signed requisitions—were obtainable from her store, books and games were supplied by her to cheer the dull hours of convalescence. The men knew from what source their comforts flowed and appreciated her kindness.

Many devoted females shared her labors, and greatly to be honored is that company of educated women who with her voluntarily exchanged the comforts and refinements of home for the dangers and privations they were sure to encounter in a military hospital. Here as every where the Catholic Sisters of Mercy did their duty bravely and well, under the superintending direction of their worthy Rev^d. Mother.

There could be no better nurses than a few of the old orderlies employed in our hospitals; they were however few and far between; the great failing was that, not forming a separate corps, they were constantly sent back to their regiments whenever required there, regardless whether they were good nurses or not; this was also the case for any offence (drunkenness being the most common reason), and not having the same inducements to remain in the hospital as the French *infirmiers,* they also frequently preferred returning to active duty; the consequence was that there was a constant moving and shifting of orderlies, and that an orderly whom a medical officer had just begun to teach his duties would be superceded by a raw recruit, who might perhaps (for such a case has been heard of) administer a poultice to a patient as a medicine.[30]

202. L. Dunne. *A Trip to Constantinople . . . and Miss Nightingale at Scutari Hospital*

[The author of this book was Foreman of Her Majesty's Stores at the Bosporus during the Crimean War.[31]]

I will now call your attention to a large building situate on the banks of the Bosporus and Sea of Marmora, which, although separated from Constantinople by the bay of the Golden Horn, being on a very elevated position is quite visible. This remarkable building, to which I wish to call your attention, is Scutari Hospital.

.   .   .   .

After remaining as long as my nerves would permit me to witness such a scene [watching the landing of the wounded from a ship], I directed my course towards the hospital, where on arriving I perceived mattresses and other substitutes for beds being hastily arranged in the corridors and every available place. On inquiry I ascertained that, in consequence of the crowded state of the hospital, Miss Nightingale had to resort to this mode of securing accomodation and comfort for the cargo of wounded and dying soldiers which was then being landed.

Hearing so much of Miss Nightingale and her noble deeds, I felt anxious to see what kind of person she was. On my way towards the kitchen of the hospital, where informed I was most likely to see her, I met three or four ladies whose mein and costume signified they belonged to some religious order; they had in their hands bandages, bottles, lint, and other necessaries, and were hurrying so hastily in the direction of the principal entrance to the hospital that I afterwards was sorry I accosted them; but fearing I had lost my way to the kitchen, I merely inquired if I was in the right direction, when one of them, as she continued almost running, replied, "That is the way, Sir, but Miss Nightingale cannot, will not, see anyone to-day except on business immediately connected with the last arrival of poor soldiers." Before I had time to inform her that I did not require or expect to have an interview with Miss Nightingale, she disappeared in one of the narrow windings of the long corridor. A little further on I met several groups of ladies hurrying in the same direction, and carrying with them all kinds of necessaries. I next met a convalescent soldier, from whom I ascertained that the ladies I first met were Sisters of Mercy, and, under Miss Nightingale's instructions, were hurrying with necessaries for the soldiers as they were carried into hospital. With the efficient aid rendered by the medical staff, in conjunction with Miss Nightingale and her noble band, this cargo of wounded and dying soldiers was attended to in that prompt and kind manner which it would be almost impossible to expect.

While the convalescent soldier and I were conversing, several groups of ladies passed and re-passed. Presently the commander of this devoted band followed, when her appearance as she hastened through the long corridor was the signal for salutes from sentinels; and although she did not seek such attention, still those who admired her could not confine their respectful feelings. No general or commander, be he ever so brave, would be received with half the voluntary pomp or honour which every grade of soldier would bestow on that unexampled lady ...

... those ladies who, also at the risk of their lives, attended to the every want of the wounded and dying, and who night or day were never absent from their post of duty, saw no golden prospect glitter in the future. ... Woman alone could successfully perform such patient and tender duties. ...

In the midst of these awful scenes of the dead and the dying, you might behold a tall, pensive-looking lady, whose expression of countenance indicated the anxiety she felt for those under her care. You might also behold other ladies seeking her for council, among whom were many who, whatever opinion some people may entertain as to their selection of a secluded religious life, they in time of need proved themselves true samaritans. I need scarcely remind you that this tall, pensive-looking lady (whose appearance among the wounded and dying soldiers was the signal for acclamation, as well as the medium of inspiring in the most despondent bosom a feeling of hope) was Miss Florence Nightingale, without whose efficient aid and kind attention not half the invalid soldiers who returned to England would have again beheld it. The prompt manner in which they were attended to under her instructions, as well as the cheerfulness and cleanliness by which they were surrounded, tended in a great measure to render them more quickly convalescent, and enabled more speedily to rejoin their regiments.[32]

203. Letter of Sir Sidney Herbert to Florence Nightingale

[This letter is of importance as explaining Mr. Herbert's views regarding the second corps of nurses sent by the government to the East. The group went out under the leadership of Mary Stanley, and their arrival caused serious practical difficulties in the situation at Scutari.[33]]

Belgrade Square, *March 5th, 1855.*

My dear Miss Nightingale,

You will long before this have seen that I am out of office altogether. I have, however, been to Panmure, and had a long talk with him, of which I will give you the result. But first I must say one or two things in explanation of matters in which I think you have been deceived or too much importance has been attached to small details which were not meant to be indications of anything. For example, as regards the latter, there is no doubt that the unwelcome batch of nurses were meant to be under your authority, and the consignment to Dr. Cumming probably arose, for I do not recollect the circumstances, for the same course being pursued with regard to the second batch as had been adopted with the first, who naturally were consigned to Cumming. At that time, moreover, these new additional and distant hospitals did not exist, and all were expected to work with and under you . . .

Liz will send you the six women. She has them all ready. The Edinburgh ones (there are no Glasgow ones) are in London. They are three in number, and Presbyterians. More were offered, but were not eligible. One nurse is ready from Devonshire Square, and two others from different parts of the country. They are all well recommended, but from all she has seen of paid nurses she has no confidence in any of them as to drinking, though nothing can exceed the testimonials these have got. They will be sent to you in a week's time.

The Smyrna Civil Hospital Staff have taken out forty nurses—half, paid nurses, half, ladies and unpaid. Dr. Meyer will after trial, pick out the lady whom he thinks most fitted to act as head at Kulali to succeed Miss Stanley. Liz thinks it will be either Mrs. Munro, Miss Winthrop, or Miss Wear. Miss Winthrop, she thinks, would do admirably. I believe the Smyrna establishment will ultimately move to Mytilene. They are entirely independent, the doctors not being under an Inspector-General, nor even under the Army Medical Board at home. The nurses, of course, independent of you . . .

2ndly. I found that his [Lord Panmure's] wish was to separate the different hospitals, so far as the nursing is concerned, now that there are so many and each so distant from the original establishments at Scutari, which were the only ones in existence when the first arrangements were made. He thinks this multiplication of hospitals at some miles distance makes any real supervision from Scutari impossible, and gives you, therefore, a responsibility without corresponding powers. But he feared to make the change, lest you should think it implied a want of confidence in you, or a want of appreciation of the great services you have rendered and are rendering. Your last letter but one (February 15th) enabled me to say that you had contemplated the possibility of such an arrangement. . . . You will, therefore, carry on your own system at the two hospitals at Scutari, supported by Dr. Cumming . . .

Pray continue to write to me for anything you want, which you don't like to say to others. I will do everything I can, I shall never forget how much I owe you for all you have done.[34]

204. Letters of Mary Stanley

[Mary Stanley (b. 1813) was the eldest daughter of Edward and Catherine Stanley and sister of Arthur Penrhyn Stanley, dean of Westminster. Her father was bishop of Norwich, and Mary aided him in all his philanthropic schemes. Among her early activities were the founding of a home for working girls and a lace school, to prepare herself for which she spent a year learning lacemaking. Miss Stanley offered her services to the government during the Crimean War and was sent at the head of a "second group" of nurses, on which matter the second letter below touches briefly. This group served chiefly at Koulali. After the war, Miss Stanley followed her strong desire to be received into the Roman Catholic Church, and went on with her charitable work.[35] Mrs. Herbert, to whom the first two letters were written, was, before her marriage to Sidney Herbert, Secretary at War during the Crimean War, Elizabeth à Court, daughter of General Charles Ashe à Court.[36]]

[Mary Stanley to Mrs. Herbert.]

Barrack Hospital, *December 21st,*
[1854].

At last we came to the guard-room, another corridor, then through a door into a large busy kitchen, where stood Mrs. Margaret Williams, who seemed much pleased to see me: then a heavy curtain was raised; I went through a door, and there sat dear Flo writing on a small unpainted deal table. I never saw her looking better. She had on her black merino, trimmed with black velvet, clean linen collar and cuffs, apron, white cap with a black handkerchief tied over it; and there was Mrs. Bracebridge, looking so nice, too. I was *quite* satisfied with my welcome. It was settled at once that I was to sleep there, especially as, being post day, Flo could not attend to me till the afternoon . . .

[Mary Stanley to Mrs. Herbert.]

Therapia, *December 24th, [1854]*.

I am now in possession of the whole state of the case, and feel anxious to write to you about it.

Florence showed me a copy of the letter she wrote to Mr. Herbert. I scarcely like to express an opinion to you about this. I can scarcely guess what answer will be sent.

I most *deeply* regret the view taken of the whole affair here. . . . I confess that I have got to be convinced that more nurses are not needed. If the experiment is a failure I concede the point; but if, as I am told here and we heard at home, it is successful, I do not understand why the comfort is to be so limited.

I grant that no one head can be individually responsible for such a number in such a position; but authority may be delegated to inferior heads who may be held responsible for a given number.

Florence requested me formally, in the presence of Dr. Cumming and Mr. Bracebridge, to succeed her at once. I refused this most decidedly, for every reason.

Another proposal she has made to me is to take charge of the General Hospital under her till she is superceded. This I have promised to consider . . .

January 17th, 1855.

She [Miss Emily Anderson] finds the work painfully interesting—such a field for labour, so few hands to do it. Last night I went her evening rounds with her. It is a solemn sight to walk through those corridors by the dim light of the lamps—at intervals stopping at the bedsides of those who were sinking, to feed them with beef-tea or jelly. Such a sad sight to see these fine men in the last stage of disease—some sunk into childishness. Round the stoves were congregated the convalescents, some reading to themselves, some reading aloud. Here and there you heard the men in the adjoining beds talking over their battles or their homes. The very sight of our passing along seemed to cheer them. "Good-night, ladies," was heard from many a bed. Certainly those who have come out to nurse them *do* undergo hardships and privations. I am fifth in the ladies' room. The only apparatus for cooking for the men (beef-tea, etc.) and for ourselves is one small charcoal stove. We have a dirty mat on the floor, three kitchen chairs, one very small tressel table. I am writing sitting on the floor, making a table of one of the trunks.

. . . .

Kulali, January 29th, [1855].

The end of our first day's work has come. The doctors have desired to have two nurses each. There are five doctors. At 10 A.M. we were called; each doctor has 125 or 130 patients. It was half-past one before we all met again in our quarters. To my great relief there were no very bad cases of frost-bite, only six very mild ones. The great majority were extreme weakness. There was nothing whatever disagreeable. As soon as we had dined, I had to go and draw the extra diets—i. e. take the diet roll and go to the store-room and receive all that my 130 patients required; then to make arrowroot and lemonade; then to go round and feed the men the last thing at night, two hours more. The Turkish carpenters were at work on the ante-room and the kitchen; Greek women scouring the floor. You can scarcely imagine the scene of work. The doctors were very grateful and pleasant, and we all met after our rounds in good spirits, feeling that *at last* we had got to work in good earnest. I shall go round the first day or two, and then I shall confine myself to the general direction. We want just double the number to do the present work as it ought to be done; and what are we to do when the number is doubled? The doctors are worn out, and simply say, "With such a diet you may use your own discretion; he must be fed, get down all you can."

. . . .

January 31st [1855].

At eight o'clock I was up mixing arrowroot for the men who require feeding early. I sent another nurse round the wards. I took the two first days. After breakfast I went to the upper hospital to see the rooms Captain Gordon and Major C. said I might have for the nuns. I came back to hear the despair of the doctors at the prospect of three hundred new patients—not a bed up for them, not a kitchen range. Each hour that passed we hoped they would not come, but I desired a wood fire to be lighted, and a cauldron of hot water prepared. At 12 Mr. Sabine and Mr. Macdonald came from Scutari. At 2.30 Lady Stratford came, and then Lord Napier, and then to my horror I saw two great steamers coming up and anchoring under our windows. However, here I am writing at 9 P.M., and none have been landed, I believe. A request was made to send some hands to sew up mattresses. I had to send the poor exhausted nuns, who, when they had done them, had to go their rounds and feed their people. Our own kitchen is scarcely finished yet, and you may imagine what a state of confusion our ante-room continues to be in, what with workpeople and messes of lemonade, arrowroot, beat-up eggs, rice pudding, etc., going on in every room. The doctors say that if the men recover it will be owing to the nurses, but the mortality is very great.

. . . I have written to *implore* Florence to send us some more nurses. . . .

As to writing for the men or reading to them, it has been out of the question, except one case. A poor man implored me to write to his mother, and I have been to him this evening and written . . .[37]

205. [Fanny M. Taylor]. *Eastern Hospitals and English Nurses: the Narrative of Twelve Months' Experience in the Hospitals of Koulali and Scutari*

[Fanny M. Taylor was a member of the second party of nurses taken to the Crimea by Mary Stanley. Her first experience was at Scutari with Miss Nightingale. Later she went to Koulali.[38]]

Two days after my arrival, Miss Nightingale sent for me to go with her round the hospital. (Miss Nightingale generally visited her special cases at night.) We went round the whole of the second story, into many of the wards, and into one of the upper corridors. It seemed an endless walk, and it was one not easily forgotten. As we slowly passed along, the silence was profound; very seldom did a moan or cry from those multitudes of deeply suffering ones fall on our ears. A dim light burned here and there. Miss Nightingale carried her lantern, which she would set down before she bent over any of the patients. I much admired her manner to the men—it was so tender and kind.

All the corridors were thickly lined with beds, laid on low tressels, raised a few inches from the ground. In the wards a divan runs round the room, and on this were laid the straw beds, and the sufferers on them. The hospital was crowded to its fullest extent. The building, which has since been reckoned to hold, with comfort, seventeen hundred men, then held nearly three thousand. Miss Nightingale assigned me my work—it was half of corridor A, the whole of B, half C, the whole of I (on the third story), and all the wards leading out of these corridors; in each corridor there were fifteen wards, except in No. 1, where there were only six. This work I was to share with another lady, and one nurse. The number of patients under our charge was, as far as I could reckon, about one thousand.

Miss Nightingale told us only to attend to those in the divisions belonging to surgeons who wished for our services. She said the staff-surgeon of the division was willing we should work under him, and she charged us never to do anything for the patients without the leave of the doctors.

When we had gone round the hospital, we came out of corridor A upon the main guard. The blast of cold air from the entrance was refreshing, after the overpowering smell of the wards. The corridors of the lower story were under the charge of Miss E———, from Miss Sellon's, assisted by nurses; the remainder of A, under Sister M. S———, of the Bermondsey nuns; corridor H, on the third story, under another nun. Several nurses were engaged in different divisions of corridor C; the rest in the diet kitchen.

Some References to the Life of Florence Nightingale

[In the meantime, Mrs. Taylor was sent to Koulali.]

Before, however, they [a party of nurses] could enter upon their work, it was necessary a Lady Superintendent, in the room of Miss Stanley, should be appointed.... Three days afterwards, Miss Hutton, one of the ladies of the new party, was nominated as Lady Superintendent, by Lord William Paulet.

Before the newly arrived nurses commenced their work, Miss Hutton laid before Dr. Humphrey, the principal medical officer, the rules for our work in the hospital, which had been drawn up by Miss Stanley previous to her departure. They were the following:

1. The nurses in charge of the wards should take care that the orders of the medical officers concerning ventilation are carried out, that everything should be clean and in order, and they should see to the cleanliness of the patients' beds.

2. They should see that the diet and medicine ordered by the medical officers be given at the appointed times, and that all their directions be strictly attended to.

3. The nurses will be in the wards when the surgeons pay their morning visits, in order to receive any directions they may give. They will be ready to wash or dress wounds, change poultices, apply fomentations, & c. as may be required.

4. The strictest attention is to be paid to the orders of the medical officers; nothing is to be given to the patients without their permission.

5. To each ward will be appointed a lady, a Sister of Mercy, and a nurse. The lady and nurse will enter and leave the wards together. They will visit the wards morning, afternoon, and evening, as they are wanted.

6. One lady will undertake the charge of the store room, giving out whatever may be needed to the ladies, sisters, and nurses for their wards. The same lady will also superintend the giving out of the extra diets for the patients.

7. Books shall not be given or lent to the patients by ladies or nurses, unless received for that purpose from the chaplain of the communion in which the patient belongs.

We will now give an account of the routine of our life. When May opened, the sickness and death had considerably abated, and our system had become more organized, and our hours regular. It should here be mentioned that on April the 21st, three ladies and seven nurses from England joined us. Our numbers were therefore twenty-three nurses (including the sick one), ten ladies, and ten Sisters of Mercy. The Sisters, as already mentioned, lived in rooms at the General Hospital.

At the ladies' home we assembled at eight o'clock for prayers, read by our superintendent; then followed breakfast. At nine, when the bell for work rang, we all assembled; each lady called the nurse under her charge to accompany her to her ward, or kitchen, or linen stores (we never allowed the nurses to go out alone, unless under special circumstances); and in five minutes, all the different groups were on their way to the hospital. At two all the ladies and nurses returned home, unless there were patients who could not safely be left altogether to the orderlies' charge; and then the lady, or sister, in whose ward the case was, either stayed herself, or appointed a nurse whom she could trust; but generally speaking, we thought it better on all accounts to be absent from the wards for an hour or two during the day.

At half-past two we dined, the ladies in one room, the nurses in another, with a lady at the head of their table. One of the ladies each week, in rotation, agreed to superintend the meals of the nurses, and sit at the head of the table. At half-past four the bell summoned us to return to the hospital. Some went sooner than this to the kitchen and the linen store. At seven we returned to tea; then one lady—we took it in turns—went out with the nurses for a walk; now and then, for a treat, in caiques, to the sweet waters, or Bebek. At nine, the chaplain of the Church of England came and read part of the Evening Service. Thus ended the work of the day, and after supper we soon retired to our rooms. Of course, such events as the arrival of sick, or extreme sickness in the hospital, would sometimes break the routine. So passed our lives for weeks and months.[39]

206. Sister Mary Aloysius. *Memories of the Crimea*

[Sister Mary Aloysius was one of the Irish Sisters of Mercy who went to the Crimea in Miss Stanley's group.[40]]

One morning, as the Sisters were assembled for morning lecture in the Community Room of the Convent of Mercy, Carlow, the Reverend Mother read the following letter, received by the morning post from the Parent House of the Sisterhood, Baggot Street, Dublin:

My dear Rev. Mother,

The Government has virtually applied for Sisters, and offered to pay their expenses; and as there is no time to be lost, I beg of you to send your candidates on Tuesday or Wednesday, to St. Catherine's and if their services be not required they can return. The eyes of the whole world will be on the poor Nuns. I know you will select those that will give most glory to God. They will want a supply of clothing, etc. Five sisters from Bermondsey have gone to the war as a private charity. Give all the aid you can, and believe me, my dear Rev. Mother, affectionately yours in Jesus Christ.

Sister M. Vincent Whitty,

Superioress . . .

I believe the whole Community offered to go; but only two could be spared, and the two selected were Sister M. Aloysius and Sister Stanislaus, both young and healthy, and well accustomed to attend the sick poor of the town, which they did when cholera had raged a short time previously . . .

Of course, we expected to be sent to the wards at once. Sister M. Agnes and the writer were sent to a store, to sort clothes that had been eaten by the rats; Rev. Mother and Sister M. Elizabeth either to the kitchen or to another store. In a dark, damp, gloomy shed we set to work and did the best we could; but, indeed, the destruction accomplished by the rats was something wonderful. On the woollen goods they had feasted sumptuously. They were running about us in all directions; we begged of the sargeant to leave the door open that we might make our escape if they attacked us. Our home rats would run if you "hushed" them; but you might "hush" away, and the Scutari rats would not take the least notice.

Where shall I begin, or how can I ever describe my first day in the hospital at Scutari? Vessels were arriving, and the orderlies carrying the poor fellows, who, with their wounds and frost-bites, had been tossing about on the Black Sea for two or three days, and sometimes more. Where were they to go? Not an available bed. They were laid on the floor one after another, till the beds were emptied of those dying of cholera and every other disease. Many died immediately after being brought in—their moans would pierce the heart—the taking of them in and out of the vessels must have increased their pain.

The cholera was of the very worst type—the attacked man lasted only four or five hours . . .

The usual remedies ordered by the doctors were stuping and poultices of mustard. They were very anxious to try chloroform, but they did not trust anyone with it except the Sisters. Rev. Mother was a splendid nurse, and had the most perfect way of doing everything. For instance, the stuping seems such a small thing, but if not properly done it did more harm than good. I will give her way. You have a large tub of boiling water, blankets torn in squares, and a piece of canvas with a running at each end to hold a stick. The blankets were put into the boiling water, lifted out with a tongs and put into the canvas, when an orderly at each end wrung the flannel out so dry that not a drop of water remained, before a preparation of choloroform was sprinkled on it, and it was applied to the stomach. Then followed a spoonful of brandy, and immediately after a small piece of ice, to try to settle the stomach, and finally rubbing with mustard, and even with turpentine. Rarely, very rarely, did any remedy succeed; and, as a rule, it was not the weak or delicate who were attacked, but the strong and healthy . . .

Ch. VII. To Balaklava.

Now I come back to Scutari, which was the principal scene of my labours. The cholera continued during the summer months, with less terrible results; but typhus fever broke out in its worst form. Every bed was occupied; I was assisted by a lady, two nurses, and orderlies. Every one knows the nursing that is required in cases of fever. The constitutions of the men were so undermined that they were not able to endure any sickness. Each day we had a number of deaths, and each day others took the dead men's places—

themselves to die. Some kind friends sent out a quantity of aromatic vinegar, of which there was some in the stores also; this was the greatest refreshment the poor patients got. When a little of it was put into water, and they were sponged with it over and over, they used to hold out their poor hands for more. My lady companion in the ward (Miss Smythe) caught the fever and lived only a week. It was hard on these ladies, many of whom, I suppose, had left luxurious homes, and were totally unaccustomed to that kind of work, some of them never having seen a dead man before. They often regretted that they had no experience, and they leaned on us in every difficulty. Sisters of Mercy have a novitiate of four and a-half years, during which they are exercised in various works of mercy; so to them it was no new thing to face disease and death. To live for the Poor had been for many years the resolve of each heart. Trained as we had been, the health and strength of the Sisters withstood the shock under which the health of the ladies sank. No wonder that Miss Nightingale should lean on Mother Mary Clare, of Bermondsey, and her four Sisters, who were with her at the Barrack Hospital.

.   .   .   .   .   .

In passing to the wards at night we used to meet the rats in droves. They would not even move out of our way. They were there before us, and were determined to keep possession. As for our own hut, they evidently wanted to make it theirs, scraping under the boards, jumping up on the shelf where our little tin utensils were kept, rattling everything. One night dear Sister M. Paula found one licking her forehead—she had a real horror of them. Sleep was out of the question . . .

Father Woollett brought us one day a present of a Russian cat; he bought it, he told us, from an old Russian woman, for the small sum of seven shillings. It made a particularly handsome captive in the land of its fathers; for we were obliged to keep it tied to a chair, to prevent its escape. But the very sight of this powerful champion soon relieved us of some of our unwelcome and voracious visitors . . .[41]

207. Margaret Goodman. *Experiences of an English Sister of Mercy*

[Margaret Goodman was a member of Miss Sellon's sisterhood when the Crimean War began.[42] After six years in the order she left it because of the strictness of the conventual rules.[43]]

In the course of the day I received a message from Miss Sellon to inquire if I were willing to go to Constantinople and attend upon the sick and wounded soldiers. It was explained to me that the work was one of peculiar danger, and Miss Sellon would not be surpised if I declined going; but I felt no unwillingness. I had previously heard but little of the war; for in a world such as ours was there are few opportunities of gathering information respecting transactions not intimately connected with it . . .

The same afternoon we proceeded to Belgrade Square, where Miss Nightingale's band assembled to receive an address from Mr. Sidney Herbert. We did not go at once to his residence, but waited in a neighbouring house until summoned; and there I first saw one on whom we were all so much to depend for guidance and support under most trying circumstances—Miss Nightingale.

Mr. Sidney Herbert, in his address, gave the two classes of nurses, Sisters of Mercy and hospital nurses, their respective cautions. To the nuns and sisters he said, "Forbear teaching, and keep yourselves to the objects for which alone Government sends you out; the administering to the bodily wants, and soothing the minds of the sick." Indeed, so careful was Government in this matter of teaching, that both the nuns and the English sisters were called upon to give their word that they would attempt no conversions. Many persons have, since my return, expressed their surprise at our giving such a promise; but I freely confess that I should never think of disturbing a deathbed by bringing controversy to its side.

On leaving Mr. Sidney Herbert's house the committee gave to each of the Devonport Sisters, half in jest, as they passed out, an immense railway rug, which proved a most acceptable gift; being used by turns as a mattress, blanket, shawl, carpet and screen. As the Scottish shepherd does for his plaid, so we conceived a sort of affection for our rugs, which duly returned with their owners. I almost felt jealous when, on coming back to Plymouth, mine passed into the hands of another . . .

The party mustered on Monday, October 21st, at Euston Square, and Mr. ――― took the command; Miss Nightingale having preceded us as far as Paris, to make arrangements for our route. The friends of the poor nurses took leave of them as of those whom they were never to see again. Many of these nurses were widows, with large families, whom they found it a severe struggle to support by their labour in England. They were too well acquainted with disease not to understand the risk they ran from contagion; but they were under the impression that if their children were left orphans, the ladies of England would make them their charge. One woman managed to conceal from the committee that she was a soldier's wife, joined the nursing staff, with the remote prospect of meeting her husband.

After a hurried journey through France, we took ship at Marseilles, in the *Vectis;* a name associated in our minds with discomforts of the most trying description . . .

Our vessel touched at Malta for a few hours. Miss Nightingale, from weakness, was unable to leave the ship, but many of us went on shore under the command of Mr. ―――. This gentleman, being a major in a militia regiment, I suppose it naturally occurred to him that it would be desirable to march the nursing staff in something like military order, about the streets of Malta. The sisters and nuns he concluded were in a higher state of discipline than the nurses, so he placed the sisters in front, to halt and advance at the word of command; while the nuns had charge of the rear. It was well for us that the special correspondent of *Punch* was not with this division of her Majesty's army, or I am afraid that we should have figured in that fun-loving periodical. We all fatigued and distressed Major ———— extremely, but especially the rear; who, after incessant straggling, were finally tempted by the Jesuits to desert their ranks altogether. The remainder of the regiment then commenced a race after them, but when found, they would not return until their own time. The major was dreadfully excited, and they quite imperturbable; he had no subordinate officer, except the courier, who on all occasions was as helpless as the rest of his class. Major ———— would rush towards the front, and shout, "Forward, black sisters!" but when he had fairly started us, came the word, "Halt," and then he condescended to explain reasons: "Those white sisters are gone again, and sometimes he even put a second adjective before "white." The people crowded around us with any-thing but reverence written in their faces; they seemed to think it extremely ludicrous to watch the bustle and anxiety of the captain; and our straggling propensities.

As I have said, the nursing staff reached Scutari the day before the battle of Inkermann; and for about a week after our arrival we were occupied in our several quarters, in making shirts, pillows, slings, & c. We thought this time very long, but at length we were summoned, and distributed each to one or other of the almost countless rooms of that gigantic hospital, to seam up the beds. A coarse wrapper, sewn up like a sack on three sides, was hastily filled with chopped straw; our work was to sew the fourth seam, and thus complete the pallet. The beds were then laid on the floor about a foot apart and the line extending round the apartment, and leaving a small space in the middle. As we laboured, the wounded were arriving from the vessels which brought them from the field of Inkermann . . .

After undoing the bandages, the nurses washed the wounds, thus laying them open for the inspection of the medical officer; when, if the case was of a simple description, the doctor gave directions and the nurse applied the dressings, and again secured the bandages. But for cleansing the wounds it was extremely difficult, in the first place, to procure water, and secondly, any vessel in which to wash them; so the copper basin was again in requisi-tion. It must be understood that those soldiers suffering slightly were attended by orderlies; our time and care were devoted to the extreme cases.

During the day scarcely a sound was heard in the wards or corridors (for the passages also were filled with patients) save the step of the orderly or the voice of the doctor. Night is especially trying to the sick and wretched; and then on all sides arose the moan of pain, or the murmurings of delirium. At this period there were no night nurses; but Miss Nightingale, lamp in hand, each night traversed alone the four miles of beds. How many lives this lady has been the means of saving during these rounds, by calling medical aid or by administering little alleviations, is fully known only to herself, and to the Unseen who watches our steps. She was peculiarly skilled in the art of soothing; her gentle, sympathetic voice and manner always appeared to refresh the sufferer. It was generally far into the night before she again reached her quarters.[44]

208. Letter of Mrs. Sidney Herbert to Mrs. S. C. Hall

[Anna Maria Hall (1800–1881) was active in philanthropic work. She was instrumental in founding the Hospital for Consumptives at Brompton, the Governess' Institute, the Home for Decayed Gentlewomen, and the Nightingale Fund. She worked for the temperance cause, women's rights, and for the friendless and the fallen. She was a friend to street musicians. Mrs. Hall wrote stories and *Sketches of Irish Character*. Her husband, Samuel Carter Hall (1800–1889), was an author and editor, a lawyer, and a critic and reviewer on art for the *British Press*. As such, he exposed the trade in old masters. He joined his wife in her philanthropic undertakings and writing.[45]]

49, Belgrade Square,
July, 1855.

Madam,

There is but one testimonial which would be accepted by Miss Nightingale.

The one wish of her heart has long been to found a hospital in London, and to work it on her own system of unpaid nursing, and I have suggested to all who have asked for my advice in this matter, to pay any sums that they may feel disposed to give, or that they may be able to collect, into Messrs. Coutts' Bank, where a subscription-list for the purpose is about to be opened, to be called the "Nightingale Hospital Fund," the sum subscribed to be presented to her on her return home, which will enable her to carry out her object regarding the reform of the nursing system of England.[46]

209. Evidence of the Duke of Newcastle Before the Roebuck Committee

[Henry Pelham Clinton, fifth Duke of Newcastle (1811–1864), was educated at Eton and Oxford. He was a member of Parliament, and became Lord of the Treasury in 1834.[47] During the Crimean War, a commission of inquiry, known as the Duke of Newcastle's Commission, was sent to the East to look into conditions there. Its report was adopted later by a committee of the House of Commons known as the "Roebuck Committee." The following evidence was given in 1855.[48]]

The employment of nurses in the hospital at Scutari was mooted in this country, at an early stage before the army left this country, but it was not liked by the military authorities. It had been tried on former occasions. The class of women employed as nurses had been very much addicted to drinking, and they were found even more callous to the sufferings of soldiers in hospitals than men would have been. Subsequently, in consequence of letters in the public press, and of recommendations made by gentlemen who had returned to this country from Scutari, we began to consider the subject of employing nurses. The difficulty was to get a lady to take in hand the charge of superintending and directing a body of nurses. After having seen one or two I almost despaired of the practicability of the matter until Mr. Sidney Herbert suggested Miss Nightingale, with whom he had been previously acquainted, for the work, and that lady eventually undertook it.[49]

210. James Henry Skene. *With Lord Stratford in the Crimean War*

[Stratford Canning, Lord Stratford de Redcliffe (1786–1880), British diplomat, was educated mainly at Eton and Cambridge. He held various government offices before being appointed ambassador to Turkey for the first time in 1824. In 1819 he was appointed minister at Washington and while there arranged with John Quincy Adams a general treaty which was later rejected by the United States Senate.[50] During the Crimean War, while he was ambassador to Turkey, Lady Stratford de Redcliffe, his wife, acted as intermediary between Lord Stratford and the hospital authorities. In this capacity she was helpful to Miss Nightingale in improving the conditions in the hospitals.[51] James Henry Skene, the writer of the book quoted, was the son of James Skene of Rubislaw, a friend of Sir Walter Scott. His sister was Felicia Skene, who nursed the sick in the cholera outbreak in Oxford in 1854.[52] One brother, William Forbes Skene, was a noted antiquarian and historian of Wales, Scotland, and Ireland. James eventually entered the diplomatic service and went to the Crimea. He became the author of several books on travel.[53]]

Miss Nightingale had arrived here [at Scutari] with her bevy of lady nurses. Her first act showed her wonderful energy and determination. The steamers laden with the wounded had cast anchor at Constantinople. There were not yet any mattresses or bed-clothes on the camp-beds in the hospital, and the latter were not nearly sufficient in number for the wounded coming. Miss Nightingale went to the quartermaster-sargeant in charge of the stores, and asked him for the stores which she required. He told her there was everything she could desire in the magazines, but that she must get the Inspector-General of Hospitals to write an official letter to the Quarter-master-General, who would send him an authority to draw the stores, and that she might then receive them on showing that authority. Miss Nightingale asked how long this would take. On being told that three days would be the shortest time necessary for the correspondence, she answered that nine hundred wounded officers and men would be in the hospital in three hours, and that she must have what they required immediately. She then went to the magazines, and telling the sargeant of the guard there who she was, asked him if he would take an order from her. He said he would, and she ordered him to drive in the door. This was done, and the wounded were provided for in time.

Her firmness at surgical operations was something marvellous. Her appreciation of her mission was grand. She stood one day with spirits, instruments, and lint in hand, during the performing of a frightful amputation. Half a dozen young lady-nurses were behind her, holding basins, towels, and other things the surgeon might want. A harrowing groan from the patient suddenly put them all to flight, except Miss Nightingale, who, turning calmly round, called to them, "Come back! shame on you as Christians! shame on you as women!" They returned holding each other's trembling hands, and some of them almost ready to faint. But they got over their nervous weakness as their novitiate advanced, and did an amount of good that yet lives in the memory of many a man rescued from death and pain by their gentle ministrations.[54]

211. *Memoir of the Rt. Hon. Sir John McNeill, G.C.B., and of his Second Wife, Elizabeth Wilson.* By Their Granddaughter

[Sir John McNeill (1795–1883) was a physician who entered political service during the Crimean War. With Sir Alexander Murray Tulloch, he was sent to the Crimea to report on conditions. Following this, he became a constant counselor to Florence Nightingale and, later, a member of the Council of the Nightingale Fund as well as a member of its subcommittee to formulate plans for establishing the school of nursing. He also collaborated with Miss Nightingale in a scheme for nursing in India.[55]]

One subject we must notice rather more especially—the Nightingale Fund, and Sir John McNeill's part in it. At a meeting to promote the National Testimonial in honour of Miss Nightingale, held in Edinburgh in February, 1856, Sir John McNeill was called to the chair. In his speech, referring to the many conversations he had had with her, he said he had never heard a "vain or thoughtless proposal" from her, that she was distinguished by "a strong practical sense...." At the Crimean Banquet in the Corn Exchange in Edinburgh on the 30th October, 1856, Sir John McNeill had the honour to propose Miss Nightingale's health. He told, as an eyewitness, of her deeds of mercy...

After a long eulogy of the British soldier and some defense of his own Report, saying that if the Government wished the Inquiry to be a sham they had selected the wrong instruments for that purpose, he spoke of the sick, and the state in which they arrived at Scutari. "Who was responsible for the omission," he said, "it would be useless to inquire. Of course, nobody is to blame." (Laughter and cheers.) "But though I am unable to tell you who was responsible for leaving the sick in that wretched condition, I am able to tell you who rescued them from it—Florence Nightingale." (Prolonged applause.) He went on to tell how she had provided linen for the numerous patients at her own expense at a cost of not less than £2,000 or £3,000; how she had arranged for having it washed; for having food well cooked; for having a large wing of the barrack hospital, which was so dilapidated as to be uninhabitable, repaired; how the workmen employed had struck because they were not paid, and the officer in charge of the work could not procure the money; how she advanced it out of her own pocket; how that building, still unfinished, was immediately filled with sick and wounded, and when the hospital authorities refused to provide furniture she again purchased it herself. "Everyone," he said, "knows the public services of Florence Nightingale, but only those who have had the honour of meeting her can know the refinement and true feminine delicacy of her mind and manner, of the unconsciousness of having done anything great or remarkable that pervades her whole deportment and conversation: Far from dwelling upon the past, or taking any pride in the applause which has followed her unsought, the whole energies of her powerful, highly cultivated, and essentially practical intellect are always directed towards further and more permanent plans of usefulness."

It was for these plans—the establishing of a training school for nurses in this country—that Sir John gave his assistance. He was one of the nine original trustees, appointed by deed in 1857, who were nominated by Miss Nightingale to form a Consultation Council to advise her how to apply the funds which a grateful nation had subscribed as a gift to herself. As is well known, it was used to found the School of Training for Nurses, now St. Thomas's Hospital.[56]

212. General Sir George Higginson, G.C.B. *Seventy-one Years of a Guardsman's Life*

[General Sir George Wentworth Alexander Higginson (1826–1915) was educated at Eton. He became an ensign in the Grenadier Guards in 1845 and served with them for thirty years. Part of this service was in the Crimea, for which he was decorated. He was Lieutenant Governor of the Tower of London from 1888 to 1893.[57]]

One figure stands out in the softened light that falls on the memory of those far-off days, nor can I close the record of them without reference to her to whose resolute indifference to routine and precedent we owed the organisation of the great hospital at Balaclava. The memoirs of Miss Nightingale, so recently published, not only disclose the defects in our hospital system which aroused so much just indignation in England, but also reveal the sweeping changes which the patient and intelligent persistence of this quiet English lady prevailed to effect in the whole of our military service. I look back with pride to the day when I was first presented to her, and established those respectful friendly relations which, up to a late period of her life, she permitted me to maintain.[58]

213. Henry Wadsworth Longfellow. "Santa Filomena"

[This poem was written in 1857 as a contribution to the first issue of the *Atlantic Monthly*.[59] Mrs. Jameson states in *Sacred and Legendary Art:* "At Pisa the Church of San Francisco contains a chapel dedicated lately to Santa Filomena; over the altar is a picture by Sabatelli, representing the Saint as a beautiful nymph-like figure, floating down from heaven, attended by two angels bearing the lily, palm, and javelin, and beneath, in the foreground, the sick and maimed, who are healed by her intercession." [60]]

Whene'er a noble deed is wrought,
Wher'er is spoken a noble thought,
    Our hearts, in glad surprise,
    To higher levels rise.

The tidal wave of deeper souls
Into our inmost being rolls,
    And lifts us unawares
    Out of all meaner cares.

Honour to those whose words or deeds
Thus help us in our daily needs,
    And by their overflow
    Raise us from what is low!

Thus thought I, as by night I read
Of the great army of the dead,
    The trenches cold and damp,
    The starved and frozen camp,—

The wounded from the battle-plain,
In dreary hospitals of pain,
    The cheerless corridors,
    The cold and stony floors.

Lo! in that house of misery
A lady with a lamp I see
    Pass through the glimmering gloom,
    And flit from room to room.

And slow, as in a dream of bliss,
The speechless sufferer turns to kiss
    Her shadow, as it falls
    Upon the darkening walls.

As if a door in heaven should be
Opened and then closed suddenly.
    The vision came and went,
    The light shone and was spent.

On England's annals, through the long
Hereafter of her speech and song,
    That light its rays shall cast
    From portals of the past.

A Lady with a Lamp shall stand
In the great history of the land,
    A noble type of good,
    Heroic Womanhood.

Nor even shall be wanting here
The palm, the lily, and the spear,
    The symbols that of yore,
    Santa Filomena bore.[61]

214. "The Nightingale's Song to the Sick Soldier," *Punch*,
       Vol. XXVII (1854), p. 184

[Many poems, songs, and articles about Miss Nightingale appeared in various periodicals while she was in the Crimea and afterward. The following is one of the best-known poems from *Punch*.]

Listen, soldier, to the tale of the tender NIGHTINGALE,
    'Tis a charm that soon will ease your wounds so cruel
Singing medicine for your pain, in a sympathetic strain,
    With a jug, jug, jug of lemonade or gruel.

Singing bandages and lint; salve and cerate without stint,
    Singing plenty both of liniment and lotion,
And your mixtures pushed about, and the pills for you served out,
    With alacrity and promptitude in motion.

Singing light and gentle hands, and a nurse who understands
    How to manage every sort of application,
From a poultice to a leech; whom you haven't got to teach
    The way to make a poppy fomentation.

Singing pillow for you, smoothed; smart and ache and anguish
        soothed,
    By the readiness of feminine invention;
Singing fever's thirst allayed, and the bed you've tumbled made,
    With a cheerful and considerate attention.

Singing succor to the brave, and a rescue from the grave,
    Hear the NIGHTINGALE that's come to the Crimea,
'Tis a NIGHTINGALE as strong in her heart as in her song,
    To carry out so gallant an idea.

CONCLUDING STATEMENT

The life of Florence Nightingale before 1860, the date of the founding of the Nightingale School of Nursing, may be thought of as having three phases: her youth which was characterized by her desire to devote her life to nursing; the beginning of the accomplishment of this wish in the various brief experiences in nursing, such as her sojourn at Kaiserswerth, and further development in her work in the Crimean hospitals, which gave her firsthand contact with nursing in an emergency situation and experience in organization and administration of great hospitals, strengthening her conviction of the necessity for improved preparation for nursing work; and finally, the third phase, the development of a new system of nursing and nursing preparation at St. Thomas's Hospital in London, and Miss Nightingale's contributions to other fields, completing the fruitful life of this great reformer of the care of the sick. This final phase is the subject of the next chapter.

Early letters and diaries, such as those of Dr. and Mrs. Howe, Elizabeth Blackwell, Elizabeth Gaskell, and Fanny Allen, give indications of Miss Nightingale's desire to become a nurse and describe her personal appearance, with which the writers were pleased. One of her letters to Dr. and Mrs. Howe refers to her sojourn at Kaiserswerth, as do letters quoted in the preceding chapter.[62]

From among the many sources on the Crimean War phase, the articles from the *Illustrated London News,* and the *London Times,* together with the letters of those who knew Miss Nightingale or observed her work in the Crimea, such as Mr. Bracebridge, Lady Hornby, Sir Sidney Herbert, and Mary Stanley, emphasize the prodigious amount of work she accomplished, her organizing ability, and her absolute devotion to the soldiers and their welfare. The accounts in the form of narratives, reminiscences, or diaries, such as those of Sydney Godolphin Osborne, Fanny M. Taylor, Sister Mary Aloysius, Margaret Goodman, James Henry Skene, Sir John McNeill, and General Sir George Higginson, reveal the adverse conditions under which the nurses devotedly worked and the transformation resulting from Miss Nightingale's untiring efforts, and narrate the work of individuals who nursed in the hospitals of Scutari and the Crimea.

Henry Wadsworth Longfellow's poem, "Santa Filomena," one of the many tributes to her at this time, pictures Miss Nightingale in the hospital idolized by the soldiers, and becoming a symbol of heroic women in wartime. The poem appearing in *Punch,* entitled, "The Nightingale's Song to the Sick Soldier," was one of many published in English periodicals at that time.

These experiences in the war were in the nature of preparation for Miss Nightingale's most important and far-reaching, though perhaps less dramatic, work—the founding of the first professional school of nursing, in London in 1860. No single event in modern times in nursing has had a more profound and revolutionary effect on the care of the sick and on the professional education of women. Although almost one hundred years in the past, the ideas involved are modern, and while they have been surpassed in part, they were the springboard of the modern art of nursing.

The sources which help to throw light on these happenings and their consequences will be presented in the next chapter.

Chapter 7

Selections from the Literature of the
New Profession of Nursing

INTRODUCTION

MISS NIGHTINGALE'S contribution to the improvement of nursing conditions during the Crimean War is perhaps her best-known work. This is probably true partly because of the dramatic quality of war nursing, and partly because this phase of her life has been emphasized in writings on Miss Nightingale, sometimes to the exclusion of her other efforts in the field of social welfare. In addition to this, at the time of the Crimean War, the character of a large proportion of the women who adopted nursing as a vocation was such that the entrance of a woman of Miss Nightingale's caliber into this field was unusual, if not unique. If the whole effect of Miss Nightingale's activities in nursing and the field of health is examined, however, it will be seen that, while her work in the war hospitals was of the greatest significance for the future, it was the establishment of a school for the education of a new kind of practitioner of the nursing art which has had the most far-reaching and lasting effect on the welfare of the sick and on the professional education of women.

The emphasis in the present chapter is on the establishment of the first professional school of nursing at St. Thomas's Hospital, London, and the effect of this on various phases of nursing in the years immediately following, particularly in the British Isles. As in Chapter 6, selections have been made, for the most part, from the less accessible materials.

From among the many source materials on the Nightingale School, the following have been selected: a letter from Dr. Elizabeth Blackwell to her sister, Dr. Emily Blackwell, describing an interview of the former with Miss Nightingale concerning the new school of nursing, and expressing concern over the latter's health (215); a letter from Agnes Elizabeth Jones to her aunt, reporting on her arrival at St. Thomas's Hospital to study nursing, together with a brief account of Miss Jones' work as a "Nightingale Missioner" at the Liverpool Infirmary, in *"Una and Her Paupers:" Memorials of Agnes Elizabeth Jones* (216); a brief outline of the main points of the program at St. Thomas's Hospital by Florence S. Lees, a Nightingale nurse (217); an article written by Miss Nightingale, which appeared in the *British Medical Journal* in 1892, describing Mrs. Wardroper as matron of the Nightingale School and St. Thomas's Hospital (218); the announcement of the opening of the Nightingale School, in the *London Times,* June 1, 1860 (219); an article by Miss Nightingale in *Good Words,* June 1, 1868, which was a memorial to Agnes Jones and which outlined many aspects of the program of the Nightingale School (220); brief excerpts from several reports of the Nightingale Fund (221); and a statement of the Nightingale Fund, published in *The Lancet* for June 22, 1872 (222).

From the writings of Florence Nightingale the following are included, in addition to those referred to above: selections from *Notes on Hospitals* (223); an excerpt from *Army Sanitary Administration and Its Reform Under the Late Lord Herbert* (224); part of the article, "A Note on Pauperism," from *Fraser's Magazine,* for March, 1869 (225); a letter to the nurses at St. Thomas's Hospital, dated May 6, 1881 (226); "Introduction to the 'History of Nursing in the Homes of the Poor,'" which is the introduction to William Rathbone's *Sketch of the History and Progress of District Nursing* ... (227); "Sick-Nursing and Health-Nursing," from *Women's Mission: A Series of Congress Papers on the Philanthropic Work of Women* (228); and *Subsidiary Notes as to the Introduction of Female Nursing into Military Hospitals in Peace and War* (229).

The emergence of the profession of nursing, initiated at the Nightingale School, was reflected in the many writings of physicians, philanthropists, and others. Many of them attributed the changes to Miss Nightingale, while other writings reveal the slowness with which the new ideas were adopted. Some of the materials highlighting these conditions include the following: an excerpt from the pamphlet *Sisterhoods; Schools for Nurses* (230); "Report of the Lancet Sanitary Commission on Night Nursing in the London Hospitals" (231); a statement of the desirable qualifications for the "monthly nurse," by Dr. Pye Henry Chavasse in his book, *Advice to the Wife on the Management of Her Own Health and on the Treatment of Some of the Complaints Incidental to Pregnancy, Labor, and Suckling* (232); Dr. James Hinton's statement of his attitude toward the profession of nursing (233); the necessary qualifications of infirmary nurses, and the requirements for nursing in the workhouse infirmaries, as stated by the Poor Law Board and the Local Government Board, and published in Louisa Twining's report, *Workhouses and*

Pauperism and Women's Work in the Administration of the Poor Law
(234); the accounts of William Rathbone and of his daughter Eleanor
Rathbone of the establishment of visiting nursing in England (235, 236);
and the account of another early use of visiting nurses in *The Story of the
Ranyard Mission,* by Elspeth Platt (237).

THE SOURCES

The Nightingale School

215. Letter of Dr. Elizabeth Blackwell to Dr. Emily Blackwell

[In the following letter, Dr. Elizabeth Blackwell relates to her sister
how Miss Nightingale attempted to interest her in the proposed school of
nursing at St. Thomas's Hospital and expressed the hope that Dr. Blackwell would come to London to practice medicine. Dr. Blackwell also
voiced concern over Miss Nightingale's health at that time.[1]]

London: February 1859.

I have just returned from an interview with Miss Nightingale at Malvern
in relation to a school for nurses which she wishes to establish; and I start
tomorrow for France en route for Mentone. My old friend's health is failing
from the pressure of mental labour. I cannot go into the details of her last
five years now, but the labour has been and is immense. I think I have never
known a woman labour as she has done. It is a most remarkable experience;
she indeed deserves the name of worker. Of course we conversed very earnestly
about the nursing plan in which she wished to interest me. She says that for
six months she shall be utterly unable to give any thought to the fund work,
and wants me meanwhile to observe English life very carefully, and make up
my mind as to whether I can give up America, which she thinks a very
serious matter. Unfortunately she does not think private practice possible in
connection with her plan. If so, it would be impossible for us to help her.
She thinks her own health will never permit her to carry out her plan herself,
and I much fear she is right in this belief.[2]

216. *"Una and Her Paupers:" Memorials of Agnes Elizabeth Jones*

[After completing her work at Kaiserswerth,[3] Agnes Jones went to
London to do missionary work among the poor there. She then, in 1862,
entered St. Thomas's Hospital School of Nursing as a probationer. After
completing her course, she became manager of a small hospital, from
whence she consented to assume responsibility for superintending the
Liverpool Workhouse Infirmary, where she died in 1868.[4] The following
letter to her aunt describes her initiation as a probationer at St. Thomas's
Hospital. The second narrative outlines briefly her experience at the

Liverpool Workhouse Infirmary as a "Nightingale Missioner," and pioneer in workhouse nursing.]

[1862]

My dearest Aunt.— ...

We reached London at 6.30, and I was fortunate about my luggage, so got off at once. I desired the cabman to drive to Surrey Gardens, and we drove on long through well-known streets, but when we passed the obelisk I came to new ground. However, not long after, we stopped, and I saw a great gateway, over which was in large letters, "St. Thomas's Hospital," so a bell was rung, and I said "Nightingale nurse;" the gate opened and we drove on a little way and then saw a long half covered way leading to a large well-lighted room. Up to this I walked; saw porter no. 2, and was admitted into a large warm hall, well panelled and partitioned, as all the house is, with well-planed deal, varnished its own colour, which looks so clean and light. I had a long wait while the cabman brought in the luggage, and then was conducted past the doors of some wards, in which I saw a few patients in bed and two nurses seated most comfortably at work at a table in the middle of the room; then we crossed a large space with trees, giving, as did all I saw, the idea and feeling of being far from any town; and though I had not yet been out, there is the perfect stillness of the country. But to go on and introduce you as I was. The porter led me into a kind of small hall, and instantly two nice-looking, almost deaconess-looking, nurses came forward and received me most kindly, saying Mrs. W. (the lady-superintendent) had been in several times during the afternoon and evening, and had just left, having given me up for that day. However, nothing could exceed the kindness of these nurses; their dress a kind of grey stuff, very neat, white aprons and caps, rather too round and coquettish I thought for sisters, but a neat pretty style of dress, which will, I am sure, be most becoming to Nurse Agnes. They brought me into a large, lofty, comfortable room, with tables, chairs, flowers, pictures, books, carpet, rug, fire, gas, like any sitting-room; off this, surrounded by the varnished boards, are the little bedroom cells; their wooden walls about ten feet high, not half-way to the ceiling, with a bed, small chest of drawers; wash-stand, chair, and towel-rail. The room was formerly a refreshment room, and is a very handsome and lofty one, lighted from the roof, and now surrounded by the nurses' cells, with the open space in the middle for their sitting-room, where I am now writing at one of the numerous little tables, with bright flowers and numbers of all kinds of magazines around me. Two things cheered me much to see: first, on entering the sitting-room, a picture of Kaiserswerth; secondly, in the bedroom, a large Bible on the drawers beside the looking-glass. I was taken to my room, provided with hot water, and after a little, called to tea, comfortably prepared in the nice light eating-room, quite separate from, but near our sitting-room. ... There is a temporary church fitted up in the house, which all attend, but every second Sunday, I shall have the whole afternoon to myself to go where I like. There are fourteen Nightingale nurses, besides sisters, and about 280 patients, when the house is full, which it is not yet, as this place was only opened a few days ago. I went to bed soon after tea, and was up for breakfast this morning at 6.30. Everything is so quiet that you more feel than know that others are moving around you. My nurse friend summoned me to breakfast where I had tea last night, and I found the whole party assembled; a nice respectable-looking set; all amiable-looking, some pretty; the sister sat at the head of the table. Bread-and-butter and toast in plenty, and each person with their own tea-pot and sugar-bowl, which they wash and keep in their own room. Each cell has its own gas, and there is some general light which seems to burn all night, for I never woke but I saw it. I could read a large print Bible in bed by it. . . . And now, darlings, do not fret yourselves about me, there seems to be every provision for comfort, and all I have yet seen or heard has given me a pleasant impression, and I feel at home already.

[May 11, 1865]

[At Liverpool Workhouse]

And now at last all was ready, and the day arrived on which the nurses were expected. . . . The party of nurses arrived from London . . . twelve Nightingale nurses and seven probationers. The next afternoon the work began in earnest. One of the great difficulties of the first year arose from the character of the ex-pauper women who were brought into the hospital from the other departments of the workhouse, to be trained under the nurses. Rough, coarse women they were, and apparently incapable of receiving instruction; besides, their habits of intemperance led them astray whenever the slightest liberty was allowed; so at last, after some months of uphill work and continual disappointment, the plan had to be given up.

[By the Editor]

Her day was, indeed, no idle one. At 5.30 A.M. she went in her dressing-gown to unlock the doors for the kitchen-women. At 6 she rang the bell for the nurses and probationers; at 6.30 all assembled for prayers in the nurses' sitting room. At 7 the breakfast began. After she made a round of the wards at 6; and if there was any anxious case, she would be up two or three times in the night. After "a race round the wards to see that all the breakfasts are correct," she came to her own at the head of the table, where nurses, probationers, assistants and scourers were seated. At 7.30 she gave the orders for the day, and then made another round of the wards. Then giving out the stores occupied her till the first dinner began at 12. She was always present herself, carved for the nurses and probationers, and dined with them. . . . Occasional visits to individual patients, giving out stores, and attending to calls innumerable, occupied the afternoon. After presiding at tea at 4, she returned to the wards, to see how the dressing was done. And here her practical knowledge of nursing-work enabled her to direct the nurses and teach the probationers, and give her weight to both, which was invaluable to her authority. At 9 o'clock the night nurses went on duty, and she visited the wards to see that each was at her post. Prayers were at 9.30, after which the day nurses went to bed; but another round of the wards was still before Agnes, and it was generally after 11 before she could go to her own room, and feel that she might lie down to rest with her work for the day done.

.   .   .   .

[Nov. 15, 1865]

I am almost distracted between sickness and anxiety and drunkenness. I have one head nurse in great danger, and much anxiety about her sister, who is with her, and almost worn out with sorrow and watching. Then these ex-pauper women whom we are training, were paid their wages on Friday, and the next day five came in tipsy. It is so disappointing; some who had done well for six months, and of whom I had hopes . . .[5]

217. Florence S. Lees. *Handbook for Hospital Sisters*

[Florence S. Lees studied nursing at the Nightingale School at St. Thomas's Hospital in 1866 and 1867. Later she studied and worked as a nurse in Berlin, Dresden, and at Kaiserswerth, after which she became a surgical sister at King's College Hospital in London. Subsequently she visited hospitals in Holland, Denmark, and France. In the latter country she participated in the nursing of many of the hospitals which she visited. She later had charge of a typhus station with the Tenth Army Corps before Metz, and was at the Ambulance for the Wounded, of the Crown Princess of Germany. She married Rev. Dacre Craven.[6]]

St. Thomas's Hospital is the seat of a well-known medical school, several of the teachers attached to which, voluntarily and without remuneration, give lectures to the Nightingale probationers on subjects connected with their special duties, such as elementary instruction in chemistry, with reference to a knowledge of the leading functions of the body; and general instructions on medical and surgical topics.

The ward-sisters are required to keep a weekly record of the progress of the "probationers," and the probationers themselves are required to keep a diary of their ward-work; in which they write day by day an account of their duties.

They are also required to record special cases of disease, injury, or operation, with the daily changes in the case, and the daily alteration in the management, such as a nurse ought to know. Besides these books, each probationer keeps notes of the lectures.

They are required to become skilful

(1) In the dressing of blisters, burns, sores, wounds, and in applying fomentations, poultices, and minor dressings.

(2) In the application of leeches, externally and internally.

(3) In the administration of enemas for men and women.

262

(4) In the management of trusses and appliances in uterine complaints.

(5) In the best method of friction to the body and extremities.

(6) In the management of helpless patients, i. e., moving, changing, personal cleanliness, feeding, keeping warm or cool, preventing and dressing bed-sores, managing position.

(7) In bandaging, making bandages, and rollers, lining of splints.

(8) In making the beds of the patients and removing the sheets whilst the patient is in bed.

(9) They are required to attend at operations.

(10) To be competent to cook gruel, arrowroot, egg-flip, puddings, and prepare drinks for the sick.

(11) To understand ventilation, or keeping the ward fresh by night as well as by day; they are to be careful that great cleanliness is observed in all the utensils, those used for the secretions, as well as those required for cooking.

(12) To make strict observations of the sick in the following particulars: —The state of the secretions, expectoration, pulse, skin, appetite, intelligence (as delirium or stupor), breathing, sleep, state of wounds, eruptions, formation of matter, effect of diet or of stimulants, and of medicines.

(13) To learn the management of convalescents. To ensure efficiency, each ward sister should be supplied with a book which corresponds with the list of duties given to the probationers. In a properly constructed ward, each sister might train four probationers.

In English hospitals it is customary for the sister of each ward to make, or see that her nurses and probationers make, the bandages, and lining for splints, &c., required in her ward.[7]

218. Florence Nightingale, "The Reform of Sick Nursing and the Late Mrs. Wardroper, The Extinction of Mrs. Gamp," *British Medical Journal*, December 31, 1892, p. 1448

[Mrs. Wardroper was Matron of St. Thomas's Hospital for thirty-three years.[8] Linda Richards, the first nurse to graduate from an American school of nursing, describes Mrs. Wardroper's appearance thus: ". . . [She was] a small lady, dressed in black. Upon her head was a cap of lace with long, flowing strings, which . . . hung down her back nearly to the waist. Upon her hands were black kid gloves. During my stay at the hospital I never saw her in any other dress. I think it was her uniform, and she was as much at home writing in gloves as is the ordinary individual without them."[9] The following article describes graphically Mrs. Wardroper's other characteristics and the development of the nursing at St. Thomas's Hospital under Mrs. Wardroper's leadership. It appeared also in the *Hospital Nursing Supplement* under the title, "A Nursing Worthy."[10]]

One has passed away without noise, without crown or sceptre of martyrdom, who was the pioneer of hospital nursing, the first lay hospital matron, at least of a great public hospital, who was a gentlewoman. Her kingdom was that of the sick. No public press heroine was she; yet countless sick will bless her name though they never heard it, and she opened a new calling for women of all classes, the Nursing Institutions for the Poor. She did this —a great work—for her country and her Sovereign, who is the mother of English-speaking womankind, thrice blessed to those for whom it initiated a divine life of common sense in nursing. No Mrs. Gamp could live in her neighborhood. Mrs. Gamp was extinct for ever. She was soon gladly acknowledged by the doctors as their chief in nursing. She led a hard life, but never proclaimed it. What she did was done silently. No herald chanted her praises.

The state of what was by ignorance called nursing when she began hospital work, the miserable state, moral and technical, of the nurses, would scarcely now be credited. Did one, who knew it, attempt to describe it, she would be, by a universal jury of her fellows, found guilty of exaggeration. But God knew it.

Reforms at St. Thomas's

I saw her first in October, 1854, when the expedition of nurses was sent to the Crimean war. She had been then nine months matron of the great hospital in London, of which for thirty-three years she remained head and reformer of the nursing. Training was then unknown. The only nurse worthy of the name that could be given to that expedition, though several were supplied, was a "sister" who had been pensioned some time before, and who proved invaluable. I saw her next after the conclusion of the Crimean war. She had already made her mark. She had weeded out the inefficient, morally and technically; she had obtained better women as nurses; she had put her finger on some of the most flagrant blots, such as the night nursing, and where she laid her finger the blot was diminished as far as possible, but no training had yet been thought of.

The Establishment of the Nightingale School

All this led to her being chosen to carry out in the hospital of which she was matron the aims, in the training of nurses, of the Nightingale Fund, which had then been subscribed. She was named first superintendent of that school, and continued for twenty-seven years till her retirement in 1887. That school under her has been more or less the model of all the subsequent nurse-training schools, of which now nearly every considerable hospital, and many an inconsiderable, has its own, but they chiefly train for themselves. She, as head of the Nightingale School trained for many other hospitals and infirmaries. The principles of this school may be shortly said to be as follows:—(1) That nurses should have their training in hospitals specially organised for the purpose; (2) that they should live in a "home" fit to form the moral life and discipline.

The New Profession of Nursing

The Work of the School

The school under this lady was opened at the old St. Thomas's Hospital, near London Bridge, in 1860. St. Thomas's and the Nightingale School were removed to the Surrey Gardens in 1862, and in 1870 to their present abode opposite the Houses of Parliament on the other side of the river. At the time of her retirement upwards of 500 nurses had completed their course in the school and entered into service on the staff of St. Thomas's and other hospitals; and of these over 50 educated gentlewomen were occupying important posts as matrons or superintendents of nurses in hospitals, infirmaries, and nursing institutions for the poor, and not only in the United Kingdom, but also abroad.

The Methods and Character of Mrs. Wardroper

This lady was Mrs. Wardroper, who passed away, quite peacefully, in her 80th year, on December 15th, 1892, and was buried quietly on December 19th. It is difficult to describe the character of such a woman, the more so as her praises were never sounded in newspaper or book. No laurel encircles her brow, no crowds assemble to do her honour. But hundreds of trained nurses, and hundreds of thousands of well-nursed sick are her meet tribute.

Her power of organisation and of administration, her courage and her discrimination in character were alike remarkable. She was straightforward, true, upright; she was decided; her judgment of character came by intuition, at a flash, not the result of much weighing or consideration, yet she seldom made a mistake; and she would take the greatest pains with her written delineations of character required for records; writing them again and again in order to be perfectly just, not smart or clever; but they were in excellent language. She was free from self-consciousness; nothing artificial about her. "She did nothing because she was being looked at, and abstained from nothing because she was looked at."

Her whole heart and mind, her whole life and strength were in the work she had undertaken. She never went a-pleasuring; seldom into society. Yet she was one of the wittiest people one could hear on a summer's day, and had gone a good deal into society in her unmarried life. She was left a widow at 42 with a young family. She had never had any training in hospital life. There was none to be had.

Her force of character was extraordinary; her word was law. For her thoughts, words, and actions were all the same. She moved in one piece. She talked a great deal, but she never wasted herself in talking; she did what she said. Some people substitute words for actions; she never. She knew what she wanted, and she did it. She was a strict disciplinarian; very kind, often affectionate, rather than loving. She took such intense interest in everything, even in things matrons do not generally consider their business, that she never tired. She would be quite late in decorating the chapel at Christmas and Easter with her own hands. She had great taste, and spent her own money. She was a thorough gentlewoman, nothing mean or low about her; magnanimous and generous, rather than courteous.

And all this was done quietly. Of late years the great nursing work has been scarred by fashion on one side, and by mere money-getting on the other—two catastrophies sure to happen when noise is substituted for silent work. Few remember her in these express-train days, dashing along at 60 years in a day.

> A perfect woman, nobly planned
> To warn, to comfort and command,

"Comfort," not in the present meaning of comfortable, easy-chair life, but comfort in the good old meaning of "Be strong with me."

And so, dear Matron, as thou wast called so many years, we bid thee farewell, and God speed to His higher world; not as the world giveth, giveth He thee.

219. The *London Times*, June 1, 1860

[When in 1860, the Nightingale School was ready to receive students, a notice was inserted in the *London Times,* setting forth the requirements and general plan of the program.]

To women desirous of being Trained as Hospital Nurses;—The Committee of the Nightingale Fund have made arrangements with the authorities of St. Thomas's Hospital for giving a year's Training to Women, between 25 and 35 years of age, for whom they will provide, free of expense, board and lodging in the Hospital, with tea, sugar, and washing, and a certain amount of outer clothing. A payment will be allowed them of £10 for the year. They will be under the charge of the Matron, and will be instructed by the Sisters and the Resident Medical Officer. At the end of a year, if their training has been found satisfactory, their names will be entered in the Committee's register, and they will be recommended for situations as hospital nurses. The first quarter will commence on the 21st inst. For further particulars apply to Mrs. Wardroper, St. Thomas's Hospital, S. E., to whom all applications for admission must be made, if personally, between 10 and 11 A.M.

A. H. Clough, Sec.

Council-office, Downing Street, S. W.

220. "Una and the Lion," *Good Words,* June 1, 1868, pp. 360–366

[This paper was written by Miss Nightingale as a memorial to Agnes Elizabeth Jones, a Nightingale nurse who was the pioneer in workhouse nursing at the Liverpool Infirmary.[11] It was reprinted with some alterations, as the introduction to *"Una and Her Paupers:" Memorials of Agnes Elizabeth Jones.* Sir Edward Cook states that this use was un-

authorized.[12] The eulogy to Miss Jones is omitted in the following
quotation.]

Writers on sick nursing have repudiated training, without saying what
training is. I perceive that I have used the word "training" a great many
times. And neither have I said what it is.

We require that a woman be sober, honest, truthful, without which there
is no foundation on which to build.

We train them in habits of punctuality, quietness, trustworthiness, personal
neatness. We teach her how to manage the concerns of a large ward or
establishment.

We train her in dressing wounds and other injuries, and in performing all
those minor operations which nurses are called upon day and night to
undertake.

We teach her how to manage helpless patients in regard to moving, changing, feeding, temperature, and the prevention of bed-sores.

She has to make and apply bandages, line splints for fractures, and the
like. She must know how to make beds with as little disturbance as possible
of their inmates. She is instructed how to wait at operations, and as to the
kind of aid the surgeon requires at her hands. She is taught cooking for
sick; the principles on which sick-wards ought to be cleaned, aired, and
warmed; the management of convalescents; and how to observe sick and
maimed patients, so as to give an intelligent and truthful account to the
physician or surgeon in regard to the progress of cases in the intervals
between visits—a much more difficult thing than is generally supposed.

We do not seek to make "medical women," but simply nurses acquainted
with the *principles* which they are required constantly to apply at the
bedside.

For the future superintendent is added a course of instruction in the
administration of a hospital, including, of course, the linen arrangements,
and what else is necessary for a matron to be conversant with.

There are those who think that all this is intuitive in women, that they
are born so, or, at least, that it comes to them without training. To such we
say, By all means send us as many such geniuses as you can, for we are
sorely in want of them . . .

   .   .   .   .

We admit at St. Thomas's Hospital Training School—subject to the judgment of the matron, and subject to certain conditions being accepted or
fulfilled by the probationer—a limited number of probationers to be trained
as nurses for the sick poor. Hitherto we have been compelled to confine ourselves to sending out staffs of nurses to hospitals or workhouses, with a view
to their becoming, in their turn, centres of training, because the applications
we receive for trained nurses are far more numerous and urgent than we
have power to answer. But did a greater number of probationers, suitable for
superior situations, offer themselves, we could provide additional means for

training, and answer applications for district nursing, and many others. These probationers receive board, lodging, training entirely free, a certain amount of uniform dress, and a small amount of pay during their year of training . . .

There are two requisites in a superintendent:—1. Character and business capacity. 2. Training and knowledge. Without the second, the first is of little avail. Without the first, the second is only partially useful; for we cannot bring out of a person what is not in her . . .

The future superintendent would be a great deal the better for two years of training for so difficult and responsible a post. But such are the calls upon us that we can often give her scarcely one.

If the lady, in training for a superintendent, can pay for her own board, it is, of course, right that she should do so (everything else is, in all cases, given free) . . .

Nursing is an art; and, if it is to be made an art, requires as exclusive a devotion, as hard a preparation, as any painter's or sculptor's work; for what is the having to do with dead canvas or cold marble, compared with having to do with the living body—the temple of God's spirit? It is one of the Fine Arts; I had almost said, the finest of the Fine Arts . . .

There is no such thing as amateur art; there is no such thing as amateur nursing. . . . Three-fourths of the whole mischief in women's lives arises from their excepting themselves from the rule of training considered needful for men.

221. From Reports of the Nightingale Fund

[The following excerpts from the reports of the Nightingale Fund indicate the requirements and the program of the school in the early years of its existence.]

[1861]
Duties of Probationers Under the Nightingale Fund.
You are required to be
> Sober
> Honest
> Truthful
> Trustworthy
> Punctual
> Quiet and orderly
> Clean and neat.

[1862]
Persons of superior manners and education, ladies in fact, are not as a rule the best qualified, but rather women of somewhat more than ordinary intelligence emanating from those classes in which women are habitually employed in earning their own livelihood. Ladies, however, are not excluded; on the contrary, where sufficient evidence is shown that they intend to pursue

the calling as a business, and have those qualifications which will fit them to become superintendents, their admission would be considered an advantage and they would readily find employment. . . . The institution undoubtedly affords an opportunity to women to fit themselves for an employment of a superior kind.

The ultimate success, however, of the scheme must depend on economical grounds. It is believed that the means are now afforded of producing examples of what a real nurse ought to be; it remains for their employers, viz., the public to display a just appreciation of their value by paying an adequate remuneration for their services.

[1869]

The candidates who are best qualified for the ordinary duties of the hospital nurse appear to be daughters of small farmers who have been used to household work, and well educated domestic servants.

Concerning the special probationers:

We want gentlewomen who come with settled purpose to do the work, free from all romance and affectation but yet not wanting in some genuine enthusiasm; possessed of that valuable and uncommon quality common sense. They must come prepared to make sacrifices without thinking themselves self-sacrificing . . . impressed with the dignity of their work, the essential importance of the way it is done, to think nothing beneath them, or too small to be well and thoroughly done. They must not be self important but remembering they are members of a community.

Women are needed able to organize and rule with an eye to the good of the cause; in sympathy with those over them as well as those under them— large minded, large hearted.

The inferior lady of moderate education, small experience, and therefore small minded is a useless commodity and is quite superceded by the educated intelligent probationer. Those again, who from want of capacity have failed in some other sphere are not suitable for this. Gentlewomen to succeed in this work must be such in truth and they are the better for having had some knowledge of the world which is gained by moving with equals and superiors.

[1872]

[The Committee appointed an assistant whose duty it was] to take charge, under the matron, of the domestic arrangements of the Home, and to conduct improvement classes for the benefit of such probationers who required such aid.

[1875]

To train and assist in supplying nurses to be employed in attending the poor at their own homes has frequently been referred to as one of the principal objects which the Committee have had in view. . . . By agreement with the above Association [Metropolitan and National Nursing Association] the Committee have now six Probationer-Nurses in training for the work of nursing the poor in their own homes and they have undertaken to admit six more.

[1881]

Memorandum as to the Qualifications Required of Candidates for Admission to the Nightingale Fund Training School for Nurses

The ordinary probationers are intelligent well educated young women of upper servant class, daughters of small farmers, tradesmen, artizans, etc. It is requisite that the ordinary probationer be intelligent and fairly well educated so as to profit by the classes for elementary technical instruction(s) which are given to train her to understand intelligently the doctor's orders, so as not to carry them out as a mere machine but to know the reason why. She must learn to observe and report accurately the state of her patients. She must be cleanly in person, and in her work, mindful of little things. She must be prepared to do as she is bid, and carry out doctor's and sister's orders implicitly. Physical health is very essential also a steady purpose, patience, and perseverance.[13]

222. Report on the Nightingale Fund in *The Lancet,* June 22, 1872, pp. 873–874

[This report, published in the medical press twelve years after the establishment of the Nightingale School, indicates the physical arrangements of the building and the situation in nursing at St. Thomas's Hospital.]

The Nightingale Fund

The Committee's report just issued for the past year embraces some interesting details connected with the Nightingale Home and the nursing at St. Thomas's Hospital. The new buildings of St. Thomas's Hospital were formally inaugurated by her Majesty in June, but not opened for the reception of patients until the end of the following September. The wards were rapidly filled, and by the end of the year the whole of the new hospital was more or less occupied, and an efficient nursing staff had to be provided. The hospital authorities were materially aided in this by the Committee of the Nightingale fund. The Nightingale Home at St. Thomas's Hospital affords a separate room to each of the 35 probationers accomodated therein. The hospital proper consists of six pavilions, containing in all 569 beds. Three of these blocks have four floors of wards, each block containing three wards of 28 beds, with a small ward of 2 beds, and one ward of 20 beds, with a small ward for 1 bed; two of the blocks have each three floors of wards, each block containing three wards of 28 beds, with a small ward of 2 beds. The sixth block is set apart for infectious cases, and contains seven wards of 8 beds each. The arrangements for the nursing staff are as follows: there are in all 16 hospital sisters, one of whom acts as superintendent of night-nurses and one as matron's assistant, besides 54 nurses, and 3 nursemaids. To 5 of the sisters are assigned two wards each, to 7 one each, and there is one sister for the infectious block. For every large ward there is one day-nurse and one night-nurse. There are, in addition, 23 ward maids and 14 scrubbers. The sisters and nurses in charge of a ward sleep in their own rooms adjoining their respective wards. The sisters receive from £35 to £50 a year as salary, the nurses from £23 rising to £25. The ward-maids are paid from £14 to £15 a year, with a shilling a week for washing. The probationers are employed as assistant nurses under the immediate direction of the sisters. During the period of the year's training they pass successively through all the different wards except the infectious block. We learn that towards the end of the last year an arrangement was entered into with the Central London Sick Asylum District for the admission of six probationers to the Highgate Infirmary, to be trained for service in workhouse infirmaries.

The Writings of Florence Nightingale [14]

[Miss Nightingale's writings reflect her many-faceted interests and show literary ability of a superior kind. For presentation in this compilation, a few have been selected from those not readily accessible elsewhere.[15] The order of presentation is, in general, a chronological one. The statements concerning the circumstances surrounding the writing of each are based on Sir Edward Cook's biography.]

223. Florence Nightingale. *Notes on Hospitals*

[Portions of this book appeared in 1858. They consisted of two papers read before the National Association for the Promotion of Social Science, at Liverpool, under the titles, "Notes on the Health of Hospitals," and "Sixteen Sanitary Defects in the Construction of Hospital Wards." When they were reprinted the following year, the book included *Evidence Given to the Royal Commissioners on the State of the Army in 1857.* Sir James Paget called *Notes on Hospitals* "the most valuable contribution to sanitary science in application to medical institutions that I have ever read." [16] This extract from the *Notes* gives Miss Nightingale's ideas of desirable numbers of head nurses and night nurses to patients in hospital wards and an outline of the types of hospital administration in existence in Europe at that time. In addition, the book contains many tables and plans.]

It may seem a strange principle to enunciate as the very first requirement in a Hospital that it should do the sick no harm. It is quite necessary, nevertheless, to lay down such a principle, because the actual mortality in hospitals, especially in those of large crowded cities, is very much higher than any calculation founded on the mortality of the same class of diseases among patients treated *out of* hospitals would lead us to expect.

Distribution of Sick in Convenient Numbers for Attendance, and Position of Nurses' Rooms.

Four wards of ten patients each, taking the average of patients as in London, cannot be efficiently overlooked by one head nurse. Forty patients in one ward can be fully overlooked by one head nurse. She ought to have her room so placed that she can command her whole ward, day and night, from a window looking into the ward . . .

Four wards of ten patients each cannot be attended by one night nurse, taking the average of London cases. Forty patients in one ward can be fully attended by one night nurse.

Appendix

In the important question of accomodation for nurses, so much depends upon the method of nursing chosen, that an Appendix is devoted to this.

The methods of nursing the sick adopted in the public hospitals of Europe may be distinguished under five classes:

1. Where the nurses belong to a religious order, and are under their own spiritual head: the hospital being administered by a separate and secular governing body.

Examples.—The hospitals of Paris, of King's College Hospital, London.

2. Where the nurses are of a religious order, the head of which administers both order and hospital.

Examples.—The Protestant institutions of Bethanien at Berlin, Kaiserswerth on the Rhine, many Roman Catholic institutions at Rome and all over Europe, also Anglican sisterhoods at home.

3. Where the nurses are secular under their own head; the hospital having its own separate and secular government.

Example.—The hospitals of London.

4. Where the nurses are secular; and under the same secular authority as that by which the hospital where they nurse is governed.

Examples.—The great general hospital at Vienna, the Charite at Berlin.

5. Where the nurses are all men and seculars, and under the same secular male authority as the hospital.

Example.—The military hospitals of Germany, and till a recent period of England, France, and Russia.[17]

224. Florence Nightingale. *Army Sanitary Administration and Its Reform Under the Late Lord Herbert*

[This paper appeared first as *Sidney Herbert,* and was privately printed and circulated among Sidney Herbert's friends after his death. It was dated August 2, 1861, the day of Lord Herbert's death. In 1862, at the urging of Lord Herbert's friends, Miss Nightingale revised and enlarged the paper under the above title. It was read at the London meeting of the Congrès de Bienfaisance in June, 1862, and printed in its proceedings in 1863.[18]]

It has been well and truly said that, in long wars, the real arbiter of the destinies of nations is not the sword, but pestilence . . .

To endeavour to prevent this destruction of life is by no means to encourage war, no more than to attend on the sick and wounded in a field hospital is to encourage war.

The object is primarily one of humanity. It is to save life, and to diminish suffering. And all who engage in this work are, in the best sense, savers of men.

Highest among such must be ranked Sidney Herbert.[19]

225. [Florence Nightingale]. "A Note on Pauperism," *Fraser's Magazine*, March, 1869, pp. 281–290

[This article was written at the insistence of Mr. Benjamin Jowett, a Church of England clergyman, vice-chancellor of Oxford, and a great educator, who was for many years a friend of Miss Nightingale. Mr. Jowett had, at this time, been urging Miss Nightingale to attempt some sustained writing. The article was the first of several contributions which Miss Nightingale made to *Fraser's Magazine*.[20]]

All paupers who can move arm or leg can more or less support themselves.

The first thing to do is:—to remove all the sick (incapable) out of workhouses and provide for their cure and care. This is, in a considerable measure, being done or about to be done.

The next is:—not to punish the hungry for being hungry, but to teach the hungry to feed themselves.

Statesmen fancy this to be done by "education,"—the three R's—teaching the laws of nature.

Now some of the very greatest rascals that ever lived are those who knew the laws of nature best.

In a country where local self government has trenched largely on the fourth R—rascaldom—everybody knows the three R's.

226. Letter of Florence Nightingale, Dated May 6, 1881, to the Nurses at St. Thomas's Hospital

[This letter, No. 104 in Cook's biography,[21] expresses some of Florence Nightingale's ideas on the personal aspects of the nurse's training. It is inscribed in Miss Nightingale's handwriting, to "Nurse Vousden St. Marylebone Infirmary with Florence Nightingale's best wishes." St. Marylebone is a northwestern metropolitan borough of London, containing many famous landmarks and a number of hospitals.]

London May 6, 1881

My very dear friends

Now once more "God speed" to you all; my very best greetings & thanks to you all, all:—to our beginners good courage,—to our dear old workers peace, fresh courage too, perseverance: for to persevere to the end is as difficult & needs a yet better energy than to begin new work.

To be a good Nurse one must be a good woman, here we shall all agree—It is the old, old story—But some of us are new to the state.

What is it to be "like a woman"? "Like a woman"—"a very woman" is sometimes said as a word of contempt: sometimes as a word of tender admiration.

What makes a good woman is the better or higher or holier nature: quietness—gentleness—patience—endurance—forbearance—forbearance with her patients—her fellow workers—her superiors—her equals We need above all to remember that we come to learn, to be taught—Hence we come to obey. No one ever was able to govern who was not able to obey. No one ever was able to teach who was not able to learn. The best scholars make the best teachers—those who obey best the best rulers. We all have to obey as well as to command all our lives.

Who does it best?

As a mark of contempt for a woman is it not said, she can't obey? She will have her own way?

As a mark of respect—she always knows how to obey: how to give up her own way?

You are here to be trained for *Nurses—attendants* on the wants of the sick—*helpers,* in carrying out Doctor's orders (not medical students) Though theory is very useful when carried out by practice, Theory without practice is ruinous to nurses.

Then a good woman should be *thorough* thoroughness in a Nurse is a matter of life & death to the Patient

Or, rather without it she is no Nurse—Especially thoroughness in the *unseen* work. Do that well & the other will be done well too. Be as careful in the cleaning of the used poultice basin as in your attendance at an antiseptic dressing.

Don't care most about what meets the eye & gains attention.

"How do you know you have grace?"—Said a Minister to a housemaid—"Because I clean under the Mats," was the excellent reply.

If a housemaid said that, how much more should a Nurse, all whose vessels mean Patients.

Now what does "like a woman" mean when it is said in contempt? does it not mean what is petty, little selfishnesses, small meannesses: envy = jealousy = foolish talking: unkind gossip = love of praise.

Careless inaccurate hearsay statements. Now, while we try to be "like women" in the noble sense of the word, let us fight as bravely against all such womanly weaknesses, let us be anxious to do well, not for selfish praise but to honour & advance the cause, the work we have taken up Let us value our training not as it makes us cleverer or superior to others, but inasmuch as it enables us to be more useful & helpful to our fellow creatures, the sick, who most want our help. Let it be our ambition to be thorough goodwomen, good Nurses—And never let us be ashamed of the name of "Nurse."

274

227. Florence Nightingale. "Introduction to the 'History of Nursing in the Homes of the Poor'"

[This is the introduction to William Rathbone's *Sketch of the History and Progress of District Nursing...*, published in 1890. Mr. Rathbone, M.P., a philanthropist of Liverpool, had appealed to Miss Nightingale for assistance in inaugurating district nursing in that city. In accordance with her suggestion that Liverpool train its own nurses for this work, the Liverpool Training School and Home for Nurses was established, providing nurses for the infirmary and for district nursing as well. Workhouse infirmary nursing in Liverpool was initiated under the leadership of Agnes Elizabeth Jones.[22]]

In hospitals and infirmaries they may say, "when everything is provided, it is easy to be clean and airy, orderly and godly, but look at us in our one room—and a sick person in it into the bargain—and with no appliances."

Here the district trained nurse steps in. Here, in the family, she meets them on their own ground. Besides nursing the patient, she shows them in their own home how they can help in this nursing, how they can be clean and orderly, how they can improvise appliances, how their home need not be broken up. She cannot make "the wilderness blossom as the rose." But now that the day of improved dwellings for the poor appears to be coming more largely, the district nurse may be the forerunner in teaching the disorderly how to use improved dwellings—teaching without seeming to teach, which is the ideal of teaching.

The trained district nurse (under the doctor) nurses the child or breadwinner back to health without breaking up the home—the dread of honest workmen and careful mothers, who know the pauperising influence of the workhouse even if only temporary. The nurse also teaches the family healthy and disease-preventing ways by showing them her own in practice in their homes.

Now, no living thing can less lend itself to a "formula" than nursing. Nursing has to nurse living bodies and spirits. It cannot be formulated like engineering. It cannot be numbered or registered like arithmetic and population. It must be sympathetic. It cannot be tested by public examinations, though it may be tested by current supervision.

A good nurse must be a good *woman*, with sympathetic insight. She cannot be a good nurse without. A good woman cannot be gauged by words. She must be *herself* the word—a name made divine to us by our great

Master, and which He expects each one of us women particularly to embody in her own duty, each in her own tiny sphere.

And one thing we may be sure, that if the poor receive good from the living, loving intercourse of the trained and educated woman, she in her turn received quite as much good from theirs.[23]

228. Florence Nightingale. "Sick-Nursing and Health-Nursing"

[This paper was published in *Women's Mission: a Series of Congress Papers on the Philanthropic Work of Women,* issued by the Royal British Commission, Chicago Exhibition, 1893. The volume was edited by Baroness Burdett-Coutts, who, throughout her life of 92 years, engaged in all sorts of benefactions. The volume included also two other papers on nursing: "Philanthropic Aspects of Nursing," by Lady Victoria Lambton and Mrs. Malleson, and "On Nursing," by the Hon. Mrs. Stuart Wortley.]

1.—A new art and a new science has been created since and within the last forty years. And with it a new profession—so they say; we say, *calling.* One would think this had been created or discovered for some new want or local want. Not so. The want is nearly as old as the world, nearly as large as the world, as pressing as life or death. It is that of sickness. And the art is that of nursing the sick. Please mark—nursing the sick; not nursing sickness. We will call the art nursing proper. This is generally practised by women under scientific heads—physicians and surgeons. This is one of the distinctions between nursing proper and medicine, though a very famous and successful physician did say, when asked how he treated pneumonia: "I do not treat pneumonia, I treat the person who has pneumonia." This is the reason why nursing proper can only be taught by the patient's bedside, and in the sick-room or ward. Neither can it be taught by lectures or by books, though these are valuable accessories; if used as such; otherwise what is in the book stays in the book.

What is nursing? Both kinds of nursing are to put us in the best possible conditions for Nature to restore or preserve health—to prevent or to cure disease or injury. Upon nursing proper, under scientific heads, physicians or surgeons, must depend partly, perhaps mainly, whether Nature succeeds or fails in her attempts to cure by sickness. Nursing proper is therefore to help the patient suffering from disease to live—just as health-nursing is to keep or put the constitution of the healthy child or human being in such a state as to have no disease.

What is training? Training is to teach the nurse to help the patient to live. Nursing the sick is an art, and an art requiring an organized, practical, and scientific training; for nursing is the skilled servant of medicine, surgery, and hygiene. . . . Training is to teach a nurse how God makes health, and how He makes disease. Training is to teach a nurse to know her business, that is, to observe exactly, to understand, to know exactly, to do, to tell exactly, in such stupendous issues as life and death, health and disease. Training has to make her, not servile, but loyal to medical orders and authorities. True loyalty to orders cannot be without the independent sense or energy of responsibility, which alone secures real trustworthiness. Training is to teach the nurse how to handle the agencies within our control which restore health and life, in strict, intelligent obedience to the physician's or surgeon's power and knowledge; how to keep the health mechanism prescribed to her in gear. Training must show her how the effects on life of nursing may be calculated with nice precision, such care of carelessness, such a sick-rate, such a duration of case, such a death-rate.

What makes a good training-school for nurses? The most favourable conditions for the administration of the hospital are:

First. A good lay administration with a chief executive officer, a civilian (be he called treasurer or permanent chairman of committee), with power delegated to him by the committee, who gives his time. This is the main thing. . . .

Secondly. A strong body of medical officers, visiting and resident, and a medical school.

Thirdly. The government of hospitals in the point of view of the real responsibility for the conduct and discipline of the nurses being thrown upon the matron (superintendent of nurses), who is herself a trained nurse, and the real head of all the female staff of the hospital. Vest the whole responsibility for nursing, internal management, for discipline and training of nurses in this one female head of the nursing staff, whatever called. She should be herself responsible directly to the constituted hospital authorities, and all her nurses and servants should, in the performance of their duties, be responsible, in matters of conduct and discipline, to her only . . .

Having then, as a basis, a well-organized hospital, we require, as further considerations: (1) a special *organization for the purpose* of training, that is, where systematic technical training is given in the wards to the probationers; where it is the business of the ward "sisters" to train them, to keep records of their progress, to take "stock" of them; where the probationers are not set down in the wards to "pick up" as they can. (2) A good "home" for the probationers in the hospital, where they can learn moral discipline— for technical training is only half the battle, perhaps less than half—where the probationers are steadily "mothered" by a "home" sister (class mistress). (3) Staff of training school. (a) A trained matron over all, who is not only a housekeeper, but distinctly the head and superintendent of the nursing. (b) A "home" sister (assistant superintendent)—making the "home" a real home to the probationers, giving them classes, disciplining their life. (c) Ward Sisters (head nurses of wards) who have been trained in the school— to a certain degree permanent, that is, not constantly changing. For they are the key to the whole situation, matron influencing through them nurses (day and night), probationers, ward-maids, patients. For, after all, the hospital is for the good of the patients, not for the good of the nurses. And the patients are not there to teach probationers upon. Rather, probationers had better not be there at all, unless they understand that they are there for the patients, and not for themselves ...

Nursing proper means, besides giving the medicines and stimulants prescribed, or the surgical appliances, the proper use of fresh air (ventilation), light, warmth, cleanliness, quiet, and the proper choosing and giving of diet, all at the least expense of vital power to the sick. And so health-at-home nursing means exactly the same proper use of the same natural elements, with as much life-giving power as possible to the healthy.

The scheme before referred to for health-at-home nursing has arisen in connection with the newly-constituted administration of counties in England, by which the local authority of the county (County Council) has been invested by Act of Parliament with extended sources of income applicable to the teaching of nursing and sanitary knowledge, in addition to the powers which they already possessed for sanitary inspection and the prevention of infectious diseases. This scheme is framed for rural districts, but the general principles are also applicable to urban populations, though, where great numbers are massed together, a fresh set of difficulties must be met, and different treatment be necessary.

The scheme contemplates the training of ladies, so called health missioners, so as to qualify them to give instruction to village mothers in: (1) The sanitary conditions of the person, clothing and bedding, and house. (2) The management of health of adults, women before and after confinements, infants and children. The teaching by the health missioners would be given by lectures in the villages, followed by personal instruction by way of conversation with the mothers in their own homes, and would be directed to: (1) The condition of the homes themselves in a sanitary point of view; (2) the essential principles of keeping the body in health, with reference to the skin, the circulation, and the digestion; and (3) instruction as to what to do in cases of emergency or accident before the doctor comes, and with reference to the management of infants and children.

What is it to feel a *calling* for anything? Is it not to do our work in it to satisfy the high idea of what is the *right,* the *best,* and not because we shall be found out if we don't do it? This is the "enthusiasm" which every one, from shoemaker to a sculptor, must have in order to follow his "calling" properly. Now, the nurse has to do not with shoes or with marble, but with human beings.

How, then to keep up the high tone of a calling, to "make your calling and election sure"? By fostering that bond of sympathy (*esprit de corps*) which community of aims and of action in good work induces. A common nursing home in the hospital for hospital nurses and for probationer nurses; a common home for private nurses during intervals of engagements, whether attached to a hospital, or separate; a home for district nurses (wherever possible), where four or five can live together; all homes under loving, trained, moral, and religious, as well as technical, superintendence, such as to keep up the tone of the inmates with constant supply of all material wants and constant sympathy. Man cannot live by bread alone, still less woman. Wages is not the only question, but high home-helps.

To sum up the dangers;

i. On one side, fashion, and want of earnestness not making it a *life,* but a mere interest consequent on this.

ii. On the other side, mere money-getting; yet man does not live by bread alone, still less woman.

iii. Making it a profession, and not a calling. Not making your "calling and election sure"; wanting, especially with private nurses, the community of feeling of a common nursing home, pressing towards the "mark of your calling," keeping up the moral tone.

iv. Above all, danger of making it book-learning and lectures—not an an apprenticeship; a workshop practice.

v. Thinking that any hospital with a certain number of beds may be a box to train nurses in, regardless of the conditions essential to a sound hospital organization, especially the responsibility of the female head for the conduct and discipline of the nurses.

vi. Imminent danger of stereotyping instead of progressing. "No system can endure that does not march." Objects of registration not capable of being gained by a public register. Who is to guarantee our guarantors? Who is to make the inquiries? You might as well register mothers as nurses. A good nurse must be a good woman.

We are only on the threshold of nursing. . . . May we hope that the day will come when every mother will become a health-nurse, when every poor sick person will have the opportunity of a share in a district sick-nurse at home. But it will not be out of a register; the nurse will not be a stereotyped one. We find a trace of nursing here, another there; we find nothing like a nation or race, or class who know how to provide the elementary conditions demanded for the recovery of their sick, whose mothers know how to bring up their infants for health.[24]

229. [Florence Nightingale]. *Subsidiary Notes as to the Introduction of Female Nursing into Military Hospitals in Peace and War*

[These notes were presented by request to the Secretary of State for War but were not issued to the public. Five hundred copies were printed at Miss Nightingale's expense.[25] The first section of the following extract comprises some of Miss Nightingale's notes on hospital nurses, the second is the government order recognizing Miss Nightingale as general superintendent of the women nurses, and the third outlines the types of nurses who were present with Miss Nightingale in the Crimean War theater.]

1. Hospital-Nurses

1. It would appear desirable to consider that definite objects are to be attained; and that the road leading to them is to a large extent to be found out—therefore to consider all plans and rules, for some time to come, as in a great measure tentative and experimental.

2. The main object I conceive to be, to improve hospitals, by improving hospital-nursing; and to do this by improving, or contributing towards the improvement, of the class of hospital-nurses, whether nurses or head-nurses.

3. This I propose doing, not by founding a Religious Order; but by training, systematizing, and morally improving as far as may be permitted, that section of the large class of women supporting themselves by labour, who take to hospital-nursing for a livelihood,—by inducing, in the long run, some such women to contemplate usefulness, and the service of God and in the relief of man, as well as maintenance,—and by incorporating with both these classes a certain proportion of gentlewomen who may think fit to adopt this occupation without pay, but under the same rules, and on the same strict footing of duty performed under definite superiors. These two latter elements, if efficient (if not, they would be mischievous rather than useless), I consider would elevate and leaven the mass.

7. The care of the sick is the main object of hospitals. The care of souls is the great province of the clergy of hospitals. The care of their bodies is the duty of nurses.

I

General Orders

March 1856

"It is notified, by order of the Secretary of State for War, that Miss Nightingale is recognized by Her Majesty's Government as the General Superintendent of the Female Nursing Establishment of the Military Hospitals of the Army. No lady, sister, or nurse is to be transmitted from one Hospital to another, or into any Hospital, without previous consultation with her. Her instructions, however, require her to have the approval of the Principal Medical Officer, in her exercise of the responsibility thus vested in her.

"The Principal Medical Officer will communicate with Miss Nightingale upon all subjects connected with the Female Nursing Establishment, and will give his directions through that lady."

II

Nurses

1. Our Nurses were of four sorts.

Nuns	Ladies
Sisters (Anglican)	Nurses

The Nuns were received not as Nuns, but as Nurses.

Their (socalled) training told sometimes against us; sometimes for us. The same with the "Sisters" (Anglican).

The Ladies were useful, exactly in proportion as they approached the professional and not the dilettante, mode of thought.

A larger proportion of paid Nurses than of Ladies did well, and this under circumstances of peculiar temptation. Paid Nurses are always the most useful . . .[26]

The Emergence of the Nursing Profession

230. *Sisterhoods; Schools for Nurses*

[This pamphlet combines two articles which appeared in the *Pall Mall Gazette* and the *Saturday Review,* in 1866.[27]]

No one who knows anything of nursing will underrate its importance, or the qualifications which it requires. No one who has ever taken the trouble to read such a treatise as Miss Nightingale's [*Notes on Nursing*] can fancy that an uneducated and ignorant woman is likely to make a good nurse, or can doubt that the profession is one in which the qualities developed by education—intelligence, observation, self-command, conscientiousness, sobriety—are of inestimable value. The duties of a nurse are by no means either mechanical or, in a true sense, menial; their proper performance demands the whole energies of a mind of more than average capacity, and a careful and thorough training. The occupation, therefore, is essentially a respectable one—unsuited to the vulgar, thoughtless, and ignorant, because they are not competent to fulfil its duties efficiently; suited to the intelligent, educated, and well-trained, because it requires the faculties, mental and moral, which they possess in the highest degree. A nurse ought to have a command of temper which few uneducated persons enjoy; a care, and minute attention to the wants and humours of the patient, which is possible only to those who have undergone considerable intellectual discipline; a refinement of feeling and manner which are seldom found among the class from which the majority of existing nurses are taken. She must be able to watch and report, with intelligence and discrimination, the symptoms of the patient; to understand and carry out, not mechanically, but with comprehension and discretion, the orders of the doctor. She should be quiet, neat-handed, skilful, gentle—as educated women mostly are, and others mostly are not.

Nor can anyone question the importance of the nurse's function. In nine cases out of ten, a first-rate nurse is of more value than a first-rate physician.[28]

231. **"Report of the Lancet Sanitary Commission on Night Nursing in the London Hospitals,"** *The Lancet,* **November 4, 1871, pp. 642–680**

[In 1871 a commission of *The Lancet,* a weekly medical journal founded in 1823,[29] reported on the conditions found in the London hospitals in the care of the sick at night. The report shows that, slow as was the change to better nursing, it nevertheless reflected to some degree the influence of the Nightingale system of education and service.]

There is no part of hospital administration in which the public has evinced a deeper interest than in that which relates to the care of the sick at night. And rightly so. During the day the sufferer is surrounded with a thousand safeguards against neglect. There are the visits of the medical officers, of the chaplains, and of friends and relations; there is also the sympathy of fellow-sufferers and the protection of broad daylight . . .

We have no need, therefore, to apologise for instituting an inquiry into the arrangements for night-nursing in the London hospitals. The fact that this department is without the sphere of public observation would alone justify us. We had no expectation of being able to discover any sensational instances of neglect. The sleepy, drunken Sarah Gamps are, happily, persons of the past. We believe that there does not exist a board of management which is not anxiously desirous of making their nursing arrangements as complete as possible; and our main object will have been accomplished if we shall be able to assure the public that the general arrangements deserve their confidence; whilst a comparison between the practice at the various establishments can scarcely fail to improve our knowledge and to eradicate defects . . .

At the Royal Free Hospital (Gray's-Inn-Road), with rather better than 100 beds, we found seven nurses on night duty, not one of whom had yet had a twelvemonth's experience of her work. They were all probationers, and most of them very young. There was not a single fully trained nurse on duty. . . . There is no regular system here for the night-supervision of the nurses. The lady superintendent is a most active and intelligent person, who labours at the calling she has chosen *con amore.* She spares herself in nothing that can in the smallest degree add to the efficient performance of the task she has taken in hand, and not only does she exercise a watchful supervision during the day, but occasionally makes a night-visit as well, in order to satisfy herself that all is as it should be. This is, of course, most praiseworthy, but we hold it to be of the greatest importance that the system of night-supervision should be systematically carried out (especially where the night nurses are, as in this case, raw recruits) by a person who is not expected to perform any day duty at all . . .

232. **Pye Henry Chavasse.** *Advice to a Wife on the Management of Her Own Health and on the Treatment of Some of the Complaints Incidental to Pregnancy, Labor, and Suckling*

[Dr. Chavasse was a Fellow of the Royal College of Surgeons of England, as well as a Fellow of the Obstetrical Society of London.[30] He credits Miss Nightingale with improving the quality of nursing of his day. The qualifications which he deemed important for the nurse will interest the present-day reader.]

Monthly Nurse

568. It is an important, a most important, consideration to choose a nurse rightly and well: the well-doing of both mother and babe often depend upon the right selection.

569. A good nurse should be taught her business. How, unless she have a regular training, can she be a proficient? You may as well expect a lady, who has never learned to play, to sit down to the piano and "Discourse sweet music,"—one is quite as absurd as the other; and yet how many women have the assurance to turn nurses who are as ignorant of the duties of a nurse as an unborn babe? It is sad that there are not in every large town proper training establishments both for monthly and for sick nurses . . .

570. Florence Nightingale has proved the great need there is for trained nurses, and has done more than ever has been done before to increase their efficiency.

571. A monthly nurse ought to be middle-aged. If she be young, she is apt to be thoughtless and giggling; if she be old, she may be deaf and stupid, and may think too much of her trouble. She should have calmness and self-possession. She must be gentle, kind, good-tempered, and obliging, but firm withal, and she should have a cheerful countenance. "Some seem by nature to have a vocation for nursing;" others not. Again, nursing has its separate branches; some have the light step, the pleasant voice, the cheering smile, the dextrous hand, the gentle touch; others are gifted in cookery for the sick. The former good qualities are essential to a monthly nurse, and if she can combine the latter—that is to say, if she is "gifted in cookery for the sick"—she will, as a monthly nurse, be invaluable. "Dr. Thyne held that sick nurses, like poets, were born, not made . . ."

573. She ought neither to be a tattler, nor a tale-bearer, nor a "croaker," nor a "potterer . . ."

574. Some monthly nurses have a knack of setting the servants at logger-heads, and of poisoning the minds of their mistresses against them . . .

576. The class of nurses is, fortunately for ladies, wonderfully improved, and the race of Sairey Gamp and Betsy Prig is nearly at an end. Drunkenness among midwives and monthly nurses is now the exception, and not the rule . . .

577. She ought to be either a married woman or a widow. A single woman cannot so well enter into the feelings of a lying-in patient, and has not had the necessary experience. Moreover, a single woman, as a rule, is not so handy with an infant (more especially in putting for the first time to the breast) as is a *married* woman.

578. She must be sober, temperate, and healthy, and free from deafness, and from any defect of vision. She should have a gentle manner, but yet be neither melancholy nor hippish. She ought to have the "softest step and gentlest tone; . . ." She ought to be fond of children, and must neither mind her trouble nor at being disturbed at night. She should be a light sleeper. A heavy sleeper—a nurse that snores in her sleep—is very objectionable; she often keeps the patient—more especially if she be easily disturbed—awake; and sleep is to a lying-in woman priceless—

> "The nurse sleeps sweetly, hired to watch the sick,
> Whom snoring she disturbs."—Cowper.

579. "Scrupulous attention to cleanliness, freshness, and neatness" in her own person, and toward the lady and the infant, are most important re-quisites.

580. A fat dumpling of a nurse—and some nurses are as fat as butter (their occupation tends to make them so)—ought not to be chosen, as she can make no proper lap for her little charge. Besides, very fat people are usually heavy sleepers, and snore in their sleep, and are difficult, when duty calls them to action, to rouse from their slumbers . . .

581. In choosing a monthly nurse, select one who has a bright sunshiny countenance; have nothing to do with a crab-vinegar-faced individual . . .

582. A fine lady-nurse that requires to be constantly waited upon by a servant is not the one that I would recommend . . .

583. As the nurse, if she does her duty, devotes her time, her talent, and her best energies to the lady and to the infant, a mistress ought to be most liberal in the payment of a monthly nurse . . .

594. A lady may, perhaps, say, "You want a nurse to be perfection?" Well, I do; a nurse ought to be as near perfection as poor human nature will allow. None but good women and true should enter the ranks of nurses, for their responsibility is great, and their power of doing either good or evil

is enormous. Hence good nurses are prizeable, and should be paid most liberally.[31]

233. Dr. James Hinton on Nursing

[James Hinton (1822–1875), English surgeon and author, went to St. Bartholomew's Hospital to study medicine and received his diploma in 1847. He wrote on physiological and ethical subjects, his works having a wide circulation on both sides of the Atlantic because of their freshness and vigor. He was appointed aural surgeon at Guy's Hospital in 1863.[32] He wrote a pamphlet on the profession of nursing, an excerpt from which is quoted below from the *Life and Letters of James Hinton,* edited by Ellice Hopkins (1836–1904), social reformer and friend of Dr. Hinton.[33] Dr. Hinton's high conception of the profession of nursing is expressed in this statement.]

An expression of surprise was once quoted in his presence "how any woman could condescend to be a doctor who had the chance of being a nurse." "Exactly so," he replied. "When a commonplace young man says, 'I want to be a doctor,' I say, 'Very well,' because I daresay he will do well enough. And if a commonplace girl wants to be a doctor, I take it for granted she will do well enough too. But if a girl says, 'I want to be a nurse,' I begin to consider whether she has the requisite qualifications. For the nurse's profession embraces all that is good in both the medical and clerical professions; the positive elements of each without the negative elements of either. She has the doctor's science without his drugs, and the parson's religion without his dogmas.' " [34]

234. Louisa Twining's Notes of Six Years' Work as Guardian of the Poor, 1884–1890

[Miss Twining's work as a Guardian of the Poor brought her into contact with workhouse infirmaries, where she gained insight into nursing conditions.[35] The latter part of the following quotation states the regulations developed by the Poor Law Board and the Local Government Board relative to nursing in these infirmaries.]

[Paddington Infirmary] When, through resignation, a new matron was required for the Infirmary, I had the satisfaction, in conjunction with the Medical Superintendent, to propose a lady, fully trained and experienced at St. Thomas's Hospital, and already known to me.

.   .   .   .

A word or two on the tone and qualifications of Infirmary Nurses.

As a matter of fact there is not the least reason why these should not compare favorably with any who are trained at the present time in our large

Hospitals. . . . The probationary system and its three year curriculum now adopted with most satisfactory results in the more advanced Infirmaries has opened out a wide field to the yearly increasing number of young women who are anxious to embrace nursing as a profession and of which a comparatively limited number only can find admission into Hospitals.

What a contrast the neat, trim probationer from whom the initial requirements of a good education and unimpeachable moral qualifications are required, presents, to the ignorant, and often times vulgar-minded, assistant nurse of ten years ago.

.   .   .   .

To the Guardians of the Poor of the several Poor Law Unions for the time being in England and Wales;—

And to all others whom it may concern.

Whereas by certain General and other Orders the Poor Law Commissioners, the Poor Law Board, and the Local Government Board have made Rules and Regulations with regard to the government of the workhouses of the said several Poor Law Unions, the nursing of the sick poor relieved therein, and as to the appointment of persons to certain offices therein, including the office of Nurse, and the qualifications, remuneration, and duties of such persons;

And whereas it is expedient that further provision should be made in the matter as herein-after mentioned:

Now Therefore, We, the Local Government Board, in pursuance of the powers given to Us by the Statutes in that behalf, do hereby Order that, from and after the Twenty-ninth day of September, One Thousand Eight Hundred and ninety-seven (herein-after referred to as "the commencement of this Order"), the following Regulations shall, except in so far as We may assent to a departure therefrom, be in force in the said several Poor Law Unions:—

Article I.—(1). Notwithstanding anything contained in any of the Orders above referred to, no pauper inmate of the Workhouse shall be employed to perform the duties of a Nurse in the Sick or Lying-in Wards of the Workhouse, or be otherwise employed in nursing any pauper in the Workhouse who requires nursing.

(2). No pauper inmate of the Workhouse shall be employed as an attendant in the sick or Lying-in Wards of the Workhouse, or upon any pauper in the Workhouse who requires nursing, unless such inmate shall be approved by the Medical Officer of the Workhouse for the purpose, and shall act under the immediate supervision of a paid officer of the Guardians.

Article II.—No person shall be appointed by the Guardians to the office of Nurse or Assistant Nurse in the Workhouse without having had such practical experience in nursing as may render him or her a fit and proper person to hold such office:

Provided that this Article shall not apply in the case of a female Assistant

286

Nurse in a Workhouse where there is a Superintendent Nurse as required by Article III of this Order.

Article III.—(1.) Where at the commencement of this Order the staff of female Nurses and Assistant Nurses in the Workhouse consists of three or more persons, the Guardians shall either appoint a Superintendent Nurse, or, with Our consent, direct that one of the Nurses shall be a Superintendent Nurse.

(2.) Where at the commencement of this Order there is not a staff of three female Nurses and Assistant Nurses in the Workhouse, but the Guardians subsequently propose that there should be such a staff, and also where any Superintendent Nurse ceases to hold office, the Guardians shall appoint a Superintendent Nurse.

(3.) Any Superintendent Nurse appointed after the commencement of this Order, shall, unless We dispense with the requirement, be a person qualified for the appointment by having undergone, for three years at least, a course of instruction in the Medical and Surgical Wards of any Hospital or Infirmary being a Training School for Nurses, and maintaining a Resident Physician or House Surgeon.

Article IV.—(1.) It shall be the duty of the Superintendent Nurse to superintend and control the other Nurses and Assistant Nurses in the Workhouse in the performance of their duties, but such superintendence and control shall, in all matters of treatment of the sick, be subject to the directions of the Medical officer of the Workhouse, and in all other matters to the direction of the Master or Matron of the Workhouse, so far as the Orders in force in the Poor Law Union and the lawful directions of the Guardians may require or permit.

(2.) The provisions of the Orders in force in the Poor Law Union applicable to the mode of appointment, remuneration, and tenure of office of a Nurse at the Workhouse shall apply to every Superintendent Nurse appointed under this Order:

Provided that no such Superintendent Nurse shall be dismissed without Our consent.

Article V.—If in an emergency it appears to the Medical officer of the Workhouse that the employment of a temporary Nurse is required for the proper treatment of any case or cases in the Workhouse, and he informs the Master of the Workhouse in writing accordingly, it shall be the duty of the Master to engage a person to act as Nurse until the next Meeting of the Guardians, and the Guardians shall pay the reasonable remuneration of the person so engaged:

Provided that where there is no Superintendent Nurse appointed under Article III of this Order, no person shall be engaged under this Article without having had such practical experience in nursing as may render him or her a fit and proper person to hold the office of Nurse.

Article VI.—This Order shall not apply to any Infirmary or School which is under administration separate from the Workhouse.

287

This Order may be cited as "The Nursing in Workhouses Order, 1897."

Given under the Seal of Office of the Local Government Board, this sixth day of August, in the year One Thousand eight hundred and ninety-seven.

Hugh Owen,   Henry Chaplin,

     Secretary   President.[36]

235. William Rathbone. *Sketch of the History and Progress of District Nursing* . . .

[In this book, to which Miss Nightingale wrote the introduction,[37] Mr. Rathbone relates how he became interested in district nursing and the steps which led to the establishment of the Liverpool Training School and Home for Nurses. The plan for nursing care, which was adopted by the various districts, is outlined. Mr. Rathbone also tells of the beginning of workhouse infirmary nursing under the leadership of Agnes Jones, of the initiation of the Metropolitan and National Nursing Association, and of the founding of the Queen Victoria Jubilee Institute for Nurses. He acknowledges the guidance received from Miss Nightingale in the early stages of these developments.]

It has become almost unnecessary at the present day, when dealing with the question of nursing, to dwell upon the great importance of a thorough professional training for nurses. People are no longer ignorant of the essential qualifications of nurses; they need no longer be assured that nursing *is* a profession, and that as such it demands a careful apprenticeship, to ensure competency. In fact, the vocation of a sick nurse has been rapidly raised from the inferior position in which it stood about thirty years ago, to one of not merely respectability, but of rare interest and attractiveness. There is even danger, in consequence of the Royal sanction and the attention lately drawn to nursing, that many may be attracted to the work who are neither strong enough for it, nor have that real interest in it which is a most necessary qualification. Many of us can remember a time when most of the nurses in hospitals were mere drudges, and too often of indifferent character; but at the present day their places can be filled by women of irreproachable character, of thorough training, and of considerable technical skill—and, as a fact, nursing has become an employment that is freely sought after by women of refinement and education—while in times gone by, a woman who had been engaged for a few weeks or months as an attendant in the wards of a hospital, or even without such training, was held to be amply qualified for the duties of a sick nurse. It is a great cause for satisfaction that at the present day the selection is much more carefully made, that the candidates for the nursing profession are now tested by a high standard, both as to moral character and aptitude for their work, and that before they are considered proficient for employment they must undergo a lengthened and systematic course of practical training as probationer nurses in the wards of a hospital, combined with scientific instruction adapted to the requirements of their calling.

Just thirty years ago (in 1859), the experience of sickness in a private family in Liverpool first suggested the establishment of a system of district nursing for the poor. The great comfort and advantage derived from trained nursing, even in a home where everything which unskilled affection could suggest was provided, led to the conclusion that among the less fortunate— the poor—untold misery, lasting disability, and death itself must ensue in cases where these comforts and appliances, as well as skilled nursing, are almost altogether wanting. It was resolved to try, even upon the smallest scale, an experiment in reducing these evils. The nurse, who had given proof of her skill in the case above referred to, was asked whether she would undertake to nurse poor patients in their own homes in a district of Liverpool. She consented to do so, and was accordingly supplied with the most necessary appliances, whilst arrangements were made providing the nourishment and medical comforts likely to be wanted. She was to afford help both by her own exertions and by teaching the poor people a better way of tending their sick. As this was only an experiment, the nurse was not engaged for more than three months. But when one month was passed, she returned to her employer and entreated to be released from the engagement. Accustomed though she was to many forms of sickness and of death, she was not able to endure the sight of the misery which she had encountered among the poor. But her employer persuaded her to persevere in the work, and pointed out to her how much of the evil which she had seen might be prevented, and that the satisfaction of abating it would in time be sure to reconcile her to the work. Thus reasoned with, the nurse persevered, and at the end of three months entirely corroborated the prediction. She found that she was able to do great and certain good, and the satisfaction of her achievement was so great that she begged to be allowed to devote herself entirely to nursing the poor, in the place of nursing in wealthy families.

The only means ... of supplying the demand for trained nurses was to form a school of nursing in Liverpool, the course suggested and recommended by Miss Nightingale ...

A training school for nurses was ... needed, not only for district work, but quite as much for the Infirmary and private nursing also. The Committee recognised this want, and Mr. Gibbon, the chairman of the Infirmary, took the preliminary step of making a personal examination of the nursing organisation at King's College and St. Thomas's Hospitals. As the result of his investigation, he was led to support an offer to erect a building to be used as a training school in connection with the Infirmary. The proposal was accepted, and in this way the Liverpool Training School and Home for Nurses was established.

.   .   .   .

The three main objects of the founders of the Liverpool Training School and Home for Nurses were set forth in the prospectus—

1. To provide thoroughly educated professional nurses for the Infirmary.
2. To provide district nurses for the poor.
3. To provide sick nurses for private families.

More interesting, and of greater importance for our present purpose, is a description of the organisation of district nursing adopted in Liverpool. This was in outline as follows:

The districts were made coterminus with parishes, or with groups of parishes, so as to facilitate the co-operation of the clergy in the work of ministering to the sick, while conducted on a purely undenominational basis so far as management was concerned. In each district a lady, or committee of ladies, was provided to superintend the work, but these ladies were not required to have any professional knowledge of nursing. They undertook to provide the medical comforts required, to find lodgings for the nurse in a good central situation, and—in beginning the work in a new district— a meeting of the clergy, of the ministers of the various religious bodies, and others living in the district, was called in order to explain to them the nature of the objects aimed at, and to request that they would interest their friends and parishioners in the work.

In each district the medical men, clergymen and ministers of all denominations were invited to recommend cases to the charity, being at the same time requested to use their power with the utmost discretion. The Lady Superintendent was herself provided with a map of the district, a nurse's register book and forms of recommendation and application. She was to visit, either in person or by deputy, all cases under treatment, so as to obtain assurance that the nurse was working faithfully and well. From time to time she was to examine the nurse's register, to consult with her on fresh cases, and to hear her report on old ones. It was her duty to arrange for the supply, custody, and distribution of medical comforts and appliances, and to keep memoranda of all expenses incurred and of articles lent.

The district nurse was expected to devote at least five or six hours a day to visiting the sick. [8 hrs. usual day's work in the Dist. Nurses Homes] She was to investigate as soon as possible all cases recommended to her by the proper persons and in proper form, to take the recommendations to the Lady Superintendent to be filed by her, and then to report upon the cases and take the Superintendent's decision upon them at the earliest opportunity. She was to report any cases in which she judged that additional nourishment would hasten the recovery of the patient; any cases which could be better dealt with in a hospital or a workhouse; any case in which the neglect or disobedience of patients or their friends made her efforts fruitless. She was to render all the assistance which the medical man might require in any operation, and to do whatever was necessary for the patient and but for her would be left undone. In the homes of the sick poor this includes, of course, many things which are not generally supposed to come under the title of nursing at all, but which, in their case, are most important accessories to it; such offices, for example, as cleaning the sickroom of lumber and unnecessary furniture, sweeping floors and lighting fires. It was the nurse's duty, moreover, to teach the patient and his family the necessity of cleanliness, of ventilation, of regularity in giving food and medicine, above all of implicit obedience to the doctor's directions, and herself to set an example of that neatness, order, sobriety, and obedience which she was to impress upon others. She was exhorted to regard as sacred any knowledge of family matters which might come to her in the course of her duties, to avoid and discourage scandal, and especially to interfere in no way with the patient's or other people's religious opinion. As a rule, the doctor and the nurse could seldom visit the patient at the same time unless by special arrangement, and to avoid the inconvenience resulting therefrom a slate and pencil were hung up in the patient's room, on which the doctor could write his instructions and make an appointment with the nurse, and on which she could enter any facts or ask any questions which she might think necessary . . .

There was . . . no lack of paying patients . . .

Perhaps no reform initiated by the new system was more beneficial than the reform in the nursing in workhouse infirmaries. In London a reform in workhouse hospitals had already been brought about by Act of Parliament [Mr. Gathorne Hardy's Metropolitan Poor Act of 1867], but the introduction into parish hospitals of trained nurses on the Nightingale system grew indirectly out of the experience and information gained in nursing the poor in their own homes.

We may safely take, as an example of the defective condition of workhouse infirmaries at the time, the infirmary at Brownlow Hill in Liverpool. It contained twelve hundred beds, which were occupied by persons in all stages of every kind of disease. Two female officers superintended the nursing; these received pay, but had not been trained as nurses, and their only assistants were pauper women who were as untrustworthy as they were unskilful. . . . But the Brownlow Hill Infirmary was certainly no worse than most other workhouse infirmaries through the Kingdom, for in none of them was a single trained nurse to be found. The Select Vestry of Liverpool, who were well known for the efficiency of their management and the purity of their administration, gladly accepted an offer which afforded some hope of amending the evils above described. This was an offer to defray the extra cost of trying for three years in their hospital the employment of trained nurses under skilled superintendence. . . . Upon the acceptance of the offer, the vestry, with the assistance of Miss Nightingale, secured as lady superintendent Miss Agnes Jones, with a staff of nurses trained in the Nightingale School at St. Thomas's Hospital, to undertake the charge of the nursing. . . . As a first step, Miss Jones was very anxious to train some of the able-bodied pauper women as nurses, who were at once put on a more liberal diet, received a small salary, and were promoted to the rank of assistant nurses. If anybody could have succeeded with such an experiment, Miss Agnes Jones would have had success. But the event showed that she entirely failed. No less than fifty-six pauper women were passed through the test, and under it every one of them broke down. The greater number used their first quarter's salary, as soon as they could obtain leave to go out of the workhouse, to get drunk. The painful fact was established that not a single respectable and trustworthy person could be found among the able-bodied women in the house; the nursing was thereupon taken entirely out of their hands . . .

. . . In less than two years after the arrival of Miss Jones and her staff, the Guardians announced their intention of never reverting to the old system, and of charging the rates with the expense of the new one. . . . Exhausted by her unremitting labours, Miss Agnes Jones sank under a severe attack of typhus fever. . . . The good results of Miss Jones' work may, indeed, be seen far beyond the bounds of Liverpool. The system has spread over the country; many of the nurses trained in her school are to be found in all parts of England . . .[38]

[Metropolitan and National Nursing Association.]

In the year 1874 the nursing of the poor received a new and important impulse from the movement which created the Metropolitan and National Nursing Association. This movement was initiated by the Council of the Order of St. John of Jerusalem, and set on foot by Lady Strangford, Sir Edmund Lechmere, and Mr. Wigram, together with other ladies and gentlemen whose names appear in the list of the Council.

The objects of the Association, as stated in its own publications, were as follows:
1. To train and provide a body of skilled nurses to nurse the sick poor in their own homes.
2. To establish in the Metropolis, and to assist in establishing in the country, district organisations for this purpose.
3. To establish a training school for district nurses in connection with one of the London hospitals.
4. To raise, by all means in its power, the standard of nursing and the social position of nurses . . .
A very important resolution was adopted on the recommendation of Miss

The New Profession of Nursing

Florence Lees [Mrs. Dacre Craven], the first Superintendent of the Central Home, namely, to recruit nurses entirely from the class known as gentlewomen.

.   .   .   .

One of the chief objects of the Metropolitan and National Nursing Association was to keep up a very high standard of nursing. This standard was set by Miss Florence Lees at the Central Home, and by her great practical skill and energy she succeeded in attaining it. The nurses were educated on the following plan. In the first place, the candidates were selected by the Superintendent-General. They remained in the Central Home for a month to learn the general nature of district nursing, after which they were placed in the hospital for a year; upon the satisfactory completion of the hospital course, the probationers returned to the Central Home and combined further training in district work with technical class instruction for six months, at the end of which time their training was usually considered complete.

.   .   .   .

[Queen Victoria's Jubilee Institute for Nurses.]

The deep interest taken by the Queen and the Royal family in the care of the sick is well known, and the English people will therefore not be surprised that Her Majesty, moved by the great benefits which her most suffering subjects have received from the care of trained nurses in their own homes, has devoted the bulk of the subscription raised by the women of England in honour of her jubilee to this great object, and has thereby made this undertaking a royal and a national one ...

In January 1888, Sir Rutherford Alcock wrote to the *Times,* enclosing the Report of the Committee. They recommended that the Jubilee Fund, which amounts to about £70,000, and may be expected to produce an income of £2000 a year, should be applied to found an institution for the education and maintenance of nurses for tending the sick poor in their homes ...

The Jubilee Fund is a splendid contribution to the work, but it is by no means adequate by itself, to the end contemplated; for the scope of the new institution embraces the whole of the United Kingdom. But Her Majesty has approved a scheme for employing the fund in connection with the ancient charity of St. Katharine's Hospital. This is an ecclesiastical corporation established formerly on the site of St. Katharine's Wharf near the Tower, but removed thence to the Regent's Park when the dock was constructed. It was founded in 1148 by Queen Matilda, wife of Stephen, with the original intention of securing repose for the souls of two of her children. In 1273 it was chartered by Queen Eleanor, the widow of King Henry III, and again in 1351, by Philippa, Queen of Edward III, when the visitation of the sick and poor in the neighbourhood of the hospital was expressly imposed as one of their duties upon the members of the Corporation.

The Queens of England have always been the patrons of St. Katharine's Hospital . . .

In thus connecting the Queen's Jubilee Institute with St. Katharine's Hospital, it is no doubt intended by Her Majesty that the visitation of the sick should again become one of the principal objects for which the ancient corporation exists.

.   .   .   .   .   .

The first duty of . . . [the] Provisional Committee was to establish or develop model training schools for district nurses in London, Edinburgh, Dublin, and elsewhere. They therefore sought to discover or make in each capital the nucleus of such a school. For London the Committee have adopted as a nucleus the Metropolitan and National Nursing Association, and invited the cooperation of the District Homes established under its auspices . . .

In Edinburgh, the energy of the president, Lady Roseberry, and of the honorary secretary, Miss Guthrie Wright, has laid the foundation of a Scottish center for the training of nurses. Glasgow, Aberdeen, and other important places are represented on the Edinburgh committee, which is already in vigorous and judicious action.

In Dublin a commencement has been made, and negotiations have been entered into with three nursing institutions, only one of which was engaged in district nursing, but no definite settlement has yet been come to . . .

Special arrangements have been made to establish a nursing institution for Wales at Cardiff.

.   .   .   .   .   .

The general scheme, which the Provisional Committee have initiated, has had for its objects—

First. The Training of nurses in the special practice of nursing the sick poor by visits at their own homes (*i. e.* district nursing) in the three centers— London, Edinburgh, and Dublin, by means, as far as possible, of the Training Schools already engaged in the work, and so maintaining a continuous supply of qualified superintendents, and nurses to local associations already existing; or to be formed for this special work throughout the Kingdom.

Secondly. As far as the income at their disposal would allow, to afford pecuniary aid towards the first establishment of such local associations; and

Thirdly. By working in unison with affiliated local associations to raise and maintain a high standard of nursing for district nurses throughout the Kingdom . . .

By a Royal Charter, bearing date the 20th September 1889, Queen Victoria's Jubilee Institute for Nurses was constituted a Body Corporate . . . to take charge of the annual income of the fund and apply it for the purposes Her Majesty had designated—viz. "The training, support, and maintenance of women to act as nurses for the sick poor, and the establishment (if thought proper) of a home or homes for such nurses, and generally the promotion and provision of improved means for nursing the sick poor ...."

The following qualifications shall be considered requisite in order to entitle a nurse to be placed on the roll of Queen's Nurses, namely—

(a) Training at some approved General Hospital or Infirmary for not less than one year.

(b) Approved training in district nursing for not less than six months, including the nursing of mothers and their infants after childbirth.

(c) Nurses in country districts ... must have at least three months' approved training in midwifery ...

Arthur L. B. Piele,

President of the Council.

St. Katharine's Royal Hospital,
Regent's Park, N. W.,
25th March, 1890.[39]

236. Eleanor F. Rathbone. *William Rathbone A Memoir*

[Eleanor Rathbone was the daughter of William Rathbone, whose account of the beginnings of district nursing is given in Reading No. 235. Miss Rathbone's narrative clarifies some points of her father's book.]

His wife had been attended during her last illness by a nurse, Mary Robinson, whose skill had done much to ease her. Seeing how much difference trained nursing could make, even in a home where every comfort and appliance that affection could suggest was provided, William Rathbone began to think what illness must mean in the homes of the poor, where comforts, appliances, and skill were alike wanting. He resolved to try an experiment. He asked Nurse Robinson to engage herself to him for three months, to nurse poor patients in their own homes in a certain district of Liverpool. She was provided with the most necessary appliances, and arrangements were made for supplying such nourishment and medical comforts as might be required to make her nursing effective. After a month had passed, she came to her employer in tears, and asked to be released from the rest of her engagement. The amount of misery she had to see was, she said, more than she could bear. With some difficulty he persuaded her to go on. At the end of the three months she declared that she would never, if he would keep her on, go back to any other kind of nursing.

· · · · · ·

In 1874, Sir Edmund Lechmere and others, connected with the English Branch of the Order of St. John of Jerusalem, desired to start an organisation for District Nursing in London. ... A meeting was held in June 1874, at which the National Association for Providing Trained Nurses for the Sick Poor came into being. The Association immediately appointed a sub-committee whose main objects, as described in the words of the resolution defining its duties, were: "To inquire into the state and need of district nursing; the training schools already existing capable of training women for nursing the poor in their own homes, and the hospitals suitable for such institutions; the district nurses already at work, and the places where need of nurses is felt.

Of this sub-committee, William Rathbone was appointed chairman, and Lady Strangford and Miss Florence Lees (now Mrs. Dacre Craven), honorary secretaries . . .

The Report of the sub-committee was issued in June 1875 . . .

The "Conclusions" note that there were only two organisations in London which employed trained nurses in nursing the poor in their own homes. The Bible and Domestic Female Mission, employing fifty-two Bible-women nurses, and the East London Nursing Society, which employed seven district nurses. There were about one hundred nurses employed in such work in London, but of these one-third were untrained, and could be of little service except in the administration of nourishment, medical comforts, and general relief. Secondly, the hospitals, as nurse training schools, did not afford such means of training nurses for the sick poor at home as ought to satisfy the requirements of the Association. Thirdly, the existing system of district nursing was open to grave objections. The chief faults observed were:—

1. Too much relief and too little nursing.

2. Too little control and direction, and consequent lapses into slovenliness and neglect, sometimes dangerous to the very lives of her patients on the part of the nurse.

3. Too little communication between the nurse and the doctor.

4. Too little instruction given to the patient's friends and family in regard to the care of the sufferer, to ventilation, cleanliness, disinfecting, etc.

The remaining "Conclusions," being the sub-committee's recommendations, may be briefly summarised.

The nurses should receive more complete and systematic hospital training, based on Miss Nightingale's suggestions, to make them real aids to the doctor.

The nurses should work under Inspectors or Superintendents, who should be themselves nurses of higher professional, social, and general qualifications . . .

The nurses should work in closer touch with the medical men, and as much as possible under their orders.

The duty of granting relief, medical comforts, nourishment, etc., should be, so far as possible, separated from the nurse's duties . . .

District nurses in large towns should be established in District Homes, under highly-trained Superintendents. In these Homes, probationers, already hospital-trained, should have special training, from three months upwards, in district work . . .

District nurses should possess some knowledge of the treatment of women after their confinements, and of their infants, which should be imparted to them, if this were possible, during their course of training . . .

There is some misconception as to the precise functions of Queen Victoria's Institute. It does not itself nurse the poor. Its objects may be shortly defined as follows:

To assist in organising, on right lines, local associations in affiliation to the Institute, who will employ district nurses, whether singly or gathered in groups in a Home and under a Superintendent.

To give district training to nurses, already hospital trained, to fit them for the service of the poor in their own homes.

To supply such nurses to affiliated Associations by whom they are paid; and also to prepare and recommend for affiliated Homes, Superintendents whose appointment must be approved by the Institute.

To maintain the standard of the nurses by periodical inspection, especially to those working singly, who are visited by an Inspector of the Institute at least twice yearly.

Generally to advise and assist those starting or carrying on district nursing, and to watch and safeguard the interests of district nurses.[40]

237. Elspeth Platt. *The Story of the Ranyard Mission*

[Mrs. Ranyard (d. 1879), who founded the Ranyard Mission in 1857, had for thirty years, as Ellen White, been a worker for the Bible Society. She has been described as a "personality who impressed herself instantly on anyone who came within reach of her." In 1868 the Biblewoman Nurses were instituted to nurse the sick in their homes. This project was discussed by Mrs. Ranyard with Agnes Jones, her friend and, for a time, her helper.[41] The name Biblewoman Nurse was an awkard one, and one doctor exclaimed, "A Biblewoman Nurse! what a name; pray tell me is she to be always preaching?"[42]]

Nurses

1. The Biblewoman Nurse is to be trained for three months as a Biblewoman only. Truthfulness, honesty and kindliness of heart are her essential qualifications, as well as true piety.

2. She is afterwards to spend three months in hospital or infirmary half in the surgical and half in the medical wards; and after that a fortnight in a lying-in hospital.

3. She is then a probationer for three months either under a competent Lady or Nurse Pioneer [43] before she is considered finally settled in a district.

5. She is expected to carry out all good sanitary principles and to do all she can to comfort and relieve suffering.

9. The salary of the Nurse is 15s. a week. She cannot collect for Bibles or hold a Mothers' Meeting though she may be able to attend one when time allows.

These were some of the rules laid down in 1868 for the first Biblewomen Nurses and, as we also read that "it is possible to be far too clean and respectable for the work to be done," and that "the nurse should have a warm, dark gown that from time to time will wash and which they do not fear to spoil," we realize afresh the marvellous transformation that has taken place in everything to do with sanitation, hygiene and the care of the sick. And if three months in hospital and three months' probation on a district seems almost worse than useless to us, we must remember that Agnes Jones, to whom Poor Law Nursing owes so much, had only one year as a paying probationer at St. Thomas's and one at the Great Northern before undertaking the charge of the Liverpool Workhouse Infirmary with 13,000 patients and the training of a corps of paid nurses ...

... only half a dozen of the Biblewomen who were considered "suitable," were willing to enter upon the Hospital training and to venture on untried paths. The word "suitable" involved a good deal, for we read that "A Christian Nurse should not be much of a talker, but a quiet, kindly, gentle and yet capable and handy woman, willing to receive instruction in her duties in a large hospital and then she will further need the mother-wit to apply the knowledge thus gained among the London poor amid surrounding difficulties. She must still follow out the original principle of the Bible and Domestic Mission in the Nursing Department, "to help the poor to help themselves," and she will need "to have a winning way of doing it."

The supervision of these very brave but sketchily trained women was to be undertaken by "a sensible and useful lady," one of those "born nurses" who, Mrs. Ranyard maintained, were to be found in "almost every upper class family." That they can have been of much use as supervisors we may doubt, but they probably did assist by encouraging cleanliness and tidiness in the nurses; as Mrs. Ranyard puts it: "The Lady will naturally prefer that the co-worker with whom she has frequent interviews, should be an example for cleanliness as well as godliness." And to assist in this cleanliness the Ladies very soon provided or encouraged the Nurses to provide themselves with washing dresses and aprons, so that in 1875 Mrs. Ranyard received a donation of £20 with this letter: "A small gift for the Biblewoman Nurses with Florence Nightingale's deepest sympathy for the noble attempt to provide nursing and cleanliness for the very poor; with gratitude to God and fervent prayer for its extension and progress. And if she might hint a wish it would be that this little sum should be expended in waterproof cloaks or washing gowns for summer, and washing linen sleeves to take on and off, and washing aprons or washing money for two or three of the Nurses in the very poorest district, where there is no local 'Lady' to look after these things for the Nurses."

·   ·   ·   ·   ·   ·

No nurse lived in the house ["Mother-house" in Regent Square] but there was a Matron and an experienced housekeeper who was always ready to give out clothing, food or comforts as well as medical stores which in those days had to be entirely supplied by the Mission.

While the house was being secured [in 1868] and prepared the first nurses were in training, two at the London Hospital, two at Guy's and two at

Westminster. These openings for probationers were often secured through the good offices of the influential Committee of the British Nurses Association who, though its chief object was to found a school for trained nurses in general, wished to have a "missionary branch of gratuitous nurses to the poor," and thought Mrs. Ranyard's Biblewoman Nurses might well form the nucleus . . .

. . . before the first year of the Nursing branch was completed a lady who had studied at the Female Medical College was appointed to supply skilled superintendence for the Nurses and "improve them by weekly advice."

By 1893 Nurses had a year's training at a General Hospital and then went to a special Hospital to gain a certificate for monthly nursing, after which they continued their training for a further period on a district, under one of the Mission's own Superintendents.

By 1907, the Mission had practically ceased to train Nurses in Hospital at its own expense. . . . So that at the end of that year new nurses were not accepted unless they had had three years' hospital training.[44]

CONCLUDING STATEMENT

The founding of the Nightingale School of Nursing in 1860 has been called by some the greatest single accomplishment of Florence Nightingale. Its influence has been widespread. Its characteristics in the early years after its founding have been described by a number of writers, most importantly perhaps by Miss Nightingale herself, as in her article on Mrs. Wardroper in the *British Medical Journal* in 1892 and in her eulogy of Agnes Jones in *Good Words* in 1868, quoted in this chapter. Probationers of the school, including Agnes Jones and Florence Lees, also described the system of nursing and nursing education there. From these it is noted that there were two groups of probationers, the "ordinary probationers" and the "special probationers," the former, intelligent, well-educated young women of the upper servant class, or daughters of small farmers, tradesmen, and the like, while the latter were "gentlewomen," women who could "organize" and "rule," and could be prepared for administration and teaching. The probationers were given a planned program which included teaching in surgical and medical nursing, the latter including "infectious" nursing, special attention being paid to their life in the nurses' residence. At the end of their course their names were entered in the register of the Committee of the Nightingale Fund.

Miss Nightingale's writings reveal her great interest in and knowledge of not only the preparation of professional nurses and conditions in nursing service but also hospital planning and construction, nursing in the homes, or "district nursing," and social problems of the day, such as pauperism. The strong emphasis on the moral aspects is understandable not only in the light of the times but also as a reflection of the character of Miss Nightingale. The positive approach to nursing and its educational emphasis are other strong characteristics of the plans advocated by Miss Nightingale.

That the new system of nursing was making inroads, however slowly, into the care of the sick in hospitals and homes is indicated by the writings of others—physicians, philanthropists, commissions—who either intentionally or incidentally frequently attribute the changes to the influence of Miss Nightingale's writings and ideas. One definite and far-reaching effect was the establishment of "district nursing," described in detail in the writings of William Rathbone and his daughter Eleanor, and in *The Story of the Ranyard Mission.*

Concurrently with the developments indicated in the chapters of Parts I and II, nursing was beginning in the New World of the Western Hemisphere. This nursing recapitulated to some degree the developments in the Old World, beginning with the preliterate societies. It later reflected the influence of the customs of migrating nationality groups which were brought to nursing in hospital and home, as well as the response of governmental groups to the needs felt in the various colonies established on the new continents. Still later, nursing in the New World was permeated by Florence Nightingale's ideas on nursing.

The sources which illustrate the developments in the Western Hemisphere will be presented in Part III in two chapters, the first of which indicates the evolution of nursing in homes and hospitals before the establishment of the first school of nursing on the Nightingale plan in 1873. The final chapter draws its material from sources having to do with the early wars of the United States.

PART III

Some Sources for the Study of Nursing in the Western Hemisphere Before 1873

Chapter 8

Some References to Early American Nursing in Homes and Hospitals

INTRODUCTION

THE earliest nursing in the Western Hemisphere developed first among preliterate peoples inhabiting North, Central, and South America. Then came groups from the Old World, migrating to various regions of the western world. A study of the migrating groups reveals that the care of the sick in each was an intrinsic part of the customs which they brought with them to the New World.

The first European group migrating to American shores and leaving permanent evidence of its care of the sick was the Spanish expedition under Cortes. After conquering Mexico City, Cortes pushed westward and made several attempts to explore the land to the north, later known as California. In this he did not succeed. The first hospital in the New World which is still in existence was founded in Mexico City by Hernando Cortes in 1524.[1] The Spanish colonists who followed were accompanied by missionaries. It is reasonable to assume that among the first hospital nurses were members of religious groups.

At about the same time, in the northeastern part of North America, other groups had explored and settled the new continent. In the sixteenth century the French Jesuit and Recollet missionaries had succeeded in penetrating, by way of the St. Lawrence River, what is now Canada, and had erected rude buildings in Quebec and Montreal for the purpose of caring for the Indians. These later grew into imposing hospitals, the Hôtels-Dieu and General Hospitals, the patients being nursed by orders of nuns and canonesses. The Sisters of St. Joseph de la Flêche, the order in Montreal, was headed by Jeanne Mance, a remarkable woman who had come from France to found the hospital.[2]

The first permanent English settlement in America was made in Jamestown, Virginia, in 1607.[3] The Pilgrim Fathers ("saints and strangers"), planned at first to settle in Virginia, but came instead to

303

New England on the *Mayflower* in 1620.[4] They brought with them a stern philosophy, not conducive to the establishment of institutions for the care of the sick. The few records of this group which mention the matter indicate that the colonists cared for each other in their homes, in the severe epidemics of smallpox and other diseases which characterized their early settlement.

In the Dutch colony of New Amsterdam, it was recommended by the surgeon of the Dutch West India Company that a hospital be established for the employees. This was eventually done, and the first institution to care for the sick in what is now the United States thus came into being in 1658.[5] This later became Bellevue Hospital. Other colonies made provision for the care of smallpox patients and, in some instances, for the mentally ill. Hospitals of a scientific character were established later. Among the earliest of these were the New Orleans Charity Hospital in 1737 [6] and the Pennsylvania Hospital in Philadelphia in 1751.[7]

In the United States various religious communities early took part in the care of the sick in hospitals and homes. Among the earliest were the Sisters of Charity established in Emmitsburg, Maryland, in 1809, by Mother Seton.[8] Protestant Episcopal sisterhoods also entered the field with the Sisterhood of the Holy Communion, founded in New York in 1845 by Pastor Muhlenberg, at what is now St. Luke's Hospital.[9] Nursing work under the auspices of the Engish Lutheran Church in the United States began when four deaconesses were brought to Pittsburgh to Pastor Passavant's Hospital in 1849, by Pastor Fliedner of Kaiserswerth.[10]

The present section (Part III) of the source book will be divided into two parts: first, the nursing in homes and hospitals of the Western Hemisphere, and second, nursing in the early wars in which the United States participated. In this chapter, references will be presented to illustrate the early nursing in the homes and hospitals before the emergence of nursing education in the first professional schools of nursing in 1873. The order of presentation is, in general, a chronological one.

The date usually given for the founding of the first hospital in the New World is 1524. The last will and testament of Cortes, dated 1547 (238), indicates that this hospital was probably not completed at that early date. The records of this hospital, the Hospital of the Immaculate Conception or, as it is also known, the Hospital of Jesus of Nazareth, enumerate the staff which existed in the seventeenth century. This included nurses (239). In the eighteenth century the "Regulations for the Management of the Spanish Royal Hospitals on the Island of Cuba . . ." (240) indicate in some detail the duties of various personnel who gave care to patients.

Early American Nursing in Homes and Hospitals

The study of early nursing in French Canada is aided by the complete reports, *The Jesuit Relations and Allied Documents,* written by the French Jesuit missionaries. The early *Relations* describe the building of the first hospitals in Montreal and Quebec and refer again and again to the work of the nuns in caring for the sick (241). The name of Jeanne Mance appears in these records. François Dollier de Casson, the first historian of Montreal, in his *A History of Montreal,* written probably in 1672–1673, tells of the arrival of Mlle Mance and of the work of the hospital there (242). Accounts of early travelers and of soldiers of the French and Indian Wars in the eighteenth and nineteenth centuries often refer to the hospitals at Quebec and Montreal and the nursing work of the nuns (243–250).

Information about the provisions made for the sick in the early colonies of the United States is found in the records, both official and nonofficial, which were kept by the colonists. Perhaps most important and interesting in this group is *Bradford's History of Plimoth Plantation,* which describes the trials of the Pilgrims when sickness struck (251). The detailed records kept by the early Moravian settlers in North Carolina refer to the members of the group who were assigned as nurses in the homes of the congregation (252). Of interest also, as indicative of the kind of nurse engaged in the homes of patients in Pennsylvania, are the notes made by Dr. Benjamin Rush in his *Commonplace Book for 1789–1813* for a "life" of a nurse which he intended to write, but which evidently never materialized (253). An 1820 report by a group of physicians in Baltimore on the disease of yellow fever mentions the nursing in an epidemic of the disease (254).

Physicians continued to interest themselves in nursing, as is indicated by the statement by Dr. Joseph Warrington in *The Nurse's Guide* (255); that of Dr. J. S. Longshore in *The Principles and Practice of Nursing or a Guide to the Inexperienced,* in which he states his point of view concerning the importance of the nurse in the recovery of the patient (256); and that of a physician, writing to the editor of the *American Medical Times* in 1861, giving his suggestions for the practical training of "monthly nurses" (257). The establishment of a group of women to visit and attend the sick in their homes in Charleston, South Carolina, is told by implication in the annual report of the board of managers for 1824 (258).

Another straw in the wind of the growing public consciousness relative to nursing is to be found in the listings of nurses in the directories of various cities. Some of those of Cleveland, Ohio, are reproduced here (259). A similar list appears in connection with a description of the New York Hospital. A traveler to San Francisco in 1848, Mary Jane Megquier, tells

305

in a letter of her intention of earning money there by attending the sick (260). Dr. Alfred Worcester's description of a "neighborhood nurse" of the early nineteenth century (261) narrates the large quantity of work accomplished by this early nurse.

The founding in the colonies of the earliest institutions for the care of the sick brought nursing into the hospitals. In some instances the documents state who was to do the nursing, and in others it is not so stated. In the territory which now comprises the United States, Bellevue Hospital in New York, originally a small company hospital of the Dutch West India Company, though designed as a shelter was the first institution where the sick received care. That a hospital was needed is indicated by the petition to the Dutch government by the people of New Netherland (262) and by the report of the company's surgeon to the director and the council in 1658, recommending that a hospital be established. The latter report is published in *Historic New York: Half Moon Papers* (263). In Pennsylvania, the Upland Court in Delaware County provided for a place to care for an insane patient in 1678 (264), while in the Colony of Connecticut, an Act, dated 1711, established a hospital to care for smallpox patients (265).

In Louisiana, at this time a French province, a hospital was early established to care for the "sick poor." This is indicated by a number of documents from among which three are given here: the preamble of the treaty between the Company of the Indies and the Ursulines in 1726 (266); the will of Jean Louis, in 1735, in which he bequeaths land and money for the building of a hospital (267); and the memorial of Bienville and Salmon in 1737, addressed to the minister in France, this document indicating that the institution thus founded was intended primarily for a hospital rather than a shelter (268).

The establishment of the Pennsylvania Hospital in Philadelphia, considered by many to be the first hospital in the modern sense, is told in a number of documents. Among these are: the petition to the House of Representatives of the Province of Pennsylvania for the erection of a hospital (269); Benjamin Franklin's *Some Account of the Pennsylvania Hospital from Its First Beginning to the Fifth Month, called May, 1754* (270); and his *Autobiography* (271). A brief note of Benjamin Franklin to Sister Elizabeth, the matron of the hospital, is also of interest (272). Another reference to this hospital is that of John F. Watson, a member of the Historical Society of Pennsylvania in 1830, written from earlier documents (273). The well-known poem by Henry Wadsworth Longfellow, *Evangeline,* describes the work of Evangeline as a Sister of Mercy in another early Philadelphia hospital, the Philadelphia Almshouse, the nucleus of the Philadelphia General Hospital (274).

The Colony of Virginia, in its *Statutes at Large* ..., in 1769 enacted a law making provision for "infected persons" and for "persons of unsound minds," as well as for the employment of nurses for the care of these patients (275). The archives of the New York Hospital, established in 1771, include the charter given by King George the Third, and reports of the hospital (276). A reference to this hospital at a very early date is also found in *Longworth's American Almanack* ... (277). The *Almanack* contains, in addition, a list of nurses practicing in New York at the time.

Hospitals and nursing are referred to in the writings and records of the founders and members of various religious groups. A selection from these is included here. The objects of the Sisters of Charity, founded in this country in 1809, in Emmitsburg, Maryland, by Mother Seton are given in the Constitutions of the Sisters of Charity, and included nursing care (278), while their arrangements for starting a hospital in St. Louis and requesting Sisters for that purpose are given in a letter of Father Rosati to Father Brute (279). Pastor Muhlenberg's narrative of the founding of St. Luke's Hospital in New York, and the Sisterhood of the Holy Communion, the first sisterhood under Protestant auspices established in America, is documented in his report for 1871 (280). The principles and rules of the Sisterhood are given by Bishop Henry Codman Potter in his book, *Sisterhoods and Deaconesses at Home and Abroad* (281). The origin of the deaconess group under the guidance of the English Lutheran Church in this country is told by Pastor Passavant in his *Life and Letters,* edited by G. H. Gerberding (282).

Finally, an article in *Harper's Weekly,* for June 6, 1857, on Florence Nightingale and Annie M. Andrews, an American nurse, describes the nursing of the latter in a yellow fever epidemic in a Norfolk hospital (283).

THE SOURCES

Mexico and Cuba

238. The Last Will and Testament of Hernando Cortes

[Hernando Cortes (1485–1547), the conqueror of Mexico, was born at Medillin, Spain. His father had been a captain of fifty light cavalry. Cortes was sent to the University of Salamanca to study law. He was, however, more interested in adventure, and departed for Cuba. Later he was entrusted with the armada which was sent by the king to explore the New World. He landed in Mexico in 1519 and conquered the country.[11] He founded and endowed the first hospital in the Western Hemisphere. The date usually given for this is 1524. Apparently, however, the hospital was not completed on the date of Cortes' will, 1547.]

In the name of the Most Holy Trinity, Father, Son, and Holy Ghost, who are three persons and one, only, and true God Whom I hold, believe, and confess to be my true God and Redeemer, and, of the most glorious and fortunate Virgin His Blessed Mother, our Lady and Advocate.

Let all who may see this Testament know that I, Don Fernando Cortes, Marques del Valle de Caxaca, Captain General of New Spain and the South Sea for the Caesarian Majesty of the Emperor Charles . . . [etc., etc.]

IX. Item: I direct that the hospital of Our Lady of the Conception, which I directed to be founded in the city of Mexico in New Spain, shall be finished at my cost according to the plan drawn. The principal chapel of its church shall be completed according to the model in wood made by Pedro Vasquez Jumetrico, and the plan described in the letter which I sent to New Spain, in this present year 1547. For these costs I set apart especially the rents deriving from my shops and houses in the said city, situated in the square and street of Tacuba and San Francisco, and in the street which unites them; this income shall be given exclusively to the said works until they are completed, nor shall my successor employ them for any other purpose. But it is my wish and will that the expenditure be made by my successor as patron of the hospital, and, when the works are finished according to the said plans, that the same rents shall be devoted to providing revenues for the wants of the administration, and the direction of the said hospital, following in this institution the order laid down by me before a notary public. Failing this, I direct that the same system of administration by adopted as that which obtains in the hospital of the Five Wounds, founded by Dona Catalina de Rivera (May she have glory), for maintaining the administration, chaplains, and other officers and servants attached to the said hospital.

XIV. Item: I destine, for the endowment of the said hospital of Our Lady of the Conception, which I am building in Mexico, two front ground plots of the houses of Jorge Alvarado, and of the treasurer Jean Alonso de Sosa, between my house and the aqueduct which extends to the houses of Don Luis Saavedra, which being now unoccupied, I assume the obligation to construct such buildings as may amply suffice for the said endowment. During such time as the said buildings are not constructed, the said hospital shall receive support from my estate to the amount of one hundred thousand *maravedis* of good money. I direct that the said endowment shall be furnished as is provided, and with the conditions I shall hereafter state, and I direct that my successor shall be free at any time to allot the said hospital some part of the said one hundred thousand *maravedis* income, in lieu of the said buildings, should he so desire, affecting this substitution in any assured manner he may wish.

[XV, XVI, XVII, and XVIII also deal with the hospital.]

Done at Seville, on the eleventh day of the month of October, the year from the birth of Our Lord and Saviour Jesus Christ, one thousand five hundred and forty seven.

Item: I say that, as, in one article of this my will, I have disposed and ordered that four thousand *ducats,* from the rent of the shops and buildings which I have in Mexico, should, after the works on the said hospital, monastery, and college I have ordered founded be entirely devoted to the endowment, property of the said college, monastery, and hospital to which I refer, should it at any time happen that the said shops and buildings should produce less than this sum of four thousand *ducats,* and my will and intention be defeated, I order that in such a year of shortage, my successor shall complete the amount from his estate, so that the said four thousand *ducats* may be paid in full without any diminution. This page is added to the other ten, done and signed on the same date. The Marques del Valle. Witness by his lordship's command, the licentiate Infante.

By his lordship's command,
Melchior Mojica.[12]

239. From the Records of the Hospital of the Immaculate Conception, Mexico City

[The following excerpt from the records of the Hospital of the Immaculate Conception or, as it is also called, the Hospital of Jesus of Nazareth, lists the personnel of the hospital in the middle of the seventeenth century. Two women nurses are mentioned—that is, if it is assumed that the assistant to the chief nurse was a nurse.]

...three chaplains, one administrator, one doctor, one surgeon, one barber, one chief nurse [*una enfermera en jefe*], one assistant to the nurse [*una ayudante de la enfermera*], a cook and three Indians coming from Coyoacan to do the cleaning of the building, and eight slaves, men and women who assisted with the different kinds of work of the hospital.[13]

240. "Regulations for the Internal, Political and Economic Management of the Royal Hospitals, Located on the Island of Cuba..."

[The continuation of this title, indicating the purposes, and types of patients cared for, is "For the purpose of healing the Troops, Criminals, and Negro Slaves of His Majesty, according to the circumstances, temperament and customs of the Country." It is dated, "Year of 1776." These regulations were specifically designed for the royal hospital at Havana and, having been ordered published, had the force of a royal decree. Undoubtedly therefore, they applied to all royal hospitals in the Indies, and since most orders for Louisiana emanated from or through Havana, the regulations may also have applied in that province.[14]]

Obligations of the Cabo de Sala [orderly]

82. It will be his care that the patients have clean and well cared for rooms because this is one of the most necessary requisites in hospitals and for this he will start with the chamber pots or services at four o'clock in the morning in the summer and at five in the winter in order that when the physician and head surgeon arrive they will find this duty performed, throwing lavendar fumes or other aromatics as soon as this is concluded.

83. The visit of the physician or surgeon being terminated, and having given breakfast to the patients he will order the nurses to sweep and clean the room which operation they will execute also after they (the patients) have been served their dinner and supper.

86. He will be a vigilant caretaker that the nurses nor anyone else introduce anything to eat or drink because this results in their ailments being increased, or that when almost recuperated they relapse into the same illness or another more dangerous.

88. As soon as the latter [the patients] have finished eating he will order the nurses to sweep the rooms and when finished the windows be closed in order that they take a nap during the *siesta* warning them [the nurses?] not to make the slightest noise.

91. It will be his obligation to order that the nurse place the large open lamp in the bed where the patient may be dying in order that the Father Chaplain may assist him up until the end.

92. He will take care that the nurses keep clean and polished all the utensils in the patient's service.

Rule and Order
Which the Physician and Head
Surgeon must follow in order
to visit their respective rooms

The Physician's Visit

In the Morning

98. The hours in which the visits are to be made in the summer and winter are already designated in order that all may be ready at those hours,

as soon as the physician arrives at the hospital the bell will toll three times and an apothecary, a practitioner of surgery, an orderly and a nurse with a light will go to the medical rooms who following the physician will do all that the latter should order them.

The Physician's Visit

In the Afternoon

103. In the afternoon visit the same four individuals will present themselves to the physician in the same order as explained in order to make a note of what he orders for the patients who might have entered after the morning visit and if the others should change they will notify him of it whether it may be to suspend what has been prescribed or whether to do again what seems suitable to him.

The Head Surgeon's Visit

In the Morning

104. The latter shall be made at the same hours as that of the physician according to the seasons of the year and as soon as the head surgeon arrives at the hospital the bell shall be rung three times in order that the head practitioners with the rest of the subordinates and nurses may present themselves to begin the treatment (for which purpose he must have forewarned the head practitioner to have ready everything which is necessary) and this finished, he will make the visit accompanied by an orderly, a surgery practitioner, a druggist, and a nurse with a light.

Approval. The King approves these rules and regulations and commands that they be printed, printing four hundred copies, and that these be sent to the other parts of the Indies for the exact observance of all its articles inasmuch as they may be adaptable on the Island of Cuba, and that the accounts of the hospitals of the Royal Patrimony be presented, taken, and audited in their respective tribunals and be sent accompanied with those of the Royal Treasury for their examination and inspection in the Office of the General Treasurer at the Council of the Indies *San Ildefonso,* August 22, 1776—Don Joseph de Gálvez. This is a copy of the original rules and regulations which remain in the office of the Secretary of State and of the *Despacho Universal* of the Indies.[15]

Canada

241. *The Jesuit Relations and Allied Documents*

[The *Jesuit Relations* are reports written by the French Jesuit missionaries in New France. They were published in Paris,[16] and cover the years 1610 to 1791. Throughout these narratives reference is made to the hospital nuns of Quebec and Montreal, and their care of the Indians. An occasional allusion is made to Jeanne Mance, the first lay nurse in North America, who established the hospital at Montreal.]

Le Jeune's Relation, 1639.

It was in this year that Madame the Duchess d'Aiguillon erected and endowed a house in honor of God in this new world, while God is preparing another dwelling for her in Heaven. And there was found an Amazon, who has led the Ursulines, and established them on these outer confines of the world. It is indeed a remarkable fact that,—at the very moment when God touched the heart of Madame the Duchess d'Aiguillon in Paris, and inspired her with the idea of building a Hôstel-Dieu for our Savages who were dying in the forests, abandoned and without any assistance, and while she was thinking of the Hospital Nuns of Dieppe for carrying out her project,—he raised up in another part of France, a modest and virtuous Lady [Mme de la Peltrie], and inspired her to undertake the Seminary for the daughters of the Savages, and to confide its management to the Ursulines.

When we were informed that a bark was about to arrive at Kebec, bearing a College of Jesuits, an establishment of Hospital Nuns, and a Convent of Ursulines, the news seemed at first almost a dream; but at last, descending towards the great river, we found that it was a reality.

Into the Hospital went the three Hospital Nuns sent by Monseigneur the Most Reverend Archbishop of Rouen . . .

For these good women, besides being very strict in discipline and in regular observance, are, beyond a doubt, excellent in the care and treatment of the sick, both in temporal and in spiritual matters. The three Ursulines withdrew to a private house, after having mutually embraced the other nuns. . . . As for the Hospital, the Nuns were not yet lodged, and their baggage had not yet arrived, when sick people were brought to them. We had to lend out straw beds and mattresses that they might perform their first act of charity. . . . The nuns . . . could not contain themselves for gladness. They had sick persons to nurse and had nothing to give them. . . . If the Savages are capable of astonishment, they will experience it here; for among them no heed is paid to the sick if they are considered sick unto death; they are looked upon as being of another world, with whom is held no intercourse, no conversation. Now, when they witness the tender care and attention that is given to their Countrymen, it causes them to entertain a high esteem for the person for whose sake this great help is given them, who is JESUS CHRIST, our Savior.

Relation of 1640.

The hospital Nuns arrived at Kebec on the first day of the month of August of last year. Scarcely had they disembarked before they found themselves overwhelmed with patients. The hall of the hospital being too small it was necessary to erect some cabins fashioned like those of the Savages in every garden. Not having enough furniture for so many people they had to cut in two or three pieces parts of the blankets and sheets they had brought for these poor sick people. In a word, instead of taking a little rest and refreshing themselves after the great discomforts they had suffered upon the sea, they found themselves so burdened and occupied that we had fear of losing them and their hospital at its very birth. The sick came from all directions in such numbers; their stench was so unsupportable, the heat so great, the fresh food so scarce and so poor in a country so new and strange, that I do not know how these good Sisters, who almost had not even leisure in which to take a little sleep, endured all these hardships.

In brief, from the month of August until the month of May, more than one hundred patients entered the hospital, and more than two hundred poor Savages found relief there, either in temporary treatment or in sleeping there one or two nights, or more. There have been seen as many as ten, twelve, twenty or thirty of them at one time. Twenty poor sick people have received holy Baptism there; and about twenty-four, quitting this house of mercy, have entered the regions of glory. All this is due to the charity and liberality of Madame the Duchesse d'Aiguillon, who accomplishes this work with a care and affection truly golden.

The savages who leave the hospital, and who come to us again at St. Joseph, or at the three Rivers say a thousand pleasant things about these good Nuns. They call them "the good," "the liberal," "the charitable." The Mother Superior having fallen sick, these poor Savages were very sorry, the sick blaming themselves for it. "It is we who have made her sick," they said: "she loves us too much; why does she do so much for us?" When this good Mother having recovered, entered the hall of the poor, they knew not how to welcome her enough. They had good reason to love these good Mothers; for I do not know that parents have so sweet, so strong, and so constant an affection for their children as these good women have for their patients. I have often seen them so overwhelmed that they were utterly exhausted; yet I have never heard them complain, either of the too great number of their patients, or of the infection; or of the trouble they gave them. They have hearts so loving and so tender towards these poor people that if occasionally some little present were given them, one could be certain that they would not taste it, however greatly they might need it, every thing being dedicated and consecrated to their sick. Their charity had to be moderated, and an order was given them to eat at least a part of the little gifts that were made to them,

313

especially when they were not strong. I am not surprised if the Savages recognized very clearly this great charity; loved, cherished, and honour them.

Relation of 1642–43.

A young savage of Tadoussac was attacked with a violent pleurisy; after six or seven days, his people brought him from Tadoussac to the Hospital Nuns at Sillery,—that is to say, from a distance of forty leagues. He is nursed with great care, and they bleed him two or three times; but the disease is stronger than the remedies.

.   .   .   .

The Hospital Mothers had lodged and fed him [a Huron Indian], with a charity which embraces all sorts of nations.

.   .   .   .   .   .

The Nuns have received and assisted in the Hospital, this year, about a hundred Savages of various nations: Montagnais, Algonquins, Atticamegues, Abnaquiois, Hurons, those of Tadoussac and the Saguéné, and of some other nations more distant.

.   .   .   .   .   .

Since their [the Indians'] rout, he [Pachirini] had always wished to live with us, together with two other patients, in the little Hospital which we had erected there for the wounded—both in order to be better cared for there, and to be more thoroughly instructed; in fact, both he and the others received in it healing for the body and for the soul.

Relation of 1643–44.

An old man of the Hiroquet Tribe—who was a notorious Sorcerer, and very well versed in all the superstitions of his Nation, which is saturated with them—could not follow his people to the chase, and was obliged to stop at Sillery, where the Hospital Mothers fed him out of the charity in their Hospital, during the whole Winter, together with many other infirm and sick persons, . . . When this poor old man saw himself so charitably waited upon and succored by the good Mothers; when he observed the attention and the great expense with which they cared for the other sick, and infirm, without any hope of reward; and when he learned that they had left their relatives and so fine a country, in order to come here to succor the indigent and the sick,—he conceived a high idea of the goodness and holiness of our Religion, and felt himself impelled to embrace it.

.   .   .   .   .   .

And, on being again asked what had converted him, he replied that it was the Charity that he had received from "the Women clothed in white," meaning the Hospital Nuns.

.   .   .   .   .   .

314

... When the Nuns left Sillery, all the Savage women came to Kebec, and erected two cabins near the Nuns' house—one for the men who were working at the building, and the other for the sick, until a ward could be prepared for them; and they did not fail at once to send thither two or three of their people who were sick, and who were afterward followed by some others. The Savages visited them at every opportunity, and urged them to complete the building of a suitable house to enable them to pass the Winter and to be protected against the snow and ice. Their [the Hospital Nuns'] Charity has this year succored over 35 sick, of whom Heaven has taken ten; and, in addition to these sick persons, many Savages have passed two or three days in this house of mercy for the purpose of undergoing purgation; and of taking medicines for the prevention of some disease with which they felt themselves threatened. Even this is not all the charity exercised by those good Mothers. The house of God does good to the poor as well as to the sick, several old men, several women, and several children have remained on their hands for two or three months during the Winter, and would have died of hardship without such assistance.

Of the House and Mission of Sainte Marie [at Montreal]
This House is not only an abode for ourselves, but it is also the continual resort of all the neighboring tribes, and still more of the Christians who come from all parts for various necessities,—even with the object of dying there in greater peace of mind, and in the true sentiments of the Faith. We have, therefore, been compelled to establish a hospital there for the sick, a cemetery for the dead, a Church for public devotions, a retreat for pilgrims, and, finally, a place apart from the others, where the infidels ... can always have some good words respecting their salvation.

... The Hospital is so distinct from our dwelling that not only men and children, but even women can be admitted to it. God has given us some good servants who are able to attend them in their sickness, while we assist them for the good of their Souls ...

Journal, 1645.
There remained at Vilmarie, of notable persons, only Monsieur d'Alibour, his wife and sister, and Mademoiselle Manse.

When I arrived at montreal [sic], they had prepared a timber dwelling for our Fathers, and it seemed that there was nothing more to be done than to raise it; but, when they were on the point of doing so, the vessels arrived, bringing word and orders from france [sic] to those who commanded at Montreal, to employ all the workmen for other things,—namely, in erecting a hospital, for which large funds had been received in the preceding years; and yet no beginning had been made.

315

On the 5th mother [sic] Marie de St. Ignace, first Superior of the hospital at Quebek, died about 5 o'clock in the morning; she was not buried until the next day.

Relation of 1645–46.

Indeed, this man [son of Francois Xavier Nenaskoumat] came to give up the ghost very piously in our arms, after having received in the Hospital at Kebec all the charitable attentions with which a poor sick man can be assisted.

. . . .

The preceding Relations have made mention of the most blessed death of a Neophyte Francois Xavier Nenaskoumat; . . . His son, who was named Vincent Xavier Nipikiwigan, was miserably wounded to death this last Autumn by the Sokoquiosis, of whom we have spoken herein above. This poor man was brought back to Kebec, and taken to the Hospital, where he was received and treated with great charity.[17]

242. François Dollier de Casson. *A History of Montreal 1640–1672*

[The date of the writing of this history cannot be precisely established, but the evidence indicates that it was written in the winter of 1672–1673. Despite the suggestion of annual letters, it seems to have been written at one time. The writer was the first historian of Montreal. He was born in Lower Brittany in 1636 and, after serving in the army, entered the Seminary of St. Sulpice in 1657. He came to the New World in 1666, where he spent time as missionary, explorer, and military chaplain before becoming superior of the Seminary of St. Sulpice at Montreal and Seigneur of the island. He was thus closely in touch with the affairs of the community, and drew much of his information for the *History* from the lips of Jeanne Mance herself, especially with reference to the latter's experiences. He wrote as an eyewitness only for the last five years of the events which he records. He warns his readers that his *History* is probably not free from errors.[18]]

Mlle Mance reached Quebec safely [Aug. 1641], where she had the comfort of learning that ten men who had been sent by the company of Montreal this same year from Dieppe had already arrived and were busy building a storehouse on the bank of the river, on a spot given by M. de Montmagny [Governor of New France 1636–48] to the company of Montreal.

. . . .

Mlle Mance had the honour to lodge this winter [1641–42] with Mme de la Peltrie at Puizeaux; M. de Maisonneuve and M. de Puiseaux wintered in the same house. During this time every one was employed in carpentry and other preparations necessary and useful to a new habitation and colony.

.   .   .   .

At length, on 19 March [1643], the Day of St. Joseph, patron-saint of the country, the framework of the main building had been raised, the cannon were mounted thereon, so as to mark the fête day by the sound of artillery, which was done with great rejoicing, everyone hoping to see all the living-places completed very soon.

.   .   .   .

[We must] ... say a word of our charitable unknown [Mlle de Bullion], who for her part sent to Mlle Mance during this year [1643–1644] a sum of 2000 livres, three pieces of church plate and some household goods, sending her all as if she were already living in the hospital. M. de Maisonneuve seeing this, decided to employ all his men, with all possible speed, to house her properly, which he did so quickly that by 8 October of the same year she was installed and able to write and date her letters from the hospital of Montreal in writing to her beloved foundress.... No sooner was the hospital finished than there appeared plenty of sick and wounded to fill it; every day the Iroquois by their massacres found new guests for it, so that everyone gave thanks to God with all their hearts for the blessed inspiration He had given to this unknown woman on behalf of the poor sick and wounded of this place.

.   .   .   .

With regard to the nuns of La Fleche, Mlle Mance and the company had written to tell them all that had occurred, and they had agreed that three members of this house or of its dependent houses should go to Montreal this year [1658–1659]. With this in view, when the spring came, Mlle Mance wrote to these nuns, arranging to meet them in La Rochelle, ... On this notice the nuns of La Fleche, to be ready by the date given them, sent at once to their houses at Bauge and Le Lude, for the Sisters Macé, de Bresolles, and Maillet, the three victims designed for Canada.... [19]

ACCOUNTS OF TRAVELERS AND SOLDIERS IN CANADA IN THE EIGHTEENTH AND NINETEENTH CENTURIES

[In the accounts of early travelers and participants in the French and Indian Wars, reference is often made to the earliest Canadian hospitals, particularly to those of Quebec and Montreal. In these, mention is sometimes made of the personnel caring for the patients.]

243. Father Charlevoix. *Letters to the Duchess of Lesdiguieres*

[Father Pierre François Xavier de Charlevoix (1862–1761) entered the Jesuit Society in 1698 and was sent to Quebec in 1705 by the King of France. He traveled in Canada and through Louisiana to the Gulf of Mexico. Following this, he was made professor of *belles lettres* in France, later returning to Canada. He published a history of Christianity and other books, including, in 1724, the life of Mother Mary of the Incarnation, the first Superior of the Ursulines at Quebec.[20]]

Letter II. Quebec, Oct. 28, 1720.

The Hospital [Hôtel Dieu] has two large Halls, one for the Men and the the other for the Women: the Beds are well kept, the Sick are well attended, and every Thing is convenient, and very neat. The Church is behind the Women's Hall, and has nothing remarkable but the great Altar, the Altarpiece of which is very fine. This House is served by some Nuns of *St. Austin,* the first of which came from Dieppe: They have begun a good House here, but it is very likely they will not soon finish it for Want of a Fund. As their House is situated on the Midway of a Hill, on a Spot that advances a little upon the River *St. Charles,* they have a very pretty Prospect.

Going down this Street, or more properly speaking, this Way, we came into the Country, and about half a Mile distant stands the General Hospital. It is the finest House in *Canada,* and would be no Disgrace to our greatest Cities of France. The *Recollets* formerly possessed this Place: M. de *St. Vallier,* Bishop of Quebec, removed them into the City, bought the Ground, and spent 100,000 Crowns in Buildings, Furniture, and a Fund for its Support. The only Defect to this Hospital is, its being built in a Marsh; however, they hope to remedy it by draining the Marsh; but the River *St. Charles* makes an Elbow in this Place, and the Waters do not easily run off, and this can never be well mended.[21]

244. *The Diary of Mrs. John Graves Simcoe*

[Mrs. Simcoe was the wife of the first lieutenant-governor of the Province of Upper Canada, 1792–1796. Elizabeth Posthuma Gwillin (1766–1850) was born at Whitechurch, Herefordshire. She was brought up by her aunt, her mother having died a few hours after her birth, and her father, a few months before, in 1766, while his regiment was stationed at Gibraltar. The diary was begun on September 17, 1791, a few days prior to her departure for Quebec from London, and the last entries were made on October 16, 1796, on the return to London of Governor Simcoe and his wife.[22]]

Thurs. 22nd [Dec. 1791]
Quebec.

I had an order from Mgr. Francois Hubert, the Catholic Bishop of Quebec, for admittance to the Convent des Ursulines, where I went to-day with Madame Bâby. The Superieure (La Mere Saint Louis Gonzague) is a very pleasing, conversible woman of good address. Her face and manner reminded me of Mrs. Gwillin (Mrs. Simcoe in this writing refers to a relative of her own, not her mother, who died at her birth). The nuns appeared cheerful, pleased to see visitors, and disposed to converse and ask questions. Their dress is black with a white hood, and some of them looked very pretty in it . . .

Another convent is called the Hôtel Dieu, for the reception of the sick, whether French or English. It is attended by the medical men on the staff, who speak highly of the attention payed by the nuns to the sick people. The General Hospital is a convent a mile out of town, where sick and insane people are received.[23]

245. Duke of La Rochefoucauld-Liancourt. *Travels Through the United States of North America, the Country of the Iroquois, and Upper Canada in the Years 1795, 1796, and 1797, with an Authentic Account of Lower Canada*

[François Alexandre Frédéric, duc de La Rochefoucauld-Liancourt (1747–1827), French social reformer and philanthropist, is perhaps best known for his establishment of a model farm on his estate, where he set up spinning machines and founded a school of arts and crafts for the sons of soldiers. He was elected to the states-general of 1789, and warned Louis XVI of the state of affairs in Paris two days before the fall of the Bastille. As the Revolution progressed, he fled to England and then to America. He later returned to France where he received small favor from Napoleon. He urged many measures for public welfare, including vaccination against smallpox, public dispensaries, and reforms of hospitals and prisons. He wrote books on these and other subjects, including industry and agriculture.[24]]

A convent of Urselines in Quebec, and another in Montreal, and a society of Charitable Sisters, who attend the hospitals and lazarettos, are the only nunneries of Lower Canada. The revenue of the hospitals consisted in part of annuities, paid by the city of Paris, the payment of which was stopped in pursuance of a decree of the French National Assembly; and this deficiency has not hitherto been made up in any other manner.

.   .   .   .

As to charitable institutions, they consist of two hospitals, one at Montreal, the other at Quebec, and a lazaretto at the latter place. They are inconsiderable and badly managed, especially in regard to the abilities of the physicians who attend the sick.[25]

246. J. C. B. *Travels in New France*

[Two copies of the original of this manuscript are known to exist: one in a private collection in Paris, and another in the Bibliotheque Nationale at Paris. The manuscript bears only the initials J. C. B., and attempts to identify the writer have failed; but in his writing the author tells certain things about himself. As a young man he left Paris to seek his fortune in Canada, where he enlisted as a gunner in the colonial troops. He was present at the founding of Fort Duquesne (1754) where he remained for three years, taking part in the battle of Monongahela. He distinguished himself at this time but was made a prisoner at the end of this campaign. He was brought to New York and from there was sent to France. His narrative is told from the point of view of a soldier. It was published in Paris after his return, after careful revision of the notes by himself. It has been said to contain many inaccuracies but is valuable as a picture of the times as they appeared to a French soldier who participated in the French and Indian Wars.[26]]

[About November, 1751, Quebec.]

... On the right, going from the Place d'Armes, is the Rue du Palais. At the right of this street is the Hôtel-Dieu, a hospital in a beautiful location overlooking the St. Charles River. There are two large wards, one for men and the other for women. The beds are clean and well kept, and the invalids are properly cared for.

The General Hospital, built half a league from the city at the end of an inlet of the St. Charles River, is the most beautiful building in the country. It was built by the efforts and at the expense of the Bishop of Quebec, St. Valier, who succeeded Sieur de Laval in 1674, at the time the Church of Quebec was made a bishopric.[27]

This establishment originally founded to care for the disabled, has since been used for invalid soldiers. They are cared for by thirty-six canonesses, instituted by Bishop de St. Valier, the founder, and all chosen from the nobility of the country. This hospital is very healthful and airy, though built in a swamp near the inlet. In my time, the hospital had one hundred and fifty beds, all endowed by the wealthiest people of the country.

[January, 1753, Three Rivers.]

It was not fortified, and it had a parochial church, a Recollet convent, and a convent of Ursuline nuns dependent on the Quebec convent, who served in a hospital ...

. . . .

The population of this pleasant city in my time did not exceed eight thousand inhabitants. It had its own governor, a staff, officer, garrison troops, a beautiful Place d'Armes, stores dealing in commodities and food, a cathedral, a parish church, a seminary, two convents for men, one Jesuit and the other Recollet, another for the nuns of the congregation, a general Hospital, and an Hôtel-Dieu.[28]

247. John Knox. *An Historical Journal of the Campaigns in North America*

[John Knox (d. 1778) was a captain in the service of the English in the French and Indian Wars. He was the third son of John Knox, merchant, of Sligo, Ireland. In 1741 he purchased a lieutenancy in the 43rd Regiment of Foot, and took part in the expedition against Louisbourg in 1757. He continued to serve in America until after the capitulation of Montreal in 1760. The *Journal* begins in February, 1757, and ends in 1760. It was published in 1769. The editor states that on the whole, it is accurate, errors of fact being very few and unimportant.[29] Although the quotation below refers to the period of the French and Indian Wars, it is placed here because the chief reference is to a Canadian hospital, the Quebec General Hospital, described by Captain Knox as it appeared in the middle of the eighteenth century. Brief mention is also made of an English regimental hospital in Albany.]

Albany [July 31] 1759.

As no women are permitted to go with the regiments, four per company of the regiments of one thousand men, and three per company of the regiments of seven hundred men, may receive provisions at Albany; a list of the said women to be signed by the Commanding Officer of the regiment, and sent to the Major of brigade, who will give their names to the Matron of the hospital, that she may call them for the service of the hospital; which if they refuse, when wanted, they are to be immediately struck off their allowance.

· · · · · · ·

October 1759

The general hospital stands near a mile from the town [Quebec] on the N. N. W. side of it, and is a very stately building: it is situated on the south side of the river Charles, which meanders agreeably under its walls, and consists of a spacious dome, looking to the east, with two great wings, one fronting the north, and the other the south;—in this house is a convent of nuns of the Augustine order, who have lands particularly appropriated for their maintenance; and the sisters, from religious motives, have assigned the principal parts of this habitation for the reception of sick and wounded Officers and soldiers, to whom they are exceedingly humane and tender; the French King has hitherto endowed this hospital with a bounteous salary for the support of a Physician, Surgeons, Directors, Clerks, Stewards, Inspector, & c. for whom there is a very decent table, as likewise for such Officers of the troops as happen to labour under any infirmity. These women are subject to the direction of a Mother-Abbess, who is sister to M. de Ramsay, the late Governor; and, according to their monastic custom, assumes the name of "Sainte Claude." Every soldier pays a weekly stipend, while he is here, besides his allowance of salt provisions; and then he is not at any farther expence. They eat and drink well of such things only as are fit for them, in the soop and spoon-meat way; whatever beverage the Surgeons think proper to direct is provided for them, and no men can lie more clean or comfortable than they do. Our soldiers were taken equally good care of; for the nuns make it a point of conscience, and perform every menial office about the sick as unconcerned, and with the same indifference, that one man would attend another; when our poor fellows were ill, and ordered to be removed from their own odious regimental hospitals to this general receptacle, they were indeed rendered inexpressibly happy; each patient has his bed with curtains allotted to him, and a nurse to attend him; sometimes she will take two, three, or more, under her care, according to the number of sick or wounded in the house. The beds are ranged in galleries on each side, with a sufficient space, between each, for a person to pass through; these galleries are scraped and swept every morning, and afterwards sprinkled with vinegar, so that a stranger is not sensible of any unsavory scent whatsoever; in summer, the windows are generally open, and the patients are allowed a kind of fan, either to cool them in close sultry weather; or to keep off the flies, which, at that season, by reason of the vicinity of some marshes, together with the river Charles, are numerous and troublesome. Every Officer has an apartment to himself, and is attended by one of those religious sisters, who, in general, are young, handsome, and fair; courteous, rigidly reserved, and very respectful; their dress consists of a black, sometimes a white, gown, with a bib and apron, a close cap on their head, with a forehead-cloth down to their brows; their breasts and neck intirely covered; the sleeves are made long, so that not above half the arm from the elbow is in sight: their cloaths sweep the ground; on the top of the head is pinned a square piece of black shalloon, which serves as a cloak, flowing carelessly over their shoulders, a little below their waist. Every woman wears a silver crucifix, about three inches in length, which hangs by a black ribband from the neck to the girdle or apron-string; and in this dress, they make a very decent, grave, and modest appearance: they are not under the same restraint as in other Popish countries; their office of nursing the sick furnishes them with opportunities of taking great latitudes, if they are so disposed; but I never heard of any of them charged with the least levity . . .[30]

248. Priscilla Wakefield. *Excursions in North America*

[The letters in this collection are not dated, but the first edition of them was published in 1806 under the name of Mrs. Wakefield (1751–1832), who had written other books of travel. They were written not by Priscilla Wakefield but by a "Gentleman and His young Companion to their friends in England." Curiosity regarding the Indians and the continent of North America induced them to visit the United States and Canada.[31]]

Arthur Middleton to his Brother Edwin from Montreal.

[Three Rivers, Convent of St. Ursula]
We . . . [rang] a bell. Upon this the curtain within the lattice was drawn

back, and we discovered an apartment surrounded with nuns, and furnished with an altar, near which kneeled several nuns, dressed in black stuff gowns, with white handkerchiefs spread over their shoulders, and drawn close up to the throat; to these were joined a kind of hood of white linen, that covers half the forehead, the temples, and ears. Each of them had, besides, a flowing veil of black gauze; and a silver cross hung from the breast. The works of these Sisters, in birch bark, embroidered with elk hair, dyed of the most brilliant colours, are very ingenious: of these materials they make pocket-books, work-bags, dressing boxes, models of Indian canoes, and a variety of the warlike weapons used by the Indians. Strangers are expected to purchase some of them, which I did willingly, and shall send them by the first opportunity to Catherine and Louisa as specimens of the art. Besides works of fancy, these good sisters employ themselves in attending on the sick in the hospital, which is close to the convent.[32]

249. Francis Hall. *Travels in Canada and the United States in 1816 and 1817*

[The writer of this account was a lieutenant in the service of the British. He sailed from Liverpool on January 20, 1816. After visiting New York, he went to Quebec and Montreal.[33]]

There are several charitable Catholic institutions in Quebec: the principal of these is the "Hôtel Dieu," founded in 1637, by the Duchess D'Aiguillon (sister to Cardinal Richelieu) for the poor sick. The establishment consists of a superior and thirty-six nuns. The "General Hospital" is a similar institution; consisting of a superior and forty-three nuns, founded by St. Vallier, bishop of Quebec, in 1693, for "Poor Sick and Mendicants." It stands about a mile from the town, in a pleasant meadow watered by the Charles. The style of building is simple, and well suited to the purposes of the establishment, consisting only of "such plain roofs as piety could raise." The present superior is a lady of Irish extraction, her age apparently bordering on thirty: in this conventual seclusion, (devoted to what might seem to the mind of a delicate female, the most disgusting duties of humanity,) she exhibits that easy elegance, and softened cheerfulness of manner, so often affected, and rarely attained by the many votaries, who dress their looks and carriage in "the glass of fashion:" she conducted us, with the greatest politeness, through every part of the building, which, as well as the "Hôtel Dieu," in point of order, neatness, and arrangement, seems singularly adapted to the comfort and recovery of the unfortunate beings, to whose reception they are consecrated. . . . There is no distinction in the admission of Catholic or Protestant: the hand of charity has spread a couch for each in his infirmities. Both houses have a small pharmacopeia in charge of a sister instructed in medicine. The several duties of tending the sick at night, cooking, & c. are distributed by rotation: employment is thus equally secured to all and the first evil of cankering thought effectually prevented. Good humour and contented cheerfulness seem to be no strangers to these "veiled votaresses . . ."[34]

250. Basil Hall. *Travels in North America in the Years 1827 and 1828*

[This writer was a Captain in the Royal Navy. In his account he
states: ... "The chief object I had in view in visiting America was to see
things with my own eyes, in order to ascertain by personal inspection;
how far the sentiments prevalent in England with respect to that country
were correct or otherwise." [35]]

Oct. 11, 1827 [Quebec].

On the 4th of October, I visited the General Hospital, a large and well-
ventilated granite building, abundantly roomy and well-ordered in every
part. Indeed, I hardly ever saw an establishment of the kind which could
pretend to rival it, except, perhaps, the Infirmary at Derby. I accompanied
one of the physicians for some hours during his round of visits, attending to
all the details of the daily routine, without which it is impossible to form
a correct idea of the internal discipline of such an institution. Of course, I
can only judge of the general merits of matters so much out of my own
particular line; but, certainly, few men-of-war are better regulated than this
excellent hospital appeared to be.[36]

United States

NURSING IN HOMES

251. *Bradford's History of Plimoth Plantation*

[William Bradford (1590–1657), second governor of the Plymouth
Colony, early joined the separatist congregation at Scrooby and emi-
grated to Leyden, Holland, in 1609. He came to New England on the
Mayflower in 1620, and was governor of the colony for most of his life.
As governor he was fairly tolerant of religious beliefs other than his own,
and in establishing good relations with the Indians.[37] The manuscript of
Bradford's History of Plimoth Plantation was first published by the Massachusetts Historical Society in 1856. The original manuscript, begun in
1630, disappeared from Boston during the Revolutionary War and was
discovered in the Fulham Library in London in 1855. It was returned to
the State of Massachusetts in 1897 by the Bishop of London.[38]]

[1620] In these hard & difficulte beginings they found some discontents
& murmurings arise amongst some, and mutinous speeches & carriags in
other; but they were soone quelled & overcome by ye wisdome, patience, and
just & equall carrage of things by ye Govr and better part, wch clave faithfully
togeather in ye maine. But that which was most sadd & lamentable was, that
in 2. or 3. moneths time halfe of their company dyed, espetialy in Jan: &
February, being ye depth of winter, and wanting houses & other comforts;
being infected with ye scurvie & other diseases, which this long vioge & their

inacomodate condition had brought upon them; so as ther dyed some times 2. or 3. of a day, in yᵉ foresaid time; that of 100. & odd persons, scarce 50. remained. And of these in yᵉ time of most distres, ther was but 6. or 7. sound persons, who, to their great comendations be it spoken, spared no pains, night nor day, but with abundance of toyle and hazard of their owne health, fetched them woode, made them fires, drest them meat, made their beads, washed ther lothsome cloaths, cloathed & uncloathed them; in a word, did all yᵉ homly & necessarie offices for them wᶜʰ dainty & quesie stomacks cannot endure to hear named; and all this willingly & cherfully, without any grudging in yᵉ least, shewing herin their true love unto their freinds & bretheren. A rare example & worthy to be remembred. Tow of these 7. were Mʳ. William Brewster, ther reverend Elder, & Myles Standish, ther Captein & military comander, unto whom my selfe, & many others, were much beholden in our low & sicke condition. And yet the Lord so upheld these persons, as in this generall calamity they were not at all infected either with sicknes, or lamnes. And what I have said of these, I may say of many others who dyed in this generall vissitation, & others yet living, that whilst they had health, yea, or any strength continuing, they were not wanting to any that had need of them. And I doute not but their recompence is with yᵉ Lord.

[1634] I am now to relate some strang and remarkable passages. Ther was a company of people lived in yᵉ country, up above in yᵉ river of Conigtecut, a great way from their trading house ther, and were enimise to those Indeans which lived aboute them, and of whom they stood in some fear (bing a stout people). About a thousand of them had inclosed them selves in a forte, which they had strongly palissoadoed about. 3. or 4. Dutch men went up in yᵉ begining of winter to live with them, to gett their trade, and prevente them for bringing it to yᵉ English, or to fall into amitie with them; but at spring to bring all downe to their place. But their enterprise failed, for it pleased God to visite these Indeans with a great sicknes, and such a mortalitie that of a 1000. above 900. and a half of them dyed, and many of them did rott above ground for want of buriall, and yᵉ Dutch men allmost starved before they could gett away, for ise and snow. But about Feb: they got with much difficultie to their trading house; whom they kindly releeved, being allmost spente with hunger and could. Being thus refreshed by them diverce days, they got to their owne place, and yᵉ Dutch were very thankfull for this kindnes.

This spring, also, those Indeans that lived aboute their trading house there fell sick of yᵉ small poxe, and dyed most miserably; for a sorer disease cannot befall them; they fear it more than yᵉ plague; for usualy they that have this disease have them in abundance, and for wante of bedding & lining and other helps, they fall into a lamentable condition, as they lye on their hard matts, yᵉ poxe breaking and mattering, and runing one into another, their skin cleaving (by reason there of) to the matts they lye on; when they turne them, a whole side will flea of at once, (as it were,) and they will be

325

all of a gore blood, most fearfull to behold; and then being very sore, what with could and other distempers, they dye like rotten sheep. The condition of this people was so lamentable, and they fell downe so generally of this diseas, as they were (in yᵉ end) not able to help on another; no, not to make a fire, nor to fetch a little water to drinke, nor any to burie yᵉ dead; but would strive as long as they could, and when they could procure no other means to make fire, they would burne yᵉ woden trayes & dishes they ate their meate in, and their very bowes & arrowes; & some would crawle out on all foure to gett a litle water, and some times dye by yᵉ way, & not be able to gett in againe. But those of yᵉ English house, (though at first they were afraid of yᵉ infection,) yet seeing their woefull and sadd condition, and hearing their pitifull cries and lamentations, they had compastion of them, and dayly fetched them wood & water, and made them fires, gott them victualls whilst they lived, and buried them when they dyed. For very few of them escaped, notwithstanding they did what they could for them, to yᵉ haszard of them selvs. The cheefe Sachem him selfe now dyed, & allmost all his freinds & kinred. But by yᵉ marvelous goodnes & providens of God not one of yᵉ English was so much as sicke, or in yᵉ least measure tainted with this disease, though they dayly did these offices for them for many weeks togeather. And this mercie which they shewed them was kindly taken, and thankfully acknowledged of all yᵉ Indeans that knew or heard of yᵉ same; and their Mʳˢ here did much comend & reward them for yᵉ same.³⁹

252. *Records of the Moravians in North Carolina 1758–1783*

[The Moravians, a branch of the Western Slavs, settled in the United States in about 1740.⁴⁰ The first Moravian settlers of North Carolina came from the agricultural center near Bethlehem and Nazareth, Pennsylvania. The first men chosen for the settlement were fifteen in number, the list including the following: "4. Friedrich Jacob Pfeil, born in Germany, aged 28, shoe-maker, sick-nurse, and moreover willing and skillful in many things." ⁴¹ The records speak of both "sick-nursing," and "sick-visiting." Only those references have been included which seemed clearly to indicate *nursing* the sick. These records of North Carolina are among the few of the early state historical documents which refer specifically to nurses and nursing.]

Bethabara Diary, 1755.
July 3. . . . As Br. Kapp has been sick some days Br. Pfeil is appointed nurse.

Memorabilia of Outward Affairs, 1756.
August. . . . A number of the Brethren were ill, so on the 13th a Sick Room was arranged in the Brothers House . . .

Diary of Salem Congregation, 1772.

May 8.... The Sisters have requested their own sick-visiting and five Sisters have been found willing to serve; therefore Sr. Bonn has again been offered and has undertaken the office for which she was destined when she married. Sr. Aust is general sick-nurse, and the Srs. Reuter, Tiersch, Utley, Beck, and Schnepf, will in turn visit the sick for a week.

Aeltensten Conferenz Minutes, 1772.

Feb. 11. Br. Spissike is now Master tailor in the Brothers House in Salem; Br. Zillman has been appointed nurse, and will also work on his own account as a tailor.

Minutes of the Grosse Helfer Conferenz, 1772.

The married Sisters have established Sick Visiting among themselves, with one general sick-nurse, and other Sisters who will serve a week at a time in turn. These Sisters will have a conference, at which Br. Bonn [community doctor] will be present to give them instructions.

Salem Diary, 1777.

Jan. 12. Br. Reuter was taken ill suddenly, and his home-going was feared. A Brother was appointed to watch with him during the night ...

Minutes of Salem Boards, 1781.

March 28. (Aelt. Conf.) Br. Bonn has raised the question of sick-nurses for the married Sisters. Eight Sisters were suggested, and on some convenient day they will have a conference with Br. Bonn and arrange the matter.

Salem Diary, 1790.

Nov. 28. There was a vacant place among the sick nurses for the Brethren and Br. Jacob Meyer was appointed.

Salem Board Minutes, 1791.

Feb. 2. (Aelt. Conf.) Br. Michael Kurchner has been installed as chief nurse in the Brothers House, and as such becomes a member of Congregation Council.

Salem Diary, 1812.

Because of poor health Sr. Landmann asks to be relieved of her duties as sick-nurse of the married women. Sr. Lehnert was appointed to take her place.

. . . .

Salem Board Minutes, 1817.
Jan. 8. (Aeltesten Conferenz.)
At present four married Brethren are seriously sick, and among them Br. Christ, who is the regular nurse for the married Brethren. It was suggested that if it became necessary Br. Bagge might be asked to serve as nurse.

. . . .

Salem Board Minutes, 1818.
Oct. 21. (Aelt. Conf.) The office of sick-nurse for the married Sisters, which the departed Sr. Stotz held for a time with much faithfulness, has been given to Sr. Kreuser who is willing to serve as long as she remains in town.

. . . .

Salem Board Minutes, 1819.
June 3. (Aelt. Conf.) Although Sr. Peter is now a widow we believe it would be well for her to retain the office of sick-nurse for the married women and widows.
In regard to the support of Sr. Peter we think that for the present one dollar a week will be sufficient . . .

. . . .

Salem Board Minutes, 1820.
April 12. (Aelt. Conf.) The married Sr. Anna Christ has accepted the position of sick-nurse for the married women.[42]

253. Benjamin Rush. *Commonplace Book for 1789–1813*

[Benjamin Rush (1745?–1813), only physician signer of the Declaration of Independence, received his medical degree from the University of Edinburgh in 1768. He became the first professor of chemistry in the colonies at the College and Academy of Philadelphia. He was a member of the Continental Congress and a surgeon in the Continental army. He became the center of a medical controversy because of his bleeding and purging of patients. His contribution to psychiatry was notable. A friend of Benjamin Franklin, he was treasurer of the United States mint at Philadelphia, and the founder of the first antislavery society in America.[43] In his *Commonplace Book for 1789–1813* he made notes for a "life" of Nurse Mary Waters, and referred briefly to other nurses. A note by the editor of the *Commonplace Book* states that Nurse Mary Waters is listed in the *Philadelphia Directory* of 1796 as "Mary Waters, widow, doctoress, Willing Alley," in 1797 as "apothecary," and in 1798 and 1799 as "doctoress," at the same address. He remarks that it is a pity that Benjamin Rush did not write his projected account, inasmuch as the story of a woman nurse at the time of the Revolutionary War, would have been a unique document in the history of nursing.[44]]

Hints for the Life of Nurse Mary Waters

Why not? Her occupation was a noble one, and her example may be interesting to thousands. Only few men can be Kings, and yet Biography for a while had few other subjects. She was born in Dublin . . . came to America in the ship . . . , Capt . . . in the year 1766. She served during the whole war in the military hospitals, where she was esteemed and beloved by all who knew her. She has been a nurse ever since. She possesses a good deal of skill and an uncommon regard for cleanliness. I never saw her out of humour. She is chatty and tells a merry story very agreeably. She dislikes nursing lying-in women, as well as all such persons as are not very ill. Nothing but great danger rouses her into great activity and humanity. She once left off nursing, but was induced to undertake it again by the advice of her minister, the late Revd. Mr. Farmer, who told her "that her skill in nursing was a commission sent to her by heaven, which she was bound never to resign, and that she might merit heaven by it." She was minutely acquainted with the characters, manners, habits & c. of all the physicians in town, and always shewed a disposition to support their influence in medicine. She was once sent for to prescribe for a lady in a consumption, for her skill was known to many people. Before she went, she found out whose patient this lady was, and upon being complimented by her when she entered the room she said "Indeed, madam, I know nothing but what I learned from Dr. ———— (mentioning the name of the physician who attended her) in the military hospitals." This at once put an end to all further application on the part of the lady, and renewed her confidence in her physician. She was truly charitable. I once knew her lend money to a patient whom she nursed, and to the family in which she lodged.[45]

254. *Baltimore. A Series of Letters and Other Documents Relating to the Late Epidemic of Yellow Fever*

[This collection comprises the correspondence of the Mayor of Baltimore, the Board of Health, the Executive of the State, and the reports of the Faculty and District Medical Society of Baltimore.[46] It also contains essays by physicians. It originated in answer to the mayor's circular requesting information on the disease of yellow fever. From the context, it is assumed that the excerpts quoted refer to nursing in the homes of the patients.]

[Fell's Point, 20 Oct. 1819 to Edw. Johnson——, M.D.]

8th, at 10 o'clock, A.M. . . . On turning round: I now beheld (for the first time, an old lady advancing towards me, and addressing me in broken English, saying, "She had came last night to nurse this poor woman, and had been up with her all night."

.   .   .   .

[Dec. 29, 1819. John Coulter to Edw. Johnson]

It is worthy of remark, and an encouraging circumstance, that the mode of treating this Fever is so well understood, by the Physicians of the present day, if immediate application is made, I verily believe not more than one in twenty, in the aggregate, would die, and where they have the chance of nursing and necessaries, a still less proportion.

.   .   .   .

[Church Street, Dec. 29, 1819. To Edw. Johnson from Richard W. Hall]

The other cases which I saw, had been removed from that part of Fell's Point near Donnell's Wharf, after the attack of disease; or had imbibed its causes while engaged in business at or near the same place, or while nursing their friends; and subsequently had the disease at their residences west of Jones' Falls.[47]

255. Joseph Warrington. *The Nurse's Guide*

[The writer, a physician, is an obstetrician who is desirous of improving the nursing care of his patients. The title of the book continues as follows: "Containing a series of instructions to Females who wish to engage in the important business of Nursing Mother and Child in the Lying-in Chamber." [48]]

Preface

Having, in common with a number of my professional friends who are also engaged in superintending the cases of parturient females, encountered many difficulties and suffered much anxiety on account of the general want of proper intelligence and qualification in *nurses* to the lying-in chamber, I have felt that it was due from some member of the profession, to place before this class of persons, (whose services, if properly performed, are highly important,) a sketch of the qualities necessary for a woman who proposes to enter upon so responsible an occupation.

.   .   .   .

Introductory Remarks.

The skill that is requisite for nursing women, during the confinement of childbirth, is best acquired by practical attendance upon persons in that condition. A middle-aged woman, of good practical education, vigorous health, and cheerful temper, capable of interesting her patient when she is alone, one who is not loquacious, nor gossiping, who is careful to avoid meddling improperly with the affairs of the family, presents many of the pre-requisites of a good nurse. To make herself useful in this important business she must carefully observe and faithfully communicate to the obstetric attendant every circumstance which has transpired relative to the woman and child, since his last visit, and must punctually execute his orders, without interposing her own opinions, lest the patient suffer by such inter-ference, as has frequently been the case with those who have been in the hands of officious and self-conceited nurses. She must neither lend her faith to the many vulgar errors about women in labour, or those who have been delivered; nor by any means communicate to the individual of whom she has, or is to have, the charge, lest she should alarm her. Since the general concession, that the duty of superintending and aiding a female at the interesting and critical period of parturition, devolves rather upon well-instructed physicians than uneducated midwives, the opinions of a nurse are not unfrequently demanded by the nervous and timid lady, and ingenuity or superstition may often be exercised in the absence of true knowledge; the nurse should, therefore, in all cases, decline any opinion as to the condi-tion of the inquirer, and refer her to the accoucheur, who should be regarded as the only person suitable to explain the condition, and direct the conduct of the pregnant or parturient female.[49]

256. J. S. Longshore. *The Principles and Practice of Nursing or a Guide to the Inexperienced*

[This treatise on nursing, by a physician, published in 1842, has as its subtitle the following: "Designed to Instruct the Nurse in the Principles of her Profession, and to Assist the Inexperienced in Performing the Various Duties pertaining to the Sick Room." An additional note states that it is "Adapted to families, nurses, and young physicians." [50]]

Important as is the office of nurse, it is a matter of no little astonishment, to reflect how few there are who assume the responsible station, that are qualified either by nature or education, to discharge its duties. If the saying be true, "That a patient stands a better chance with a good nurse and an inferior physician, than with a good physician and an inferior nurse, (and we are not disposed to doubt it,) everyone will admit that those who offer themselves to the public as nurses, or guardians of their welfare in the hour of danger, should have previously, by reading and observation, amply qualified themselves for the undertaking. But how many are there who have devoted even one month or week to preparatory study or reflection; or how many, previously to the commencement of their career, have passed one day in the sick room, for the purpose of acquiring, by observation, that

331

knowledge necessary for an efficient and agreeable nurse? Very few, very few, is the response to the inquiry . . .[51]

257. "Female Nurses in Military Hospitals," *American Medical Times,* July 18, 1861, pp. 25–26

[This periodical was published in New York City. In 1861 the editor was Stephen Smith, M.D., and the associate editor was George P. Shrady, M.D. The following editorial reveals the concern of the medical profession, at the beginning of the Civil War, about the lack of qualified obstetric nurses in the United States. It states the steps being applied in Nottingham, England, to remedy a similar deficiency, as outlined in *The Lancet.*]

Every obstetric physician experiences the want of skilled monthly nurses. In general any superannuated widow, unable to live by other means, obtains the names of several physicians as references, and issues her cards as a qualified nurse. She enters upon her profession with no practical knowledge of her duties; or just conception of her relation to the patient and the medical attendant. Her head is full of old women's remedies, with which she is constantly annoying the physician, or in his absence administering to the patient; she is foreboding if the labor is tedious, and horror-stricken if it is complicated, and requires operative interference; in short, instead of being an assistant to the accoucheur, and a source of comfort and support to the patient, she proves to be a constant annoyance to the former and an alarmist of the latter.

What we need is, a school for the practical training of monthly nurses. In a recent number of the *London Lancet* we find the following remarks upon this subject, which we commend to the attention of the profession:—

"Dr. Lory Marsh, of Nottingham, has so far successfully called attention to the deficiency of skilled, childbed nurses as to have evoked an organisation for applying a remedy. His views have been supported, we are informed, by the great majority of his local brethren, and are actively taken up by a committee of ladies. Now, since practical instruction seems to require some special institution for the reception of lying-in women, it is proposed that in every town an institution having this object in view, should be established; and that nurses should in them acquire the skill they will be called upon to exercise. In large towns there can, unhappily, be no doubt there will rarely lack a sufficient number of poor women needing charitable succor in their travail to furnish an hospital or maternity charity. In small towns this may not always be the case. But we do not think it will ever be necessary to collect these poor women together into one building. The experience of the Royal Maternity Charity of London, which annually delivers at their own homes 3500 women, is ample proof that no insurmountable difficulty exists in administering efficient medical assistance to parturient women in isolated dwellings. If for the sake of facility of administration, it should ever be found desirable to give some degree of local concentration to a maternity charity, nothing is more feasible than to found an institution on the system of cottage-hospitals. This system lends itself with the most admirable convenience to the requirements of a lying-in institution. A cottage may accomodate two or three women in separate rooms. According to the demand, another and additional cottages may be taken. These should be employed in rotation, each being kept empty for a fortnight, to allow of purification by scrubbing, lime-washing, and aëration. This arrangement would afford ample means of instructing nurses—none the worse for the greater similarity of the conditions to those of a private dwelling. Each patient might be at liberty to select any medical practitioner in the town of those willing to act, to superintend her case. Periodical lectures and demonstrations might be given; and some form of certificate or diploma of competency might be awarded to the nurses who had undergone a sufficient training. In many places it would hardly be necessary to have special institutions at all."

258. Annual Report of the Board of Managers to the Ladies Benevolent Society, September 15, 1824

[The Ladies Benevolent Society of Charleston, South Carolina, was founded in 1813. It is believed that this society and the Philadelphia Lying-in-Charity, founded in 1828, were the first efforts for nursing the sick poor in their homes in the United States.[52] The preamble of the constitution states the purposes of the society as follows: "To relieve the distresses of the poor, and administer comfort to the sick, are duties enjoined on every individual." Its motto was: "I was sick and ye visited me." [53] The tradition through the years has always been that the first ladies did some nursing when the need arose, and supplied a nurse to care for the patient in other cases. It will be noted that in the report of 1824, the board stated that it had *attended* (*italics ours*) and relieved the want and misery of 2,916 *destitute sick poor,* since the founding of the society. This tradition is documented by the statement of Ella Crandall, Executive Secretary of the National Organization for Public Health Nursing, on February 11, 1913, when the society celebrated its one hundredth anniversary, and she said of it, "We who are interested in Modern Visiting Nursing, should be especially interested in this old society, for, it represents the first effort in this country for systematic nursing among the poor." [54]]

Ladies,

Your Board respectfully congratulate you on this being your eleventh Anniversary and with infinite pleasure perform their duty of reporting to you the transactions of the past year as follows:

Receipts			Disbursements		
To Balance from last Year	$	4.17	By Cash p. on last year's account	$	27.80
To Amt. of Annual Sub- scriptions		1665	" Amt. Spent on 208 sick persons		1725.82
To Life Do — —		50	" Cash p. for Blankets Flannel		89.25
To Donations — —		500.56	" — " Sheets & Pavilions		96.19
To Int. on Stock		464.75	" —Domestic Coffee, Drag. & Landuy		7.93
		2684.48			
			" —Cardozo, editor of the Southern Patriot for Printing Annual Report & Quarterly Meetings		17.31
			" —3 Shares U. S. Bank		330
			" —Carting Wood to V. Committee		5.50
			Balance		384.68
Total	$2684.48		Total		2684.48

The $50—paid by a Life Member, and the $464.75 Interest arising from stock, belong to the Permanent Fund.—Of the Donations, $125 are in part payment of a Note of $250, *given the last year,* and payable this—

All the articles received—1 Piece of London Duffel Blankets—10 y^{ds} of Flannel—7 Cords of Wood—2 Bundles of Baby Linen—and 9 lbs of Arrow Root.—Donations in Dry Goods, Groceries, Wood, Rice & ᶜᶜ, aid our funds very acceptably.—The Blankets, Flannel, & Wood, which have been frequently sent us, have comforted and warmed the sick destitute Sufferers; until reaching their hearts, have lighted them up into a blaze of gratitude and praise to that Being, who inspired their Benefactors with Compassion and generosity towards them;—and in the same breath, have implored blessings on their heads.—

Your Board are happy that the expenditures of the past year, have not exceeded the receipts of the Society, but have left a Balance in its favour.—

Since our last Anniversary, 16 Ladies have joined our Institution, 12 Annual and 4 Honorary Visiting Members; and one of your old Ann.[1] Subscribers, has become a Life Member.—19 Subscribers have withdrawn, some have quitted the State; and 6 have died—we mourn the loss of all.— When those who have left the State bade us a long adieu in this Room, where for upwards of ten years we so often met together in the cause of suffering humanity; we then lost some of our most valuable Members, who had been Officers and Visitors from the commencement of the Institution: —"The chain was severed with regret, and hallowed by a tear."—

In consequence of the prevailing Epidemic, we have appointed a Committee to communicate with the Board of Health, if it should be requisite.—

We think it will be satisfactory to the Members and Donors generally, and to the Visiting Committee in particular, to have the aggregate number of Sufferers presented to their view, who have been relieved by their bounty during the lapse of eleven years.—From the instituting of our Society on the 15:th Sept. 1813, to the present day, we have attended, and relieved the want and misery of 2916 *destitute sick poor:*—from the Infant in the Cradle, to the old Man of an *hundred* and five!—

We cannot close this Report, without returning to the Visiting Com^{tees} our warmest acknowledgments, for having so obligingly served at our request.—We feel ourselves much indebted to you Ladies;—as without your humane hearts and judicious distributions, Officers, Managers, and money, would all have been useless.—You have visited the sick and forlorn in their wretched Hovels, without once shrinking from the inclemency of the weather.—In this world you receive a reward *in the act*—and in the next, you will receive a greater, according to it.—It is unnecessary for *us* to recommend to the Society, that they should return their grateful acknowledgments to the faithful Dispensers of their Charities—"Out of the abundance of their hearts, their mouths will speak."

Your Board find the conducting of your Society a pleasing duty, and will strive so to act, as to continue to recommend it to your's, and the public's fostering care:—it has hitherto been liberally supported.—We assure you, that as Managers we find but one difficulty.—That difficulty has long existed, and is noticed in our Journal as far back as 1814, namely—*the difficulty of obtaining Visiting Committees.*—It has been said, "The pleasure of the Law consists in overcoming difficulties," but we wish to give up that pleasure exclusively to the Gentlemen of the Bar; it does not suit the Managers of the *female* Board.—Permit us then respectfully to recommend, nay, entreat, that all of you who have not young, or large families, with a few other exceptions, will come forward, and visit in Committees as it may suit your convenience—In that case, you would be called upon but seldom, as your Society consists of 346 Members.—Visitors being our Distributors, are quite as necessary for carrying on the usefulness of the Society as money:—each without the other, would be nothing worth.—Subscribers & Donors may throw liberally into your Coffers, and your Treasurer may securely lock them; but the Keys of the *Visiting Committees* must open them—or, the sick must languish and die, crying in vain to us for that very money which was given them, but which would remain locked up.—This is a most *serious* consideration! one, that we respectfully hope will be impressed on your minds, and carried home with you.—Christ has set us an example of visiting the sick and needy.—He has pointed it out to us as the Christian's duty, equally obligatory on all; and to fulfil *this* duty was our Society expressly instituted.—Christ has promised blessings, and eternal life to the performance of this duty.—He has said he will consider it as done unto *himself!* How honorable is it then to visit our sick, destitute fellow Beings!—How great the blessing and reward! Let us all adopt the following sentiments of the Rev. Dr. Scott.—"Did we but understand and consider, how divinely significant it is to supply the necessities, and contribute to the happiness of others; would it as our highest preferment, and bless God for deeming us worthy of such an illustrious employment; and that among the numerous blessings he has heaped upon us, he has vouchsafed to admit us to share with himself the glory of doing good—*for Man hath in nothing so much of God; as in doing Good.*—" [55]

259. Lists of Nurses in Early Editions of the *Cleveland Directory*

[The first *Directory of Cleveland* was issued in 1837–38.[56] The early issues listed only heads of families. In the Directory of 1850–51, nurses are listed separately, and in succeeding years lists of nurses are found. The lists are given here as an indication of the recognition of nurses as a separate group in cities of eastern United States. A similar list will be found for New York City in Reading No. 277.]

Cleveland Directory, 1850–51.

Nurses

Mrs. Montgomery, 62 Prospect St.
Mrs. Sutton, r. 161 Lake Street.
Mrs. Wilson, r. York Street.[57]

Cleveland Directory, 1856.

List of Nurses

Armstrong, Lettie, h. 37 Fulton. (widow)
Downs Nancy, h. 13 Harmon.
Frederick Mary, h. 116 Pearl. (Widow)
Grahams Catherine, h. Long.
Greenvault Phebe, h. Courtlandt n. Detroit. (widow)
Holden Christiana, h. 89¼ Kinsman.
Hubar Frances, h. 15 York. (midwife)
Knowlton Sarah F., h. Sibley n. Perry, (midwife)
Pfur Elizabeth, h. St. Clair n. Erie
Pool Roxana, h. 26 Birch.[58]

Cleveland Directory, 1857.

Nurses

Armstrong Lettie, h 37 Fulton WS [west side]
Bellmuth Susan, (ladies) Green n Chatham WS
Blackford Maria, (ladies) 177 St. Clair
Frederick Mary, (ladies) 118 Pearl WS
Grossman Christine, (ladies) 5 Orange
Huber Caroline, (ladies) 15 York WS
Koch Dores F. Mrs., (ladies) 18 Burwell
Koerner Anna, (ladies) 137 Garden

Setchfield Mary, 11 St. Clair
Slosson Jane M., 75 Lake
Walker Margaret, (ladies) 33 N Brownell [59]

260. *Apron Full of Gold The Letters of Mary Jane Megquier from San Francisco, 1849–1856*

[Most of these letters were written from San Francisco or en route to California. The writer was the wife of Dr. Thomas Lewis Megquier of Winthrop, Maine, and the letters were addressed to their children, close relatives, or friends. Tradition states that Mrs. Megquier was the first American woman to cross the Isthmus, and it is certain that Dr. Megquier was the first American physician to establish a practice in San Francisco.[60] Whether Mrs. Megquier ever carried out her intention of doing nursing is not revealed by the letters.]

[From Panama]. May. 20. [1849]

... The news from the gold regions far exceeds our expectations; every man that goes to the mines picks up a fortune. I have had a lump of pure gold, weighing two pounds in my hand, just as it was dug, as ladies are very scarce I except to make money in the way of odd jobs such as cooking and attending the sick ...[61]

261. Alfred Worcester. *Nurses and Nursing*

[Alfred Worcester, physician (b. 1855), was educated at Harvard University and at Tufts College. He was the founder of the Waltham Training School for Nurses, and became a controversial figure because of his views on nursing education. He was the author of several books on nursing and of selected medical papers.[62] The following is a description of a "neighborhood nurse" of the middle of the nineteenth century.]

As the untrained nurses have been so often maligned, it seems only fitting in this sketch of New England nursing to describe at least one of them as she was known and loved in our neighborhood. Her name was Mary K. Green, and her little gravestone says she died in 1884, aged seventy-three years. She was born in one of the up-country villages of Massachusetts, the oldest of seven children, on a poor farm where it was a hard struggle to get food enough for the family. When Mary was only twelve, her mother died, leaving a baby daughter, Ruth, with five brothers in between. For four years Mary did all the housework for this family. She then started out to earn her own living and to help support the old home. She found work in a farmer's family in Waltham, where she slaved from four in the morning until well into the evening ...

... and then she went to live with another family ...

In her new situation she had an easier time of it. But, besides the ordinary work of the farmhouse, she had the care of the old grandfather in his dotage,

337

and of many of the little grandchildren who were sent back from their city home to build up in the country, and she was also often called upon for a few weeks' special service in one after another of the daughters' homes where there was sickness or any extra stress. . . . Her service to this one family was . . . given to five generations.

For the last half of her life Mary Green was an "untrained" nurse. How did she become one, and of what sort was her nursing? During her early years the only nurses were the neighbor nurses already described. Often in the families where she was working she served as an assistant watcher; but it was not until she was of middle age that she was taught the art of nursing. Nor was she in any hurry to undertake the responsibility. But finally she was persuaded to do so by an expectant mother, who promised to teach her what nursing she herself would need, and then to recommend her, and teach her at these cases what nursing was needed for them.

In this way Miss Green, as she then came to be called, was launched upon her nursing career. After her long preparation of helpful service, it was no wonder she soon became a famous nurse. Fortunate, indeed, were the families that found her in their times of need. For not only would she do the strictly nursing work in tending the patient, but she also delighted in doing the family washing before breakfast, the ironing in the forenoon, and the mending before or after nightfall, with the baby on her lap. Much of the cooking and general housework she would do between-times. The amount of her day's work was astonishing; nor were her patients ever neglected.

While faithful to the old doctors whom she knew, and always punctilious in giving the medicine as ordered, she was a terror to the younger physicians, for whom she had little use. To one of them, who incautiously asked, "How is your patient?" her snappy answer was, "That is for you to find out;" and again when he asked if the fine breast bandage he had so proudly applied the day before had proved a comfort, she admitted that she had taken it off directly after he left the house. She "didn't like them things," she added.

For the clinical thermometer and for modern antiseptics she had supreme contempt. Soapsuds were cleansing enough for anybody sick or well, she would say; "and as if any fool ought not to be able to tell without thermometers whether the patient or the chamber were too cold or too warm." It was no use to allow fruit or any other "outlandish diet" to her patients. She believed in gruels and broths, fresh air and perfect quiet. What she believed in would be given, and nothing else. "If you want any other kind of nursing, get it," was her ultimatum.

Though she died many years ago, she is still missed, and she deserves a more fitting memorial.[63]

NURSING IN HOSPITALS

[The hospital now known as Bellevue Hospital in New York City, the first institution which cared for the sick in what is now the United States, was established on December 20, 1658. Before this date, during Peter

Stuyvesant's administration as governor of the Dutch colony, means were sought to supply care for those who were unable to provide for themselves when ill. This culminated in the establishment of a hospital and shelter.[64]]

262. "Remonstrance of New Netherland, and the Occurrences There"

[These papers were a petition to the Dutch government addressed to it by the people of New Netherland, on July 28, 1649. They contained a complaint concerning the absence of a hospital, the complaint being renewed the same year. The feeling seems to be expressed here that the hospital should not be financed by the Dutch West India Company but by the Dutch government.[65]]

There is occasionally, a flying report of an hospital and of asylums for orphans and for old men, & c., but as yet not a sign of an attempt, order or regulation has been made about them.

.   .   .   .

[1650] The question is, are the Company or the Directors obliged to have constructed any buildings for the people out of the duties paid by the trader in New Netherland on exported goods, particularly as their High Mightinesses granted those duties to the Company to facilitate garrison, and the payment of the expenses attendant thereupon, and not for building Hospitals and Orphan Asylums, Churches and School-houses for the people.[66]

263. *Historic New York: Half Moon Papers*

[These papers take their name from the ship of Henry Hudson, the English navigator (fl. 1607–11) who, in the employ of the Dutch East India Company, discovered the river named for him, giving the Dutch their claim to this region.[67] In the latter years of Stuyvesant's administration, Master Jacob Hendrichsen Varvanger, the surgeon of the Dutch West India Company, through whose agency New Netherland had been founded, in his report to the Director and the Council, December 12, 1658, recommended the establishment of a hospital for soldiers and employees of the company.[68] The hospital was established on December 20, 1658. Hilletje Wilbruch, the wife of Condil Tubias Wilbruch, was appointed its matron at a yearly salary of 100 florins.]

[He is] . . . sorry to learn that such sick people must suffer much through cold, inconveniences, and the untidiness of the people who have taken the poor fellows into their houses where bad smells and filth counteract all health producing effects of the medicaments given by him, the surgeon. Death has been the result of it in several cases and many deaths will follow.

He requests, therefore, that by order of the Director and Council a proper place may be arranged for the reception of such patients, to be taken care of by a faithful person, who is to assist them bodily with food and fire and allow soldiers to pay for it out of their wages and rations, Company's negroes to be attended at Company's expense or as thought most advisable.[69]

264. Records of the Upland Court, Delaware County, Pennsylvania

[Upland, the seat of justice of Delaware County was said to have derived its name from being situated on high or "up land." Another account states that the word was derived from the Swedish word *upsala*.[70] The court was authorized in 1672, and the first court was held at Upland in 1676. The name Upland was changed to Chester by William Penn. The following notation is in the records of 1678.[71]]

Jan Cornelissen of Amesland complayning to ye Court that his son Erick is bereft of his naturall sences & is turned quyt madd and y^t: hee being a poore man is not able to maintaine him;—ordered: that three or 4 p^{r}sons bee hired to build a Little Blockhouse at amesland for to put in the s^d madman, and att the next Court, order will bee taken y^t: a small Levy Laid to pay for the building of ye house and the maintayning of ye s^d mad man according to Lawes of ye government.[72]

265. *Public Records of the Colony of Connecticut from October, 1706, to October, 1716 . . .*

[The Act quoted below was passed by the Assembly in 1711, to make some provision for the control of diseases in the colony, particularly of smallpox.]

153. An Act providing in cases of Sickness.
Be it enacted by the Governour, Council and Representatives in General Court Assembled, and by the authority of the same, That for the better preventing the spreading of infection, when it shall happen, any person or persons coming from abroad, or belonging to any town or place within this Colony to be visited, or that late before having been visited with the small pox, or other contatious sickness, the infection whereof may probably be communicated to others; the selectmen of each town be, and hereby are impowered to take care, and make effectual provision in the best manner they can for the preservation of the inhabitants, by removing and placing such sick or infected person or persons to and in a separate house, and necessaries for them, at the charge of the parties themselves, their parents, or masters, (if able,) or otherwise at the charge of the town or place whereto they belong.[73]

266. Treaty of the Company of the Indies with the Ursulines

[Early in the history of the Western Hemisphere, the Company of the Indies contracted with the Ursulines in France to come to the New World to establish a hospital in New Orleans and to educate young girls. The preamble of the treaty indicates these purposes. The hospital was not established until a later date. The treaty is taken from the Register of the Accounts of the Indies.[74]]

The Company considering that the most solid foundations of the colony of Louisiana are the establishments which tend to the advancement of the glory of God and the edification of the people, such as those made by the Reverend Capuchin Fathers, and the Reverend Jesuit Fathers, whose zeal and charity assure spiritual succor to the inhabitants and give great hope for the conversion of the savages; wishing moreover, by a new establishment as pious, to succor the poor sick, and provide, at the same time, for the education of young girls, it has agreed to and accepted the offers made by the Sisters Marie Tranchepain de St. Augustin and Marie-Anne Boulanger de Ste Angelique, Ursulines of Rouen, to take in charge the hospital of New Orleans . . .

Made in Paris, in the Hotel of the Company of the Indies, on the 13th day of September, 1726.

Signed: L'Abbe Raguet, J. Morin, D'Artaguette, Diron, Castanier, Deshayer, P. Saintard.

Soeur Catherine de Bruscoly de St. Amand, premiere Superieure des Ursulines de France.

Soeur Marie Tranchepain de St. Augustin, Superieure.

Soeur Marie des Anges Boulanger de Ste Angelique, Depositaire.[75]

267. Holographic Will of Jean Louis, 1735

[Among the interesting documents concerning the Charity Hospital of New Orleans is the will of Jean Louis, at one time a sailor in the employ of the Company of the Indies. Having no family, he bequeathed all he possessed to found a hospital. His estate amounted to about 10,000 livres.[76]]

Holographic Testament Written by My Hand

In the name of the Father, and of the Son, and of the Holy Ghost, Amen.

Nothing being more certain than death and nothing more uncertain than its hour, being stricken with a dangerous bodily malady, but sane of mind, I desire to settle my affairs, explaining how I intend that my last will be carried out by my testamentary executor who will be named hereafter, without anyone being able to contravene, being of age, having neither father nor mother, one having died in my childhood, and my mother thirteen years ago; besides what I possess I have earned in this country irreproachably.

As to what may come to me from France of any nature whatsoever, I set in order before leaving and willed it where I should.

I recommend my soul to God the Father, Son and Holy Ghost, to the Holy Virgin, to my angel guardian, to all the Saints of Paradise, particularly to my holy patrons, praying them to receive my soul amongst the Blessed when it shall pass from this world to the other, Amen.

I give my (soul) to God, my body to the earth, asking my Executor to have me buried simply. Before my funeral a high mass will be said during which, if there are priests, others will be said. During one year, on every first Monday of the Month, there will be a service for my intention in the parochial church and fifty low masses said.

Item—I beg those whom I have offended in any way whatever to be willing to forgive as I forgive. I desire that my notes or debts, if any are found, to be acquitted and paid preferably to anything else.

Item—I give to the parochial church for some ornament or embellishment which my executor will be kind enough to have made, such as a large crucifix or something else at his will, two hundred livres to be used by him for that purpose according to the most pressing needs.

Item—I give to the poor of this city who are ashamed to beg two hundred livres and one hundred livres to procure clothes for the most needy orphans, at my executor's pleasure.

My debts having been paid and the above provisions having been executed, a sale shall be made of all that remains, which, together with my small lot, I bequeath to serve in perpetuity to the founding of a hospital for the sick of the city of New Orleans, without anyone being able to change my purpose, and to secure the things necessary to succor the sick.

I will and direct that the said sale be made by my testamentary executor, whom I name as director and inspector of said foundation, during his life, and in case of his death or of his removal from the colony he will, at his choice, name a person to execute my wishes.

I beg the Curé of the parish to kindly work with my testamentary executor for the establishment of the said hospital and the execution of my will.

This present will, written by my hand, in full possession of my faculties and judgment, revoking all wills and codicils that I may heretofore have made, the same to be null, willing and intending that this present be executed according to its form and tenor, and this rather increased than diminished, referring to my testamentary executor's good will, and to execute all that is herein contained I pray and name Monsieur Raguette, Councillor of the Superior Council of this province, to kindly take it in charge and act thereon as if it were his own, without being obliged to render an account to any one whomsoever, nor shall any offices of justice take cognizance of it, trusting entirely in his probity and faithfulness.

At New Orleans, this sixteenth of November, one thousand seven hundred and thirty-five.

Signed: Jean Louis [77]

268. Memorial Addressed to Comte de Maurepas in France, by Bienville and Salmon, May 20, 1737

[Evidence exists in the Cabildo Archives which establishes the fact that there was a hospital in New Orleans before St. John's, now Charity Hospital. Sieur de Bienville (Jean Baptiste le Moyne) (1680–1768) was governor of the province, while Salmon was intendant-commissary. Bienville founded the city of New Orleans on its present site in 1718. The document quoted seems to indicate that the hospital was established primarily for the care of the sick, but that it might serve also as a shelter.[78]]

Louisiana   20. May 1737

Messrs de Bienville and Salmon
Extract

Foundation of a
hospital at New Orleans.

Sir

One Jean Louis formerly a sailor in the employ of the Company of the Indies and who formerly had a small business died last year, and being a bachelor he leaves by olographic will all his property to found a hospital. This estate after all debts are paid will amount to about 10,000 livres cash. We are of the opinion together with the Curé and the Executor of his will that no better use could be made of it than to purchase the house of Madame de Kolly which is on a large tract of land at the extreme end of the City and which was occupied formerly by the Nuns. It will cost only 1200 livres because it needed many repairs which amounted to 2500 livres: there have been bought at the same time some beds, some linen and other utensils necessary for the hospital. The remainder amounting to about 5000 livres; which with the help furnished by the inhabitants will be used to build a large brick hall to shelter the sick later on because the house which is on the ground will not last much longer. There are at this time 4 or 5 patients there. In this way there will no longer be any beggars, they will all be confined there and their skills will occupy them after that. This will contribute at the same time to diminishing the number because the majority of those who beg and who are healthy seeing themselves thus confined will prefer work in order to have their freedom. This beginning of the establishment will make it possible to persuade the inhabitants to subscribe and furnish some materials and some days of work with which to continue the strong building which will become necessary when the old house will no longer stand. This will release at the same time the Royal hospital where they were often forced to receive the poor inhabitants who without this help should have perished in misery.

We are with a very profound Respect
Sir
Your very humble and very Obedient servants

Bienville
Salmon [79]

At New Orleans
The 20 May 1737

343

269. "Petition to the Honourable House of Representatives of the Province of Pennsylvania"

[The Pennsylvania Hospital in Philadelphia is considered by many to be the first hospital in the United States in the modern sense of the term. It was started mainly through the efforts of Benjamin Franklin and Dr. Thomas Bond. The charter was granted by the Assembly and approved by Lieutenant Governor James Hamilton on May 11, 1751.[80]]

The Petition of Sundry Inhabitants of the said Province Humbly sheweth,
That with the Number of People, the number of Lunatics or Persons distempered in Mind and deprived of their rational Faculties, hath greatly encreased in this Province.

That some of them going at large are a Terror to their Neighbors, who are daily apprehensive of the violences they may commit; And others, are continually wasting their Substance, to the great injury of themselves and Families, ill disposed Persons wickedly taking Advantage of their unhappy Condition, and drawing them into unreasonable Bargains, & c.

That few or none of them are so sensible of their Condition, as to submit voluntarily to the Treatment their respective Cases require, and therefore continue in the same deplorable State during their Lives; whereas it has been found, by the Experience of many Years, that above two Thirds of the Mad People received into Bethlehem Hospital, and there treated properly, have been perfectly cured.

Your Petitioners beg Leave further to represent, that tho' the good Laws of this Province have made many compassionate and charitable Provisions for the Relief of the Poor, yet something farther seems wanting in Favour of such, whose Poverty is made more miserable by the additional Weight of a grievous Disease, from which they might easily be relieved, if they were not situated at too great a Distance from regular Advice and Assistance; whereby many languish out their Lives, tortur'd perhaps with the Stone, devour'd by the Cancer, deprived of Sight by Cataracts, or gradually decaying by loathsome Distempers; who, if the Expence in the present manner of Nursing and Attending them separately when they come to Town were not so discouraging, might again, by the judicious Assistance of Physic and Surgery, be enabled to taste the blessing of Health, and be made in a few Weeks, useful Members of the Community, able to provide for themselves and Families.

The kind Care our Assemblies have heretofore taken for the Relief of sick and distempered Strangers, by providing a Place for their Reception and Accomodation, leaves us no Room to doubt an equal tender Concern for the Inhabitants. And we hope they will be of Opinion with us, that a small Provincial Hospital, erected and put under proper Regulations, in the Care of Persons to be appointed by this House, or otherwise, as they shall think meet, with Power to receive and apply the charitable Benefactions of good People towards enlarging and supporting the same, and some other provisions

344

in a Law for the Purposes above mentioned, will be a good work, acceptable to God and to all the good People they represent.

We therefore humbly recommend the Premises to their serious consideration.

A. Morris, Jun.	Nath'l Allen	S. Shoemaker
Jona. Evans	Wm. Coleman	Samul Sansom
Joseph Shippen	Wm. Atwood	Saml. Hazard
John Inglis	Anth. Morris	Wm. Plumsted
Reese Meredith	Thos. Graeme	Luke Morris
Jos. Richardson	John Mifflin	Stephen Armitt
Jos. Sims	Geo. Spotford	Samuel Rhoads
Edward Cathrall	John Reynell	Will Branson
Amos Strettell	Chas. Norris	Israel Pemberton
John Armitt	William Griffitts	Johnson Crosby
Jos'h Fisher	Samuel Smith	Will Allen [81]

270. Benjamin Franklin. *Some Account of the Pennsylvania Hospital from Its First Beginning to the Fifth Month, called May, 1754*

[Benjamin Franklin (1706–1790), American statesman, printer, scientist, and writer, was born in Boston. He acquired an interest in the *Pennsylvania Gazette* in 1729 and published *Poor Richard's Almanac* from 1732 to 1757. He organized the American Philosophical Society and helped to establish an academy which later became the University of Pennsylvania. He was a great statesman of the American Revolution and a delegate to the Continental Congress. He spent several years in England and France in relation to the American cause. He wrote many books, among them the history of the Pennsylvania Hospital of which he was a founder.[82]]

The following papers were published in the Pennsylvania Gazette, of August the eighth, and fifteenth, 1751, viz...

"The difference between nursing and curing the sick in a Hospital, and separately in private lodgings, with regard to the expense, is at least as ten to one. For instance, suppose a person under the necessity of having a limb amputated, he must have the constant attendance of a nurse, a room, fire, & c. which cannot for the first three or four weeks be procured at less expense than fifteen shillings a week, and never after at less than ten. If he continues two months, his nursing will be five pounds, his surgeon's fee, and other accidental [sic] charges, commonly amounts to three pounds, in the whole near ten pounds; whereas, in a Hospital, one nurse, one fire, & c. will be sufficient for ten patients, the extra expense will be inconsiderable, and the surgeon's fees taken off, which will bring the above calculations within the limits of truth . . ."

The managers hired the most convenient house that could be procured, with gardens, & c. agreed with a matron to govern the family, and nurse the sick, and provided beds and other necessary furniture; and prepared the following rules respecting admission and discharge of patients, a number of which were printed and dispersed among the contributors, viz.

Rules agreed to by the managers of the Pennsylvania Hospital for the admission and discharge of Patients . . .

. . . .

Fifteenthly, That such patients as are able, shall assist in nursing others, washing and ironing the linen, washing and cleaning the rooms, and such other services as the matron may require.

The foregoing rules were agreed to by a board of managers of the Pennsylvania Hospital, the twenty third day of the first month (January) 1752.

Benjamin Franklin, Clerk.

We do approve of the foregoing rules,

William Allen, Chief Justice.

Isaac Norris, Speaker of the Assembly.

Tench Francis, Attorney General.[83]

271. *Autobiography of Benjamin Franklin*

[This edition of the autobiography was edited from the manuscript by John Bigelow (1817–1911), minister to France from 1865 to 1866 and Secretary of State of New York from 1875 to 1877. He shared with William Cullen Bryant the ownership and editorship of the *New York Evening Post*. He is given much credit for preventing French recognition of the Confederacy.[84]]

In 1751, Dr. Thomas Bond, a particular friend of mine, conceived the idea of establishing a hospital in Philadelphia (a very beneficial design, which has been ascrib'd to me, but was originally his), for the reception and cure of poor sick persons, whether inhabitants of the province or strangers. He was zealous and active in endeavouring to procure subscriptions for it, but the proposal being a novelty in America, and at first not well understood, he met but with small success.[85]

272. Note of Benjamin Franklin to Sister Elizabeth

[Elizabeth Gardner was appointed Matron of the Pennsylvania Hospital on November 6, 1751, and resigned on May 14, 1760. She also acted at times as steward of the hospital.[86] The following note in Franklin's hand is in the library of the hospital.]

346

June 4, 1753

Sister Elizabeth

Please to receive the Bearer into the Hospital, & entertain him there till the Physicians have considered his Case

Your Friend & Serv[t]
B Franklin [87]

273. John F. Watson. *Annals of Philadelphia, Being a Collection of Memoirs, Anecdotes, & Incidents of the City and Its Inhabitants from the Days of the Pilgrim Founders*

[The compiler of these *Annals* was a member of the Historical Society of Pennsylvania. The account is said to have been taken from the original documents, but it differs in some respect from others. The publication date of the book was 1830.]

The earliest Hospital, separate from the Poorhouse, to which in early times it was united, was opened and continued for several years in the house known as "Judge Kinsey's dwelling and orchard,"—the same two story double front brick house now on the south side of High Street, third door west from Fifth Street. The Hospital there, nearly eighty years ago, was under the general government of Mrs. Elizabeth Gardiner as matron.

In the year 1750, several public spirited gentlemen set on foot a proposition for another and more convenient building than was before possessed for the sick at the Poor-house—then on the lot occupying the square from Spruce to Pine street, and from Third to Fourth street.

By the MS. Diary of John Smith, Esq. I see noted that on the 5th of 5 mo. 1751, he with other managers of the Hospital Fund, went out to inspect several lots for a place for an Hospital, and he states that none then pleased them so much as one on the south side of Arch street between Ninth and Tenth streets. But afterwards, on the 11th of 8 mo. 1751, he notes, that he with Dr. Bond and Israel Pemberton, inspected the late dwelling house of E. Kinsey, Esq. and were of opinion it would be a suitable place to begin the Hospital in. The year 1751, therefore marks the period at which the Hospital in High street began. It there continued ten or twelve years.

The Pennsylvania Hospital was founded in the year 1760. At the occasion of laying the corner stone, the celebrated John Key, "the first born," was present from Chester county. The inscription on the corner stone, composed by Doctor Franklin, reads thus:

"In the year of Christ
MDCCLV
George the Second happily reigning
(For he sought the happiness of his people)
Philadelphia flourishing
(For its inhabitants were public spirited)

This Building
By the bounty of Government,
And of many private Persons,
Was piously founded
For the Relief of the Sick and Miserable
May the God of Mercies
Bless the Undertaking." [88]

When the Hospital was first placed there it was deemed very far out of town, and was approached not by present rectilineal streets, but across commons the length of several squares. The only building then finished for several years was the present eastern wing, then entered by its front gate on Eighth street.

At and before the year 1740 it was the practice when sick emigrants arrived, to place them in empty houses about the city. Sometimes diseases were imparted to the neighborhood, as once occurred, particularly at Willing's Alley. On such occasions, physicians were provided for them at public expense. The Governor was induced, in 1740, to suggest the procuring of a Pesthouse or Hospital; and in 1742, a Pest Hospital was erected on Fisher's Island, called afterwards Province Island, because purchased and owned by the province, for the use of sick persons arriving from sea. [89]

274. Henry Wadsworth Longfellow. *Evangeline, A Tale of Acadie*

[The poem *Evangeline* tells the story of the forcible removal by the British in 1755 of a colony of French settlers from Nova Scotia. A young couple, on the day of their wedding, were separated and sent in different directions, losing all trace of each other. Evangeline wanders for many years in search of Gabriel, and finally discovers him, an old man on his deathbed in a public hospital in Philadelphia (the Almshouse, now the Philadelphia General Hospital), where she had been in the habit of going as a Sister of Mercy. In this, the last scene of the poem, Evangeline sees the "assiduous, careful attendants" moving about among the patients.

The Philadelphia General Hospital received its name in 1902. In 1731 the City of Philadelphia had established an "Almshouse and House of Employment" for its old and infirm poor, and in 1836, this was designated the Philadelphia Hospital and Almshouse. For a time the sick of the almshouse were cared for at the Pennsylvania Hospital. [90]

Henry Wadsworth Longfellow (1807–1882), the composer of the poem, graduated from Bowdoin College in 1825, in the class with Nathaniel Hawthorne. He taught modern languages at Harvard College, writing his own textbooks. He distinguished himself as a poet, writing *Evangeline* in 1847. Longfellow was the first American poet whose bust was placed in the Poets' Corner of Westminster Abbey. [91]]

Gabriel was not forgotten. Within her heart
　　was his image,
Clothed in the beauty of love and youth, as last
　　she beheld him,
Only more beautiful made by his deathlike
　　silence and absence.
Into her thoughts of him time entered not, for
　　it was not.
Over him years had no power; he was not
　　changed, but transfigured;
He had become to her heart as one who is dead,
　　and not absent;
Patience and abnegation of self, and devotion
　　to others,
This was the lesson a life of trial and sorrow
　　had taught her.
So was her love diffused, but, like some odor-
　　ous spices,
Suffered no waste nor loss, though filling the
　　air with aroma,
Other hope had she none, nor wish in life,
　　but to follow
Meekly, with reverent steps, the sacred feet of
　　her Saviour.
Thus many years she lived as a Sister of Mercy;
　　frequenting
Lonely and wretched roofs in the crowded lanes
　　of the city,
Where distress and want concealed themselves
　　from the sunlight,
Where disease and sorrow in garrets languished
　　neglected.
Night after night, when the world was asleep,
　　as the watchman repeated
Loud, through the gusty streets, that all was well
　　in the city,
High at some lonely window he saw the light
　　of her taper.
Day after day, in the gray of the dawn, as slow
　　through the suburbs
Plodded the German farmer, with flowers and
　　fruits for the market,
Met he that meek, pale face, returning home
　　from its watchings.
Then it came to pass that a pestilence fell
　　on the city,

Presaged by wondrous signs, and mostly by
    flocks of wild pigeons,
Darkening the sun in their flight, with naught
    in their craws but an acorn.

Only, alas! the poor, who had neither friends
    nor attendants,
Crept away to die in the almshouse, home of
    the homeless.
Then in the suburbs it stood, in the midst of
    meadows and woodlands;—
Now the city surrounds it; but still, with its
    gateway and wicket
Meek, in the midst of splendor, its humble walls
    seem to echo
Softly the words of the Lord: "The poor ye
    always have with you."
Thither, by night and by day, came the Sister
    of Mercy. The dying
Looked up into her face, and thought, indeed,
    to behold there
Gleams of celestial light encircle her forehead
    with splendor,
Such as the artist paints o'er the brows of saints
    and apostles,
Or such as hangs by night o'er a city seen at
    a distance.

Thus, on a Sabbath morn, through the
    street, deserted and silent,
Wending her quiet way, she entered the door
    of the almshouse.

Something within her said, "At length thy
    trials are ended;"
And, with light in her looks, she entered the
    chambers of sickness.
Noiselessly moved about the assiduous, careful
    attendants,
Moistening the feverish lip and the aching brows,
    and in silence
Closing the sightless eyes of the dead, and con-
    cealing their faces,
Where on their pallets they lay, like drifts of
    snow by the roadside.[92]

275. *The Statutes at Large . . . of Virginia . . .*

[In the early years of the Colony of Virginia and, after the Revolutionary War, of the Commonwealth, laws were enacted to make necessary provision for institutions for the welfare of the people. These laws were sometimes included in the acts passed for the incorporation of cities, and mentioned, among other institutions, hospitals for "infected persons," and "persons of unsound mind." They provided usually for doctors and nurses for the care of the patients in these hospitals.]

January 1764—4th George III.
An act to empower the corporation of the city of Williamsburg to assess taxes on the inhabitants thereof for the purposes therein mentioned, and for repealing a certain act of Assembly therein also mentioned.

II. *Be it therefore enacted by the Lieutenant-Governour, Council and Burgesses of this present General Assembly, and it is hereby enacted by the authority of the same,* That it shall and may be lawful for the mayor, recorder aldermen, and common-council, of the said city of Williamsburg, for the time being, in common-hall assembled, to levy and assess by the poll, on the tithable persons inhabiting within the said city, all such sums of money as shall be sufficient for defraying the charges and expenses of building a court-house, market-house, and prison, for the said city, when those now in use shall happen to fall to decay, or be otherwise destroyed, and to keep the same in repair; also for building, purchasing, or renting, one or more house or houses, to be made use of as hospitals, for the reception of any person or persons, who may be hereafter found within the said city infected with contagious distempers and for paying the charges of removing such persons to the hospital, and providing doctors, nurses, and other necessary attendants, as also guards, to prevent the spreading of such distempers . . .

November 1769—10th George III.
An act to make provision for the support and maintenance of ideots, lunatics, and other persons of unsound minds.

II. *And be it further enacted, by the authority aforesaid,* That the said court of directors be, and they are hereby impowered to purchase a piece or parcel of land, not exceeding four acres, the most healthy in situation that can be procured, and as convenient as may be to the city of Williamsburg, and to contract for the building thereon a commodious house or houses, fit for the reception and accomodation of such disordered persons as are described by this act, and to provide a proper keeper and matron of the said hospital, with necessary nurses and guards, and, as occasion may require to call in any physicians or surgeons for the assistance and relief of such poor persons . . .

May 1782—6th of the Commonwealth.
An act for incorporating the town of Richmond, and for other purposes.

II. *And be it enacted,* That they and their successors, by the name aforesaid, shall especially have power to rent, erect or repair work-houses, houses of correction, a court-house, prison, market-house, and hospitals for the reception of persons infected with contagious disorders, and other public buildings for the benefit of the said city, to pay the charge of removing such infected persons to the hospital, to provide doctors, nurses and other necessary attendants, as well as guards to prevent the spreading of such disorders . . .

October 1782—7th of the Commonwealth.
An act for further continuing and amending the act to make provision for the support and maintenance of idiots, lunatics, and persons of unsound minds . . .

II. . . . *Be it enacted,* That the treasurer . . . is hereby empowered and required to pay annually, out of the treasury, such sum or sums of money as shall be by law appropriated for the repairing the said hospital, the payment of salaries to the keeper and matrons, and also to the nurses, guards, physicians, or surgeons . . .

October 1786—11th of Commonwealth.
An act to amend the act, instituted an act to provide for the poor of the several counties within this commonwealth.

III. *Be it further enacted,* That the overseers of each district shall provide for the poor, lame, blind, and other inhabitants of the district not able to maintain themselves, and may also provide houses, nurses and doctors, in such cases as they, or a majority of them, shall think necessary; the expenses of which, if the contingent fund shall be insufficient, shall be provided for in the succeeding levy.[93]

276. Official Records of the New York Hospital

[The New York Hospital was founded in 1771 through the initial efforts of certain public-spirited physicians. The Mayor, recorder, aldermen, and assistants of the city government, the rector of Trinity Church, the ministers of several Protestant churches, the president of King's College (now Columbia University), and a number of the principal citizens of the city were named as members of the corporation.[94]]

[From the Charter of the New York Hospital, Section III.]

George the Third, by the Grace of God, of Great Britain, France, and Ireland, King, Defender of the Faith, and so forth.

To all to whom these Presents shall come Greeting:

Whereas our loving Subjects, Peter Middleton, John Jones, and Samuel Bard, of our city of New-York, physicians, by their humble petition presented unto our trusty and well-beloved Cadwallader Colden, Esq. our Lieutenant-Governor . . . of our province of New York . . . on the ninth day of March, which was in the year of our Lord one thousand seven hundred and seventy . . . set forth that there had been a subscription set forth by them . . . [for a] public hospital . . . know ye, therefore, that we, of our special grace . . . have granted [said request].

[From address of Dr. Middleton, at King's College, Nov. 3, 1769.]

The necessity and usefulness of a public infirmary, had been so warmly and pathetically set forth, in a discourse delivered by Dr. *Samuel* Bard, at the commencement, in May last, that his excellency, Sir Henry Moore, immediately set on foot a subscription for that purpose, to which himself, and most of the gentlemen present liberally contributed . . .[95]

By-Laws and Regulations;

Ordained and established by the Governors of the New-York Hospital, for the better government of the Officers, Members, Patients, and Servants of the Hospital.

Passed the 6th June, 1811.

Of the Matron

I. The matron shall visit the wards in the house and asylum, every day, and see that they are properly attended by the nurses.

II. She shall oversee all the female patients and servants, and take care that the wards, apartments, beds, clothes, linen, and other things are kept clean. All the patients, nurses and servants, must be obedient and submissive to her.

III. The female nurses must not be absent without leave of the matron.

IV. She must take care of all the household goods and furniture.

Of the Patients

V. Such patients as, in the opinion of the attending physician or surgeon, are able, shall assist in nursing others, washing and ironing the linen, washing and cleaning the rooms, and in such other services, as the superintendent or matron may require.

Of the Lying-in Ward

VI. Such patients as are able, shall assist in nursing others; in washing and cleaning rooms; and in such other services as the matron or nurses shall require.

VII. The nurse in the lying-in ward shall take the utmost care to preserve cleanliness and decency.[96]

277. *Longworth's American Almanack, New-York Register, and City Directory: For the Thirtieth Year of American Independence*

[The title of this book is self-explanatory. The volume contains reference to the New York Hospital and a list of nurses residing in New York and practicing there.[97]]

It is to the capital that individuals resort from every part of the State to seek employment in their various occupations, to improve their fortunes and to engage in pursuits more congenial to their dispositions or better adapted to their capacity. Destitute of property, depending on their daily labor for gaining a subsistence, persons of this description who are the most exposed to casualty and sickness, when attacked by disease, often become, from improvidence or misfortune, reduced to extreme indigence and distress. In this helpless condition, they must miserably perish, did they not find, in a public hospital, that prompt relief, from nourishing diet, good nursing, and the best medical assistance, which may restore them again to health, strength and usefulness. In the rapid circulation between the city and the country, and from the multiplied relations of society, every citizen in the most distant part of the state feels, in a greater or less degree, the benefits of this institution.

NURSES

——— "O, thou are tender all!
Gentle and kind, as sympathizing nature!"

Barcley, Jane	Hunt, widow Elizabeth	Tremper, Mary
Bortis, Ann	Johnson, Jemima	Vandervoort, Sarah
Buckmaster, widow S.	Lowerre, Jane	Wade, Edward
Caswell, Sarah	Lewis, Mrs.	Willer, Ann
Dunbar, widow	Mager, Mary	Wheeler, Ann
Earland, Eleanor	Neasmith, Mrs.	Wilson, Joanna
Fleming, Mrs. Blair	Rozier, widow	Worden, widow Cath.[98]
Harter, Elizabeth	Tremper, Leah	

278. The Constitutions of the Sisters of Charity

[The Constitutions of the American foundation of the Sisters of Charity of St. Vincent de Paul were formulated by the community of the Sisters and approved by Archbishop John Carroll of Baltimore on January 1, 1812. They touch upon the care of the sick in hospitals and in homes and upon the education of the young.[99]]

The object of the Institution of the Sisters of Charity in America, according to the plan laid down by St. Vincent of Paul, being to honour the sacred infancy of our Lord Jesus Christ as the source and model of all charity by rendering to Him every temporal and spiritual service in their power, in the persons of the poor, either sick, children, prisoners, or others in distress;

to honour the sacred infancy of Jesus Christ in the young persons committed to their charge, whom they are called upon to form to virtue, whilst they sow in their minds the seeds of useful knowledge;

accordingly the care of the poor of all descriptions and ages, sick, prisoners, invalids, foundlings, orphans, and even insane in hospitals, and private houses shall be the object of the solicitude of the Sisters and they will exercise their zeal gradually, as circumstances, openings and means of doing either shall be afforded them.[100]

279. Letter of Father Rosati to Father Brute

[Bishop Brute, in 1816, as President of St. Mary's College, Baltimore, had received and entertained the first members of the order of St. Vincent de Paul to land on American shores. In this group had been Father Rosati, later Bishop of Saint Louis. Bishop Rosati, remembering his old acquaintance, appealed to Bishop Brute to use his influence to obtain sisters for the hospital at St. Louis.[101]]

St. Louis, June 23, 1828.

I come to obtain through your intervention three Sisters of Charity for a Hospital in St. Louis. When I wrote to you the first time I had no certain information on which to build hopes of seeing an establishment of that kind in the city. I felt its necessity and I desired to find some means to execute that which I wished to undertake. How admirable is Providence! Without having said one word, a very rich man offers me a very beautiful piece of ground with two houses in the city of St. Louis. He will give besides another lot with other houses that will bring a revenue of six hundred dollars a year. He will give one hundred and fifty dollars for the journey of the Sisters, three hundred and fifty to furnish the house. But, he will not leave it in the hands of mercenaries, if we do not get the Sisters of Emmitsburg this establishment will fail.

Perry County, Missouri.   ✜ Joseph, Bishop, of St. Louis &
Speak, pray, exhort, etc.   Administrator of New
                                       Orleans [102]

280. Pastor Muhlenberg's Report of 1871

[Pastor Muhlenberg founded the Sisterhood of the Holy Communion in New York in 1845. This was the year in which the Park Village Community began, and before the establishment of Miss Sellon's sisterhood, which came into existence in 1848. The Sisterhood of the Holy Communion was the beginning from which came the nursing in St. Luke's Hospital in New York.[103] In the following quotation from Pastor Muhlenberg's Report of 1871, he tells of the founding of the sisterhood and the hospital.]

On St. Luke's Day, 1846, the want of a church hospital in this city was laid before the congregation of the Church of the Holy Communion ...

Before this, however, much thought had been given to the plan and practical working of the projected institution. In order that it might have a genuine Christian character, it was felt that its beneficiaries must be chiefly in the care of volunteers of charity, and they, Christian women, waiting upon the sick and needy for the lord's sake.... Why could we not have ... Sisters here, and in our *own* church?

... The question was presented to an earnest Christian woman, who alone of all my acquaintances was likely to listen to it with any thought of acting upon it. The result ... was the devotion of a life to the voluntary ministrations of Christian love, especially among the poor.... This single volunteer, in the course of a twelvemonth or more, was joined by two others as probationers, and thus there was the germ of a community ...

      .   .   .   .   .   .

During this and several succeeding years the Sisters, though few in number, were actively engaged in carrying on the church school and in the care of the poor and sick of the parish, to which, after a time, they felt they might add the inception of that special work to which they longingly looked forward. They entered upon it in two apartments of a rear building in Sixth Avenue, near the church, whence, before long, they had the pleasure of transferring their patients to a commodious house on the Avenue, fitted up for them with seventeen beds, and designated "The Infirmary of the Church of the Holy Communion." ... This was the infant St. Luke's ...[104]

281. Principles and Rules of the Sisterhood of the Holy Communion

[These rules were in effect in 1873, and it is assumed that they resemble closely those of the original group. They are found transcribed in the book, *Sisterhoods and Deaconesses at Home and Abroad,* by Bishop Henry Codman Potter (1835–1908), appointed Protestant Episcopal Bishop of New York in 1887.[105]]

I. From the Principles of Association.

The members of the Community are of two classes, United Sisters and Probationers.

The United Sisters are those who, after a satisfactory probation, are elected full members of the society.

The Probationary Sisters are those under training for full membership and are not ordinarily under twenty-one nor over forty years of age.

The vote of the United Sisters is necessary for full membership.

The probationary term is never less than six months, and may be prolonged at discretion.

The services of the Sisters are gratuitous, but they have their board and lodging free of expense.

The term of engagement for a United Sister is three years, renewable, if desired, at the expiration of the same, by the vote of the other Sisters, as at first.

The government of the Community devolves upon one of the United Sisters, known as the First Sister, to whom the others are expected to yield a cheerful obedience in all things pertaining to the ordering of the Community and the work given it to do.

II. From the Rules.

The Sisters are required to conform exactly to the appointed order of the day.

They dress alike, and as plainly and inexpensively as possible ...

The Sisters have daily an allotted time for recreation, and during the summer months a vacation each of four weeks ...[106]

282. G. H. Gerberding. *Life and Letters of W. A. Passavant, D.D.*

[William Alfred Passavant (1821–1894), writer and Lutheran pastor of Pittsburgh, was born in Pennsylvania. The Passavant line in Germany is said to have reached back to 1200. Pastor Passavant was called, in 1844, to take charge of the organization in Pittsburgh known as the "First English Evangelical Lutheran Church." In 1846 he visited Kaiserswerth, after which arrangements were made for the establishment of a branch of the Kaiserswerth Institution in Pittsburgh. In 1849 Pastor

Fliedner himself accompanied four deaconesses to Pittsburgh, and the institution was opened.[107]]

London, Oct. 18th, 1846,
Sunday morning.

Dear brethren and sisters,—

Having visited Kaiserswerth on the Rhine, where the first Protestant institution of this kind was commenced from which all others are copied, both in Germany, Holland, France and Prussia, I shall on my return give myself the pleasure of giving the brethren an opportunity of learning more of this wonderful institution. In my whole course of observation, I saw nothing anywhere which so commends itself to the better feeling of the heart as the order just referred to.

They [the deaconesses] make no vows for life, but can return to their friends if so disposed. And yet very few ever use this privilege, but live and die in the service.

[From *The Missionary,* April, 1848, by Pastor Passavant.]

It was, after having studied the practical working of this office of the Hospitals, Insane, Orphan, and other Asylums of Prussia, France and Germany and elsewhere, seeing the humanizing and Christianizing influence of these Christian women in the different fields of human suffering, that arrangements were entered into with the Director of the Parent Institution of Kaiserswerth, for the establishment of a Branch in the United States. For various reasons, Pittsburgh was selected as the best location for the American Institution, and should no intervening Providence delay their coming, four deaconesses are expected to arrive in New York in the month of June. They will work by the rules of the Parent House in Prussia, and for the present will remain in connection with it. Should the way be opened in the future, it is understood that every encouragement will be given by the Parent Establishment to the organization of an Institution, entirely independent of foreign connection. In the meantime, however, ladies of suitable character and qualifications, who wish to devote themselves to the work of mercy and charity, will be received as inmates of the Institution, according to the rules of Parent House.

[From Pastor Passavant's Report of 1849.]

The arrival of Rev. Theodore Fliedner from Prussia, on the fourteenth of July, accompanied by four deaconesses from the Parent Institution in

Kaiserswerth on the Rhine, seemed to indicate Sunday the seventeenth, as the most suitable time for consecrating it [the new institution] to the service of God, and to the merciful purpose for which it was designed.

. . . . . .

Rev. Fliedner addressed the congregation in German, explaining the design of the Institution as an Infirmary for the sick, and a Mother-house for the training of Christian Deaconesses for hospitals, asylums and congregations in other parts of the United States.

. . . . . .

[From Report, dated 1850, by Pastor Passavant.]

In consequence of many and unforseen difficulties the house was not opened for patients until January, 1849. . . . The general public knew next to nothing of its existence at first; no one applied for admission, and a whole month elapsed before a single patient was admitted.

[By the editor of the letters.]

The Mexican War had just come to an end. A boat load of discharged soldiers was brought up the river and landed in Pittsburg. . . . Mr. Passavant of course knew of their coming . . . he went down and searched the bunks of the boat. He found two poor, neglected, sick soldiers, suffering from ship-fever. A carriage was procured to convey them to the empty hospital. But the building was not yet ready for patients. The reception room was furnished and ready. The kitchen had a cookstove and a table. One nurse's room had been fitted up. The sick rooms had one bed and several chairs. Several cots and bedding were hastily ordered from the store, and so the patients, the embryo outfit and the two men, started for the empty house on the other side of the two cities.

The sick soldiers, after their long journey in the crowded and stuffy boat, were badly in need of a bath. But the only nurses present were Mr. Passavant and Mr. Waters [friend, helper, and student]. Each of these inexperienced hands took a dirty soldier, washed him from head to foot, put on a clean bed robe and put him into a clean bed. The poor sick men gratefully recognized the work done for them and in a few weeks were discharged well and happy.

. . . . . .

[From *The Missionary,* June, 1853, by Pastor Passavant.]

Hitherto the principal labor of the Sisters had been the care and relief of the sick. For this purpose a hospital has been established, grounds purchased and the building erected, which offer every accomodation, comfort and facility in the treatment of the suffering. There are forty beds in the Infirmary, though the number of sick is generally from twenty-five to thirty . . .

In addition to the above about forty have been nursed by the Sisters in their own homes in this vicinity and other places, principally in the cases of cholera or other contagious and dangerous diseases . . .

. . . .

[From Pastor Passavant's Report of 1854, during the cholera epidemic.]

Our dear Sisters were indefatigable in their labors of love, and although at times almost prostrated by the exertions and watching of this time, they were yet wonderfully sustained by the grace of God and the blessing of those who were ready to perish. In the language of one of the city papers: "They labored night and day, when hired nurses could not be obtained, and performed the most disgusting offices for the poor sick under their charge with the greatest readiness and cheerful pleasure.[108]

283. *Harper's Weekly*, Saturday, June 6, 1857, p. 353

[This article, entitled "Two Noble Women," [109] states that Annie M. Andrews was the daughter of a physician of New York, then residing in New Orleans. His daughter, reared by her aunt, early showed an aptitude for nursing. The experience described occurred during a yellow fever outbreak in Norfolk, Virginia.]

. . . When the fever at Norfolk broke out, she was living with her uncle, Judge Hall, of Syracuse, New York; she instantly announced her desire to go and offer her services as nurse. The need of nurses was so pressing, it will be remembered, that the most enormous prices were paid for very sorry attendants: still, the danger was so obvious that Miss Andrews' relations were much opposed to the scheme. By much entreaty she prevailed on them to allow her to write to the Mayor of Norfolk, tendering her services; they consented—mainly from the persuasion that the Mayor would decline the offer.

He, like a prudent man, neither declined nor accepted. He stated the pressing want of nurses, and described the terrible suffering of the people, but gave no opinion on Miss Andrews' application. His description of the destitution of the poor sufferers was enough for her; she stipulated that she was to pay her own expenses, and departed alone. For two days and nights she traveled alone by rail. On approaching Norfolk she met three Sisters of Charity, bent on the same errand as herself; in their company she reported herself to the Mayor, and received permission to serve as a nurse. It was late in the evening when this formality was fulfilled; the Sisters of Charity, with professional experience, prudently retired for the night; Miss Andrews went directly to the hospital, and waited on the sick that night.

Previous to the outbreak of fever, Norfolk had no hospital; an old race-stand was temporarily converted into an infirmary and baptized the Julappi Hospital. It was a miserable building; through the roof the rain poured in bad weather; every moment Miss Andrews could steal from her duties as nurse was devoted to calking the seams in the building . . .

Those who have had experience of a yellow fever hospital can alone appreciate the danger and the discomfort of Miss Andrews' position. . . . Miss Andrews shrank from no trial of the kind. Many and many a poor sufferer, in his last delirious moments, was recalled to consciousness by feeling her cool hand on his fevered forehead, and by hearing gentle words of a future life uttered in her kind voice.

The patients, as we all know, far outnumbered the capacity of the hospital; the nurses were far too few . . .

Even death did not limit the cares which her self-imposed mission devolved upon Miss Andrews. When patients died of yellow fever, it was almost impossible to find persons to lay them out for burial; this also fell to her lot, and when the number of corpses made it necessary for her to hire assistance, she paid for the services of a negro out of her own funds.

It only remains to say that the Howard Association of Norfolk, grateful as well for the eminent services of Miss Andrews as for the noble example she set, have presented her with the gold medal usually awarded to physicians . . .

CONCLUDING STATEMENT

Contemporaneously with the events of the end of the Middle Ages and the centuries following in the Old World, came the exploration and development of the lands of the Western Hemisphere. It is assumed that the primitive peoples of the New World cared for their sick and wounded according to their customs and mores, as did those of the Old World. When the first explorers arrived on western shores, they brought with them their group habits, including those of caring for the sick.

The last will and testament of Cortes, the conquerer of Mexico, indicates the founding, in the sixteenth century, of the first hospital in the Western Hemisphere, which is still in existence at the present day. The Spanish later established regulations for all royal hospitals under their control in Cuba, and it is assumed that these regulations applied eventually to all royal Spanish hospitals. In these regulations mention is made of nurses and nursing.

In the north the French, in colonizing lower Canada, utilized the services of religious groups, as is narrated in *The Jesuit Relations and Allied Documents,* which tell of the establishment of hospitals in Montreal and Quebec in the seventeenth century, and of the kind and considerate nursing by the sisters of the religious orders. The earliest historian of Montreal, François Dollier de Casson, and travelers of later days corroborate these facts.

The writings of the early Pilgrims in Massachusetts lead us to believe

that the colonists cared for each other in their homes in the early epidemics which visited them. The records of the Moravians in North
Carolina in the early eighteenth century are among the few of the migrating groups which are specific concerning how the sick were to be
provided with nursing care. In this case, members of the congregation,
both men and women, were appointed for the purpose.

In the writings of early physicians such as Benjamin Rush and others,
there are inklings of the attitudes of physicians about the characteristics
of nurses and of the importance of the nurse in the recovery of the patient. It is apparent that some of the nurses possessed practical skill and
knowledge which rendered them useful for this occupation. Physicians
also suggested remedies for the lack of qualified nurses, among which
was the proposal that they be trained as in England, in "cottages" accom-
modating two or three maternity patients, under the supervision of ob-
stetricians, who would give lectures and demonstrations, and finally issue
certificates or diplomas to the nurses, setting forth their qualifications.
The early city directories indicate that many nurses were widows acting
in the role of "monthly nurses." An official report of an epidemic of
yellow fever in Baltimore indicates the use of nurses in that disaster.

The official records of the early colonies disclose the necessity of providing hospitals for persons suffering from smallpox and from mental
disease. The earliest institution caring for the sick, founded in what is
now the United States, was that in New Amsterdam, the forerunner of
Bellevue Hospital, which came about partly at the suggestion of the
surgeon of the Dutch West India Company.

Among other early hospitals were the Charity Hospital of New Or-
leans, the Philadelphia Almshouse, and the Pennsylvania Hospital in
Philadelphia. Many documents tell of the founding of these hospitals.
The New York Hospital, established twenty years after the Pennsylvania
Hospital, provided the citizens of New York City with additional facili-
ties.

Religious groups early played an important part in supplying nurses
for the sick, as is shown in existing documents. Among the earliest were
the Sisters of Charity, founded by Mother Seton in Emmitsburg, Maryland, the statement of the objects of which refer to the nursing of the
sick; the Episcopal Sisterhood of the Holy Communion, established by
Pastor Muhlenberg, told in an early report by the pastor himself; and
the Lutheran deaconesses, founded by Pastor Passavant of Pittsburgh,
in the English Lutheran Church, through the assistance of Pastor Fliedner, described by Pastor Passavant's letters and periodical articles.

An enlightening and interesting chapter in the early nursing history of
the United States is that concerned with the care of the sick and wounded

in wartime. The study of this phase leads to the belief that in the French and Indian Wars, the sick were nursed by families and individuals residing in the areas where the battles were being fought, and in some instances, in hospitals, where these existed. In the early part of the Revolutionary War the American Congress made plans for a system of army hospitals, with necessary personnel, including women nurses. The Civil War was characterized on both sides by the provision of nurses for the care of the sick and wounded.

The documentation of early war nursing in this country adds to our understanding of this phase of nursing history. Some of the sources have been selected for presentation in the next and final chapter.

Chapter 9

Selected Documents of Early War Nursing in the United States

INTRODUCTION

THE care of the sick in wartime is perhaps the most dramatic of all aspects of nursing history, furnishing it with many highlights. Examples of this occurred in the Crusades of the Middle Ages and in the work of Florence Nightingale in the Crimean War during the nineteenth century, to mention but two instances. In the early wars in which the United States of America participated, there are many cases of nursing care given to the sick and wounded.

Of the many wars in which the United States has taken part, not all yield readily to the search for information concerning nursing care. In the beginning of the colonization of the continent, wars occurred with the Indians. During the conflict among certain European powers for control of the colonies, as between the English and the Dutch for control of New York, and in the struggles of European nations such as France and Spain for control of Florida, the Carolinas, and Georgia, wars on a small scale were fought in the territory which now is part of the United States.

The French and Indian Wars (Seven Years' War), from 1754 to 1763, involved not only Canada but parts of what is now the United States. Then came the American War of the Revolution and the War of 1812, which again involved Canada and the Indians as well as the early colonists. The War with Mexico for California, from 1846 to 1848, and finally the great struggle between the North and the South from 1861 to 1865, complete a partial list of wars fought in the period with which this book is concerned and about which information would be valuable for the study of nursing history.

The question with which this chapter is concerned relates to the nursing care of the sick and wounded in some of these wars. With reference to the very earliest struggles, it is impossible to answer the query with any certainty or accuracy. It is assumed that in these first wars the sol-

364

diers cared for each other, and that families in the neighborhood nursed the soldiers brought to them and, in some instances, went out on the field of battle to rescue them. In the French and Indian Wars, this is indicated by the bills rendered for care given. In these wars also, the sick and wounded were sometimes taken to hospitals in the vicinity, as for example, the soldiers mentioned by Captain John Knox, an officer in the Forty-third Regiment, as having been cared for in the General Hospital in Quebec.[1] In the Revolutionary War, bills were rendered to the American Congress for care given to soldiers in private houses, and the Congress also made provision for military hospitals to be connected with the Army. Nurses were mentioned, both men (soldiers) and women. In the Civil War, measures were early taken by the United States Sanitary Commission to establish hospitals, provide nurses, and appoint a superintendent of nurses. Similar conditions did not exist in the South, but thousands of women volunteered to care for the sick and wounded in hospitals.

In this chapter examples will be drawn from the literature illustrating the nursing in the French and Indian Wars, the Revolutionary War, and the Civil War.

In the French and Indian Wars the chief documentary evidences of nursing presented here are the bills for nursing service, rendered by various individuals. The Massachusetts phase of the war yielded a number of such bills (284).

At the time of the Revolutionary War, definite steps were recommended and carried out to provide hospital care for the soldiers. *The Journals of the American Congress from 1774 to 1788* outline the organization of the Medical Department of the Army, and in addition note payment to individual nurses who rendered service to the sick and wounded (285). William Shippen, Jr., who was appointed director general of the military hospitals, recommended the organization of his department and provided, in his plans, for nursing care (286). From among the writings of General George Washington, references to nursing care are included as follows: *Official Letters to the Honorable American Congress . . . ,* 1776, in which he urges the employment of women nurses and an increase in their pay (287), and his *Orderly Book,* in which a notation directs commanding officers of regiments to assist regimental surgeons in procuring women nurses (288). The state papers of certain states also record payment to individuals who nursed soldiers. Some of those from the "Journal of the Committee of Safety of Virginia" are given here (289).

Two personal accounts touching on the nursing in the Revolutionary War are included. One is from the journal of Mary Slocumb, whose husband was a lieutenant in the American Army (290), and the other is from the *Letters and Memoirs Relating to the War of American Independence, and the Capture of the German Troops at Saratoga,* by Madame de Riedesel, wife of the commander of the Brunswick forces in the British Army (291).

The war between the North and the South produced almost innumerable documents of various kinds in which nursing is described. From among the many, a selection has been made representing both Northern and Southern nursing. From the group of official or semiofficial documents: a petition to the Secretary of War urging the formation of a sanitary commission (292); Henry Whitney Bellows, *Report Concerning the Woman's Central Association of Relief at New York to the U.S. Sanitary Commission at Washington* (293); and various other excerpts from the collected documents of the Sanitary Commission. Included are: *Report of the Committee Appointed on the 29th inst. to Visit the Military General Hospitals In and Around Washington* (294); J. G. Forman, *The Western Sanitary Commission* (295); Dr. John Strong Newberry, *The United States Sanitary Commission in the Valley of the Mississippi during the War of the Rebellion, 1861–1866* (296), and *A Visit to Fort Donelson, Tenn. for the Relief of the Wounded of Feb'y 15, 1862: a Letter* (297); and *Hospital Transports . . . ,* compiled by Frederick Law Olmsted (298).

References from two periodicals are also reproduced—from the *American Medical Times* for July 18, 1861 (299), which discusses the controversial question of women nurses in the war hospitals, and from *The Medical and Surgical Reporter,* November 8, 1862, and September 10, 1864 (300, 301), dealing with the requirements and payment of women nurses.

In the group of letters and memoirs, the following have been chosen: *Letters of a Family during the War for the Union 1861–1865* (302); Jane Stuart Woolsey, *Hospital Days* (303); and Katherine Prescott Wormeley, *The Cruel Side of the War, With the Army of the Potomac* (304). From the writings of Louisa May Alcott, two are reproduced here: *Life, Letters and Journals of Louisa May Alcott* (305), and *Hospital Sketches and Companion Fireside Stories* (306), the latter written for children. Jane Grey Swisshelm, the pioneer woman journalist, wrote for publication a number of articles on the war (307) and later gathered together some of her experiences in an autobiography, *Half a Century,* in which she refers to her nursing activities (308). *South After Gettysburg Letters of Cornelia Hancock from the Army of the Potomac 1863–1865* (309) narrates her activities as a nurse during the period indicated.

Mary Livermore's *My Story of the War: A Woman's Narrative of Four Years' Personal Experience* is the account of another newspaperwoman (310). The point of view of one Army surgeon concerning women nurses is found in *Personal Memoirs of John H. Brinton, Major and Surgeon, U.S.V., 1861–1865* (311). The writings of Walt Whitman on the war are represented in this chapter by the following: articles which appeared in the *New York Leader* (312), *Specimen Days and Collect* (313), and brief excerpts from two articles published in the *New York Times* (314). The correspondence of Pastor Passavant refers to the nursing by the deaconesses of Pittsburgh (315), while the diary of Sister Anthony O'Connell (316) and a letter to the *Baltimore Catholic Mirror* for February 25, 1862 (317), refer to the work of the Sisters of Charity of Cincinnati. The point of view of a patient, a colonel, concerning the effect of the care which he received from his nurse is briefly told in his diary (318).

Six accounts of nursing by women of the South are included: Kate Cumming, *A Journal of Hospital Life in the Confederate Army of Tennessee from the Battle of Shiloh to the End of the War* (319); Susan Leigh Blackford, *Letters from Lee's Army* (320); a brief extract from *Diary of a Southern Refugee During the War,* the diary of Judith Brockenbrough McGuire (321); a short letter from the pen of Ella Newsome Trader (322); a letter from Louise Wigfall Wright, the daughter of a Southern senator, in *A Southern Girl in '61* (323); and, finally, an account by a North Carolina woman, Annie K. Kyle, a nurse in a hospital at Fayetteville (324).

THE SOURCES

French and Indian Wars

[The "French and Indian Wars" is the name given by American historians to the North American colonial wars which took place from 1754 to 1763 between Great Britain and France. They were, in reality, campaigns in the world-wide struggle for empire, and were roughly linked to European wars. The American phase involved Massachusetts, Ohio, Virginia, New York, Pennsylvania, and other eastern states, and southern Canada.[2] The following quotations are bills rendered for the nursing of soldiers in the Massachusetts phase of the wars.]

284. Bills Rendered for Nursing Soldiers in Deerfield, Massachusetts

#1   Province of the Massachusetts Bay Debtor to William Arms for Extraordinary Charges of Bedding, firing candles, tendance & c for Ezekiell Wells Whilst Sick and Wounded at his house from Nov 6, to January 17, 10 weeks and 2 days at 10s per week

       N T £5 0 0

       HAMPSHEAR SS DEERFIELD March 27 1748-9 William Arms appeared and made oath to the truth of the above account and that he had not received any reward for the same before me

                         Thos Wells Just peace

Deerfield March 27 1749 Alow^d by the Com^r

#2   Province of the   }   to Samuel Bardwell of
Massachusetts Bay {   Deerfield D^r 1749

To Nursing & Attendance of Sam'l Trumble one of Cap't Phinehas Stevens's men In his Long & very Grevious Sickness from Apr'l ye 8th to August 30th Twenty Weeks & Four Days at 1s pr Day   £ 7   4   0

		£	s	d
To Twenty one pounds of Butter	@ 15 per lb	1	1	0
To Twenty Six pounds of Suger	@ 1s 3d per lb	1	12	0
To Six pounds of Candles	@ 1s 2d		7	0
To Fire Wood 30s		1	10	0
To Damage Done my Beding 30s		1	10	0
		£13	4	6

The above acct Is Justly Charged Excepted by me

                 Samuel Bardwell

        Hampsh^r Sc^t 3 Nov: 25th 1749

Mr. Sam^ll Bardwell made oath That the abov Acct Is a Just & True Acct: & That he has Never Received any Consideration of the Province or any other theirfor

           before me Thos Wells

               Just Peace

Read and alow^d by ye Com^tee
to be p^d Col Hinsdal

       J Osborne

#3   Deerfield Nov 5th 1748

Province of the Massachusetts Bay to Sarah Wells Dr

	£	s	d
To Nursing & Attendance Jonathan Stone whilst Sick & In the Province Service *vizt* 3 Weeks at 7s 6d pr week	1	2	6
To Sundry Necessaries *vizt* Sugar 1 lb 2s 6d 2s Butter 1 lb 2s Wood ¼ load 12s 6d		19	
Damage done Bed & Beding 5s		5	
	£ 2	6	6

Aug 30 1749 To Nursing & Attendance on Samuel Trumble
whilst Sick *vizt* Six Weeks at 7s 6d per week 2 5
To Sundry Necessaries *vizt* Candles lb 1 2s
  Sugar lb iv 5s Butter
  & Lard lb 12 12s Wood ⅔ of Load 7s 6d 1 6 6
Damage done Bed & Beding 10s 10

4 1 6
Brot Down 2 6 6
N. Tenor 6 8

L. M. 3 8 3

True amt Error Excepted   Sarah Wells
      Hampshire SS DEERFIELD Mar. 12, 1749
Then Sarah Wells Subscriber to yᵉ above Amt personally appear
ing made Solemn oath to yᵉ Truth of the Same & that she had recᵈ
no Consideration for any Part thereof
Alowᵈ by the Comᵗᵉᵉ   J Osborne   Comᵐ Wm Williams
                                           Justˢ Paceᵉ [4]

#4   Deerfield
     Novᵉʳ   Province of yᵉ Massechusetts Bay to David Field Dr
     1755   To Nursing Peter Ledue a Soldier in
                   Col Ephraim Williams Reigment four
                   weaks & 4 days when sick   £   0   10   0
                   for Slops Shuger & Rhum   1   5   0
                   to feuel Candles bed & necesarys ⎱
                   for watchers ─────────────⎰ 0   16   6

                     a true account Error Excepted £ 2   11   6
Hampshire Sc   David Field
   Janʸ 3ʳᵈ 1756 Then Mʳ David Field made oath to the Truth
                 of yᵉ above acᵗ. Corᵐ Elijʰ Williams Jusᵒ Pacˢ.
                 David Fields
                   Account
                 Committed
                 Warrant Advised
                 March 3-1756
                     2. 11. 6

                           Alowᵈ p the Comᵗⁱᵉ £
                             2-11-6 [5]

Revolutionary War

285. *Journals of the American Congress from 1774 to 1788*

[The *Journals* of the Congress in this period refer to the organization
of the Medical Department of the Army and to payment to individuals

for nursing sick and wounded soldiers. The latter notations occur with great frequency in 1776, and less often in 1777. It will be noted that both men and women did the nursing.]

July 27, 1775.

The Congress took into consideration the report of the Committee on establishing a hospital, and the same being debated, was agreed to as follows:

That for the establishment of an hospital for an army, consisting of twenty thousand men, the following officers and other attendants be appointed, with the following allowance or pay, viz.:

One director general and chief physician, his pay per day four dollars.

Four surgeons, ditto, one and one third of a dollar.

One apothecary, ditto, one and one third of a dollar.

Twenty surgeons' mates, each, ditto, two thirds of a dollar.

One clerk, ditto, two thirds of a dollar.

Two store-keepers, each four dollars a month.

One nurse to every ten sick, one fifteenth of a dollar per day, or two dollars per month.

The duty of the above officers,

The director to furnish medicines, bedding and all other necessaries, to pay for the same, superintend the whole and make his report to, and receive orders from the commander in chief.

Surgeons, apothe- ⎱ To visit and attend the sick, the mates to obey
cary and mates ⎰ the orders of the physicians, surgeons and apothecary.

Matron. To superintend the nurses, bedding, & c.

Nurses. To attend the sick, and obey the matron's orders.

Clerks. To keep accounts for the director and store-keepers.

Store-keeper. To receive and deliver the bedding and other necessaries by order of the director.

The Congress then proceeded to the election of officers for the Hospital. . . .

Resolved, . . .

That one clerk, two store-keepers, and one nurse to every ten sick, be appointed by the director.

Wednesday, Apr. 24, 1776.

To Margaret Smith, for nursing two men in the small pox, belonging to Captain Benezet's company, the sum of 24 dollars.

Saturday, May 11, 1776.

To Walter Drummond, for nursing several persons belonging to Captain Benezet's company, the sum of 27 dollars.

Wednesday, June 19, 1776.

To Mary Thomas, for nursing and boarding two of captain Benezet's men in the small-pox, the sum of 12 dollars.

Thursday, June 20, 1776.

To Abraham Mills, for nursing and boarding six soldiers in the smallpox, the sum of 33 86-90 dollars.

Thursday, June 27, 1776.

To Elizabeth Slaydon, the sum of 24 dollars, for nursing and boarding two soldiers, of which sum Steward is to be charged with 13 3-60 dollars, for nursing and boarding the man he wounded in the state-house yard; the remainder to the continent; the said 24 dollars to be paid to colonel T. Matlack:

Saturday, July 20, 1776.

That there is due to Michael Brecht, for provisions and attendance of sick soldiers at Reading, the sum of 17 42-90 dollars:

Thursday, July 25, 1776.

To Elizabeth Slaving, for boarding and nursing a sick soldier, 4 dollars:

Thursday, September 26, 1776.

To John Shultz, for boarding and lodging sundry continental troops, 201 60-90 dollars; and for boarding and nursing sundry sick troops, 29 40-90 dollars, both sums making 231 19-90 dollars:

Wednesday, October 9, 1776.

That each of the hospitals be supplied by the respective directors with such a number of surgeons, apothecaries, surgeons' mates, and other assistants, and also such quantities of medicines, bedding, and other necessaries as they shall judge expedient:

That the wages of nurses be augmented to one dollar a week.

Wednesday, November 13, 1776.

That there should be paid to the Pennsylvania hospital, for the support and clothing of J. Hughes, a wounded soldier, 36.54 dollars:

Friday, November 15, 1776.

To Dr. Nicholas Way, for medicine, attendance, lodging, nursing, & c. of sick soldiers of the 5th and 6th Virginia regiments, 467 36 dollars.

.   .   .   .   •   .   .

Thursday, February 13, 1777.

To Jacob Myers, for entertaining the Virginia Light-horse, on their march to join general Washington, and for wagonage, his extraordinary expenses and trouble, and taking care of the sick, 439.75 dollars.

.   .   .   .   .   .

March 29, 1777.

Resolved, . . .

That a matron be allowed for every hundred sick or wounded, who shall take care that the provisions are properly prepared; that the wards, beds, and utensils be kept in neat order, and that the most exact economy be observed in her department:

That a nurse be allowed for every ten sick or wounded, who shall be under the direction of the matron: . . .

That each physician and surgeon-general of the armies, shall appoint such a number of surgeons, nurses, and orderly men, as the director or deputy-director-general shall judge necessary for the more effectual care and relief of the sick and wounded . . .[6]

286. William Shippen's Plan for Organization of the Military Hospital

[William Shippen, Jr. (1736–1808) received his medical degree from Edinburgh University in 1761. His father, also a physician, was a member of the Continental Congress. The son, in his medical work, utilized the dissection of the human body, and thus aroused great animosity. He gave courses to medical men and to women who intended to practice midwifery. He was appointed to the staff of the Pennsylvania Hospital, and was one of the founders of the College of Physicians of Philadelphia, which became the medical school of the University of Pennsylvania. In 1791 he was appointed to the chair of anatomy, surgery, and midwifery.[7] The *Journals* of the Congress for Friday, April 11, 1777, record his appointment as the director general of all military hospitals of the army.[8] In that year he submitted a plan to Congress for the organization of the hospitals. It is written out in Shippen's own handwriting, and was transmitted to Congress on February 14, 1777.[9]]

Three Districts Northern, middle and Southern.

To each one . . .

A Matron to every 100 sick who shall see the provisions are properly prepared, the Wards, Beds, & Utensils shall be kept in neat order, & that ye greatest Oconomy be observed in her department. A nurse to every 15 Sick at the direction of ye Matron . . .[10]

. . . . . .

For the Flying Hospital
There shall be a director and Surgeon Genl. whose Duty in subordination to ye Dir. Genl. shall be to superintend & receive from him a suitable number of large strong Tents—Beds, Bedd[ing,] Medicine, & Hospital Stores for such sick & wounded persons as cant be transported to ye general Hospital. . . .
He shall have under him . . .
A suitable number of mates to dress, & of Nurses and orderly men ye number to be determined and they appointed and paid by ye Dir.
All the above officers to be appointed & recieve [sic] such Salarys as the Congress shall please to direct.[11]

287. *Official Letters to the Honorable American Congress . . .*

[Among matters which caused concern to George Washington as Commander-in-Chief of the Continental Army was the welfare of sick soldiers. He refers to this in various writings, among which are his letters to Congress, and his *Orderly Book*. His *Official Letters* to the Congress were published from the original papers preserved in the Office of the Secretary of State in Philadelphia when Washington was President of the United States.[12]]

Headquarters, New York,
Sept. 14, 1776.

Sir,
I have been duly honored with your favor of the tenth, with the resolution of Congress which accompanied it, and thank them for the confidence they repose in my judgment respecting the evacuation of the city.

. . . .

Before I conclude, I would beg leave to mention to Congress, that the pay now allowed to nurses for their attendance on the sick is by no means adequate to their service; the consequence of which is, that they are extremely difficult to procure: indeed they are not to be got; and we are under the necessity of substituting in their place a number of men from the respective regiments, whose service by that means is entirely lost in the proper line of their duty, and but little benefit rendered to the sick. The officers I have talked with upon the subject all agree that they should be allowed a dollar per week, and that for less they cannot be had.
Our sick are extremely numerous, and we find their removal attended

with the greatest difficulty. It is a matter that employs much of our time and care; and what makes it more distressing is the want of proper and convenient places for their reception. I fear their sufferings will be great and many. However, nothing on my part, that humanity or policy can require, shall be wanting to make them comfortable, so far as the state of things will admit of.

I have the honor to be, & c.

G. W.[13]

288. *Orderly Book of General George Washington ...*

[The original of the *Orderly Book* is in the Boston Athenaeum. The handwriting is for the most part that of Major Samuel Shaw.[14]]

31 [May, 1778] ...

Commanding Officers of Regiments will assist the Regimental Surgeons in procuring as many women of the Army as can be prevailed on to serve as nurses to them, for which they will be paid the usual price ...[15]

289. "Journal of the Committee of Safety of Virginia"

[Committees of safety in the various colonies were formed on the recommendation of the Second Continental Congress on July 18, 1775, to carry on the all-important functions of government and to augment the work of the Revolutionary Committees of Correspondence. The latter were organized as part of the transitory Revolutionary machinery to facilitate the spread of propaganda and to coordinate the patriot party. In the "Journal of the Committee of Safety of Virginia" are found a number of references to payment to individuals for the care of sick and wounded soldiers.[16]]

Thursday, *15th February, 1776.*
Ord., a warrant to Sarah Spotswood for £2.10.0 for nursing sick soldiers.

Tuesday, *April 30th, 1776.*
Same [a warrant] to Sally Spotswood for £1.00.0 for nursing two Gent. of the Culpepper minute batt'n.

Monday, *June 3d, 1776.*
A warrant to Gab. Galt for £5.4.0 for nursing and attend'e, prov's, &c., to two sick soldiers of Capt. Patteson's comp.; and for use of John McKeand £3.16.3 for Linen furnished the prisoners at Richmond.

Monday, *June 10th, 1776.*

Same [warrant] to John Mayo, Esq'r, for use Anto. Christian for 22s for nursing sick soldier of Patterson's comp. 6th Reg't.

.   .   .   .

Friday, *June 28th, 1776.*

Same [warrant] to Mrs. Cooley for £12.10.0 for attendance of herself and negro as nurse to 1st Regiment.[17]

290. The Journal of Mary Slocumb

[Mary Slocumb was the wife of Lieutenant Slocumb of the American Army on whose plantation in Carolina Colonel Banastre Tarleton and his British forces encamped during the invasion of that area by Lord Cornwallis in 1780.[18]]

A few yards from the road, under a cluster of trees were lying perhaps twenty men. They were the wounded. I knew the spot; the very trees; and the position of the men I knew as if I had seen it a thousand times. I saw it all at once; but in an instant my whole soul was centered in one spot, for there, wrapped in his bloody guard-cloak, was my husband's body! How I passed the few yards from my saddle to the place I never knew. I remember uncovering his head and seeing a face clothed with gore from a dreadful wound across the temple. I put my hand on the bloody face; 'twas warm; and an *unknown* voice begged for water. A small camp-kettle was lying near, and a stream of water was close by. I brought it; poured some in his mouth; washed his face; and behold—it was Frank Cogdell. He soon revived and could speak. I was washing the wound in his head. Said he, "It is not that; it is that hole in my leg that is killing me." A puddle of blood was standing on the ground about his feet. I took his knife, cut away his trousers and stocking, and found the blood came from a shot-hole through and through the fleshy part of his leg. I looked about and could see nothing that looked as if it would do for dressing wounds but some heart-leaves. I gathered a handful and wound them tight to the holes; and the bleeding stopped. I then went to the others; and—Doctor! I dressed the wounds of many a brave fellow who did good fighting long after that day! . . .[19]

291. Madame de Riedesel. *Letters and Memoirs Relating to the War of American Independence, and the Capture of the German Troops at Saratoga*

[The Baroness Frederica de Riedesel (b. 1746) was the wife of the commander of the Brunswick forces in the British Army during the Revolutionary War, General de Riedesel being at that time in Canada. While in America, the Baroness addressed a detailed account of her life to her mother, the widow of the Prussian Minister of State, Mr. de Massow. Soon after the general's death, the account was published in Germany.[20]]

I endeavoured to dispel my melancholy, by continually attending to the wounded. I made them tea and coffee, for which I received their warmest acknowledgments. I often shared my dinner with them . . .

I also took care of major Blomfield who was wounded by a musket-ball which passed through both cheeks, knocked out his teeth and injured his tongue.[21]

Civil War

292. Petition to the Secretary of War

[The United States Sanitary Commission was founded on May 18, 1861, at the instance of three groups in New York. One of its primary purposes was the nursing of the sick and wounded, which was the especial concern of the Woman's Relief Association of New York.[22]]

To the Secretary of War:

Sir,—The undersigned, representing three associations of the highest respectability in the City of New York,—namely, the Woman's Central Association of Relief for the Sick and Wounded of the Army, the advisory Committee of the Boards of Physicians and Surgeons of the Hospitals of New York, the New York Medical Association for furnishing Hospital Supplies in aid of the Army, beg leave to address the Department of War in Behalf of the objects committed to them as a mixed delegation with due credentials . . .

The undersigned are charged with several distinct petitions, additional to that of asking for a Commission for the purposes above described [of giving relief to the Army], although they would all fall under the duties of that Commission.

2. The Committee represent that the Woman's Central Association of Relief have selected, and are selecting, out of several hundred candidates one hundred women, suited in all respects to become nurses in the general hospitals of the army. These women the distinguished physicians and surgeons of the various hospitals in New York, have undertaken *to educate and drill in a most thorough and laborious manner;* and the Committee ask that the War Department consent to receive, on wages, these nurses, in such numbers as the exegencies of the campaign may require. It is not proposed that the nurses should advance to the seat of war *until directly called for by the Medical Bureau here,* nor that the Government should be at any expense until they are actually in service.

Feeling themselves directly to represent large and important constituencies, and, indirectly, a widespread and commanding public sentiment, the Committee would most respectfully urge the immediate attention of the Secretary to the objects of their prayer.

Very respectfully,

Henry W. Bellows, D.D.

W. H. Van Buren, M.D.

Elisha Harris, M.D.

J. Harsen, M.D.

Objects of the Proposed Commission

3. Relief.—The Commission would inquire into the organization of military hospitals, general and regimental; the precise regulations and routine through which the services of the patriotic women of the country may be made available as nurses; the nature and sufficiency of hospital supplies; the method of obtaining and regulating all other extra and unbought supplies contributing to the comfort of the sick; the question of ambulances and field service, and of extra medical aid; and whatever else relates to the care, relief, or cure of the sick and wounded—their investigations being guided by the highest and latest medical and military experience, and carefully adapted to the nature and wants of our immediate army, and its peculiar origin and circumstances.[23]

293. Henry Whitney Bellows. *Report Concerning the Woman's Central Association of Relief at New York to the U.S. Sanitary Commission at Washington*

[At the beginning of the Civil War, it became necessary to make plans for the care of the sick and wounded. To this end the women of New York formed the Woman's Central Association of Relief, the purposes of which included the provision of nurses for the Army.

Henry Whitney Bellows (1814–1862) was the pastor of the First Unitarian Church of New York from 1839 to his death, was one of the founders of Antioch College, editor of *The Christian Enquirer* and *The Christian Examiner,* and the first president of the first Civil Service Reform Association in the United States. His greatest contribution is said to have been the organization and administration of the United States Sanitary Commission, of which he was the only president.[24]]

October 12, 1861.

At a meeting of fifty, or sixty ladies, very informally called at the New York Infirmary for Women, on April 25th, 1861, the providential suggestion for attempting to organize the whole benevolence of the women of the country into a general and central association, was ripened into a plan, and took shape in . . . [an] appeal, which at the instance of the following Committee—

Mrs. Dudley Field	Miss E. Blackwell, M.D.
Mrs. Henry Baylis	Dr. Harris
Mrs. Cyrus W. Field	Dr. Bellows, Ch'n.,

was procured to be signed by the ladies whose names are appended. It was published in all the principal New York papers of Monday, April 29, 1861.

To the Women of New York, and especially to those already engaged in preparing against the time of wounds and sickness in the Army.

. . . .

To make the meeting practical and effective, it seems proper here to set forth briefly the objects that should be kept in view. The form which woman's benevolence has already taken, and is likely to take, in the present crisis, is, first, the contribution of labor, skill, and money in the preparation of lint, bandages, and other stores, in aid of the wants of the Medical Staff; second, the offer of personal service as nurses.

. . . . . .

Articles of Organization:

Woman's Central Association for the Sick and Wounded of the Army.

. . . . .

III. The objects of this Association shall be to collect and distribute information, obtained from Official sources, concerning the actual and probable wants of the Army; to establish a recognized union with the Medical Staff of the Federal and State Troops, and to act as auxiliary to their efforts; to unite with the New York Medical Association; for the supply of lint, bandages, & c., in sustaining a central depot of stores; to solicit and accept the aid of all local associations, here or elsewhere, choosing to act through this Society, and especially to open a bureau for the examination and registration of candidates, for medical instruction as nurses, and to take measures for securing a supply of well-trained nurses against any possible demand of the war.[25]

294. *Report of the Committee Appointed on the 29th inst. to Visit the Military General Hospitals In and Around Washington*

[This report, dated July 31, 1861, is signed by Dr. William H. Van Buren, Dr. G. R. Agnew, and Frederick Law Olmsted. The first two were New York physicians who helped to promote the organization of the United States Sanitary Commission. Frederick Law Olmsted (1822–1903) was an American landscape architect and writer who was appointed secretary of the United States Sanitary Commission.[26]]

The female nurses [in the General Hospitals] ... as far as your committee could ascertain, were of great comfort to the sick. They were tolerated without complaint, and, in several instances, their services were even highly spoken of by the medical officers in charge. In regard to male nurses, on the contrary, there was much complaint as to their inefficiency and want of aptitude and disposition for their duties; this was especially remarked of the volunteers.[27]

295. J. G. Forman. *The Western Sanitary Commission* ...

[Rev. Forman was secretary of the Western Sanitary Commission for three months, after which he resigned to fill his position as chaplain of the Third Missouri Volunteers. In May, 1863, he again became permanent secretary of the Commission.[28]]

The organization of the Western Sanitary Commission was the result of circumstances growing out of the war in Missouri; the necessity for it was both sudden and unexpected, and its earliest labors were entirely spontaneous and unpremeditated. The city of Saint Louis had become the Headquarters of the Military Department of the West. During the summer of 1861 the battles of Boonville, Dug Spring, Carthage, and Wilson's Creek, were fought in Missouri ...

Arrivals of sick and wounded combined and other accomodations had to be obtained without delay. All the available wards of the Saint Louis Hospital, kept by the Sisters of Charity, and of the City Hospital were immediately taken and filled, and still there was need of more hospitals ...

It was at this juncture that the Western Sanitary Commission was suddenly called into existence. Miss D. L. Dix, the philanthropist, was then in Saint Louis, and in communication with the new Commander of the Department, Major General Fremont; Mrs. Fremont was also deeply interested in everything relating to the welfare of the sick and wounded soldier.... [An] order [was] issued by General Fremont on the 5th of September, appointing the Western Sanitary Commission, in which its duties and sphere of action were thus defined:

Its general object shall be to carry out, under the properly constituted military authorities, and in compliance with their orders, such sanitary regulations and reforms as the well-being of the soldiers demands.

This Commission shall have authority—*under the direction of the Medical Director*—to select, fit up and furnish suitable buildings for Army and Brigade Hospitals, in such places and in such manner as circumstances require. It will attend to the selection and appointment of women nurses, under the authority, and by the direction of Miss D. L. Dix, General Superintendent of the Nurses of Military Hospitals in the United States. It will co-operate with the surgeons of the several hospitals in providing male nurses, and in whatever manner practicable, and by their consent.

379

The employment of female nurses, and their assignment to duty in the hospitals, was another important service rendered by the President of the commission—a delicate trust—and one attended with many difficulties. The example of Florence Nightingale and her corps of female nurses in the Crimea, and the patriotic sympathies of the women of America with their brothers in arms, led large numbers of them to offer themselves for this service. The natural superiority of women, as nurses, was felt by all, and the government, therefore, determined to make room for a certain proportion of female nurses in the hospitals. Miss D. L. Dix, a lady widely and favorably known by her humanitary labors for prisoners and the insane, was appointed Superintendent of Women Nurses, "to determine upon their qualifications and grant certificates, either from her or her agents," were to be employed by the surgeons in charge of general hospitals. The President of the Western Sanitary Commission was made the agent of Miss Dix for the Western Department, and on him the duty devolved of receiving all applications for this branch of the service, determining the qualifications of the applicants, granting the certificates of appointment, and assigning them to duty in the hospitals, on the request of the surgeons in charge for the number required.

The qualifications of women nurses were, that the applicants should be of suitable age, (from 25 to 50 years,) that they should be persons in good health, with sound constitutions, capable of bearing fatigue; that they should be free from levity and frivolity, of an earnest but cheerful spirit; that they should dress in plain colors, and in a manner convenient for their work; that they should be persons of good education; and that they should be recommended by at least two responsible persons, (their clergyman and physician being preferred,) as to their fitness for this service.

At a later period Surgeon General Wm. A. Hammond issued an order regulating the number of women nurses to be employed in the general hospitals, to one for every twenty beds afterwards modified to one for every thirty beds, and requiring that no nurses should be employed without the certificate of Miss Dix, or her agents, except in emergencies.

Under these regulations a large number of women nurses were employed in the hospitals of the Western Department, and were allowed a compensation of $12 per month and transportation from their place of residence, and to it again on their being relieved from duty, with quarters and a ration (or board) in the hospitals.[29]

296. Dr. John Strong Newberry. *The United States Sanitary Commission in the Valley of the Mississippi during the War of the Rebellion, 1861–1866*

[Dr. John Strong Newberry (1822–1892), American geologist and paleontologist, received his education at Western Reserve University and Cleveland Medical College. He was appointed surgeon and geologist to an exploring party in northern California and Oregon, and later made other studies of the West. Because of his recognized organizing ability, he was appointed to the United States Sanitary Commission, on which he served throughout the war. He was subsequently appointed professor of geology and paleontology at the Columbia School of Mines, and state geologist of the state of Ohio.[30]]

Steamer "Lancaster No. 4."
    Paducah, Ky., May 10, 1862—3 A. M.
Fred. Law Olmsted,
    General Secretary Sanitary Commission, Washington, D. C.
My dear Olmsted—The sick are all sleeping, or quiet, and now while I am watching over them, let me improve this rare moment of respite from the pressure of my cares and duties to jot down hastily for your benefit a few of the more important items of my experience since I last wrote you!

With the help of Drs. Read and Fulton—the latter a surgeon who volunteered for the trip—and an efficient corps of nurses, (including two ladies, experienced and unexceptionable women, members of the Aid Society of Northern Ohio, and friends of mine, who have been at Pittsburg Landing, in care of the sick and in our depot, for some time,) we are doing for the sick all that their wants require, and all that their friends at home could ask.[31]

297. John Strong Newberry. *A Visit to Fort Donelson, Tenn. for the Relief of the Wounded of Feb'y 15, 1862: A Letter*

[This letter was written by Dr. Newberry,[32] Associate Secretary of the United States Sanitary Commission, to Rev. H. W. Bellows, D.D., President of the Commission.[33]]

Feb. 15, 1862.

The eighty-one wounded men who were taken on board the Allen Collier were sadly in want of immediate surgical attendance, which was thoroughly and systematically given them. Each was placed in a clean and comfortable bed; their soiled and bloody clothing removed; they were washed with warm water throughout, including their feet, new and clean underclothing; with socks, and, when needed, slippers were furnished to all; food, nourishing and palatable, and delicacies to which they had long been strangers, were supplied to them. In short, in all things they were nursed and served as though they had been our own brothers and sons.[34]

298. *Hospital Transports: A Memoir of the Embarkation of the Sick and Wounded from the Peninsula of Virginia in the Summer of 1862*

[This document was compiled by Frederick Law Olmsted (1822–1903),[35] American architect and writer. Mr. Olmsted, who had been a wanderer from his early years, made a walking tour through England

and a horseback trip through the Southern states. He and Calvert Vaux prepared the plans which were adopted for the formation of Central Park, New York. He also planned parks and grounds in other localities, such as Boston, Philadelphia, Montreal, Washington, Chicago, Buffalo, Leland Stanford University, the Niagara Frontier, and the Yosemite. During the Civil War he was Secretary of the United States Sanitary Commission.[36]]

> (A.) Hospital Transport *Daniel Webster,* Cheesman's Creek, April 30, 1862.

... We had six medical students, twenty men nurses (volunteers all), four surgeons, four ladies, a dozen contrabands (field hands), three carpenters, and half a dozen miscellaneous passengers ...

(M.) By dark the *Wilson Small* came alongside with our first patients, thirty-five in number, who were carefully lifted on board and swung through the hatches on their stretchers. In half an hour they had all been tea'd and coffeed and refreshed by the nurses, and shortly after were all undressed and put to bed clean and comfortable, and in a droll state of grateful wonder; the bad cases of fever furnished with sponges and cologne-water for bathing; and wine and water or brandy-toddy for drinking, and a man to watch them, and ward-masters up and down the wards, and a young doctor in the apothecary's shop, and today (May 3d) they are all better ...

Meantime additional supplies arrived from Washington, Baltimore, and Fortress Monroe, and a surgeon and nurses of our company were busy daily on shore at the Ship Point Hospital, dispensing stores, and doing what they could for the poor fellows there, who seemed to us in want of everything ...

... The ladies are all, in every way, far beyond anything I could have been induced to expect of them. The dressers (two-year medical students) are generally ready for whatever may be required, and work heroically. The male nurses are of all sorts. The convalescent soldiers have been the most satisfactory, because there was not among them the slightest taint of the prevailing sentiment of the volunteer nurses, that they were going upon an indiscriminate holiday scramble of Good-Samaritanism ...

Regulations for Floating Hospital Service of the Sanitary Commission for the Campaign of Virginia ...

Nurses.

Two or more nurses are to be constantly on duty in each ward [50 to 100 patients]. They will perform any and all duties necessary in the care of the patients, under the instructions from the surgeons received through the ward-masters ...

Watches.

Ward-masters and nurses, and all who have put in duty of a constant character, will be divided into two watches, which will be on duty alternately, as follows:

1.	From 7 A. M. to 1 P. M.	A	
2.	" 1 P. M. to 4 P. M.	B	(dog watch.)
3.	" 4 P. M. to 7 P. M.	A	
4.	" 7 P. M. to 1 A. M.	B	
5.	" 1 A. M. to 7 A. M.	A	
6.	" 7 A. M. to 1 P. M.	B	(second day.)

All Hands.

In receiving and discharging patients, or in any emergency which makes it necessary, ward-masters and nurses may be required to do duty in their watches off. In cleaning, fitting, or repairing the vessel for hospital purposes, they will act under orders of the administrative agent . . .

Fred. Law Olmsted, Gen'l Sec'y.

White House, Virginia, May 20, 1862.[37]

299. *American Medical Times,* July 18, 1861, pp. 25–26, 30

[This periodical was published in New York City. The editors at this time were Dr. Stephen Smith and Dr. George F. Shrady.]

"Female Nurses in Military Hospitals"

Our readers are already aware in what light we regard female nurses. But our attention is again forcibly called to the subject by a letter which appears in another column, from an intelligent correspondent, a distinguished surgeon of the army, who expresses decided opinions against the present effort to introduce them into the public service. Believing that he represents a class of army surgeons who will not regard with favor the substitution of female for male nurses, in our military hospitals about to be opened, we take the occasion to call their attention to some of the more obvious reasons for this change, and the circumstances under which it should be made.

It is conceded that women may be employed "as the regular administrator of the prescribed medicines," and that she is more capable than the opposite sex of those "delicate, soothing attentions which are always so grateful to the sick." This has already been proved in the hospitals. At Cairo, Ill., where Mrs. Yates and her well trained nurses are winning the good opinions of the very physicians who at first opposed their admission, says an observer:—"The presence of these ladies has demonstrated that there are numberless little things essential to the comfort of the sick, which not one man in a thousand ever thinks of, but which woman sees by intuition, and supplies as if by magic."

We doubt not it will also be admitted that she is better adapted than man to prepare food for the sick, to preserve cleanliness of the wounds, and of the beds, and to regulate and keep in order whatever relates to the domestic appointments of a hospital. Miss Nightingale has aptly said on this point:— "I think the Anglo-Saxon would be very sorry to turn women out of his own house, or out of civil hospitals, hotels, institutions of all kinds, and substitute men housekeepers and men matrons. The contrast between even naval hospitals, where there are female nurses, and military hospitals where there are none, is most striking, in point of order and cleanliness." There can be few who will not agree with her in the opinion, that "the woman is superior in skill to the man in all points of sanitary domestic economy, and more particularly in cleanliness and tidiness;" and further, that "great sanitary, civil reformers will always tell us that they look to the women to carry out practically their sanitary reforms."

What then are the objections to the employment of female nurses in military hospitals? Our correspondent has stated several, but they are more imaginary than real. We are not aware what plan will be adopted in our new military hospitals, nor what special duties will be assigned to female nurses, if they are employed; but we know from personal experience, that he has assumed the existence of difficulties which will never occur in a hospital that has a proper organization. Let us recur to this experience, as showing that female nurses are already successfully substituted in certain general civil hospitals in this country, and by inference that the system may be extended to the military hospitals soon to be organized.

It was our fortune to spend a portion of our medical pupilage as resident in a hospital which was entirely under the supervision of females. This hospital was general in its character, admitting all classes of patients, medical and surgical, and of both sexes. During this period cholera prevailed in the town, and the sick of this disease crowded the wards. The general management was under the direction of a matron who had for years been an experienced hospital nurse. Subordinate to her were six chief nurses. These nurses were educated, intelligent, and refined, and many of them were from the highest ranks of society. They were skilled nurses. They adopted this employment from strong religious convictions of duty, and, entering upon it as a lifework, submitted to thorough preparation by systematic training. The division of labor was as follows: one had entire charge of the culinary department, a second of the laundry, and the remaining four of the several medical and surgical divisions of the wards. Under their immediate supervision, therefore, was the preparation of the diet, the washing of the clothes and bedding of patients, the administration of medicines, and all minor dressings. There was also the usual number of visiting physicians and surgeons, and a resident medical student. Although there was but a single male, there was always ample assistance to be obtained among the convalescents. The administration of the medicines was never committed to assistants, not indeed, any of the details of nursing. Surgical dressings of a delicate character were, of course, under the immediate charge of the Resident Physician, and the assistance of male patients from their beds was the proper duty of the orderly. During the residence of a year in this institution we never knew the slightest indecencies on the part of male patients towards their nurses, nor were the latter ever placed in a position embarrassing to one accustomed to the daily duties of hospital wards. On the contrary, the patients entertained the most profound respect for the nurses, the convalescents volunteering with the utmost alacrity to aid them in their duties. In regard to that hospital we speak but the unanimous sentiment of every physician and surgeon connected with it when we affirm that in cleanliness of wards and beds, in the preparation of the food for the sick, in precise administration of medicines, in watchful care at the bedside, in a word, in everything pertaining to the management of the domestic and medical department of a hospital, this was a model institution, and one which has no equal in this country. And if we add to these excellencies, the thousand little offices of kindness which woman alone knows how to bestow upon the sick and suffering, we need not be surprised that many a patient from that hospital was heard in after years to utter a benediction upon his former nurses, the good *Sisters of Charity!*

The testimony of those who have seen the practical working of the system of female nursing is of the same purport; and as such evidence is that upon which we must rely in coming to a rational conclusion, we shall refer briefly to the opinions of those who have had opportunity for extended observation.

At Guy's Hospital, London, there were *no male nurses* in 1857, according to the evidence of Mr. Steele, its Superintendent. There were eighteen chief nurses, having charge of the day and night nurses; of the former there were twenty-seven, and of the latter twenty-three. The duties of the chief nurses are thus stated:—"They have the general superintendence of the wards, and they are responsible to the physicians for the medicines and wines, and for the cleanliness of the patients; they have charge of the ward furniture and the bed-linen." The other nurses had the immediate charge of the patients. In reply to the question, Does your system of nursing work well? he answered:— "Remarkably well." The only improvement suggested was the employment of one or two orderlies for the venereal, and bad surgical cases. The same system was in operation in London Hospital.

After an extended investigation of the working of the hospital systems on the continent, Mr. Alexander gave evidence before a Parliamentary Commission as follows: "From what we saw and heard of female nursing in Paris and Brussels, there cannot be a doubt that good results would follow the introduction of a certain number of well-selected educated nurses to our hospital establishments. In Jamaica, in 1837, I recommended female nursing to be employed, from what I saw of the evil effects, and even risk of life, by orderly or soldier nursing in severe cases, but no attention was paid to my recommendation; and from my more extended experience, I am still more convinced of the advantages that would be derived from the

judicious introduction of female nursing into our permanent hospital establishments."

It appears also that, at the time this investigation was made, the French
emperor was forming a corps of female nurses for military hospitals, the
selection being made from the Sisters of Charity in the civil hospitals.

During the Crimean war female nursing in Military Hospitals was put to
a practical test, and the opinions of those who witnessed its efficiency are
worthy of especial consideration. Dr. Parkes, who had charge of the Renkioi
Hospital, says: "I have a very high opinion of female nurses, if they have
been trained and are proper nurses." Mr. Meyer, Medical Director of the
Civil Hospital at Smyrna, states that "they worked uncommonly well; out
of twenty-two female nurses only one was removed for any misconduct. . . .
Several of the ladies that we had did the work uncommonly well, and it would
have been very difficult to have got as large a class of severe cases of fever
attended so well by night and day except by the agency of those ladies, who
were thoroughly to be relied on, not only from their superior intelligence
but their devotion to the work."

But we need not multiply this evidence, for happily our Government and
the intelligent Chief of the Medical Bureau require no further arguments
or evidence to prove the importance of employing qualified female nurses in
the military hospitals. This question has already been settled by the Surgeon-
General, and the good fruits of the new system are beginning to be manifest
at Cairo and Fortress Monroe. And it is still more gratifying to learn that
this question is about to receive the sanction of the Legislature. The bill
introduced into the Senate by Senator Wilson, for the "better Organization
of the Military Establishment," provides for the substitution of female nurses
in military hospitals, with pay and rations.

We can cite no more convincing proof of the flexibility of a free Government and its power of adapting itself to unforseen emergencies, above that
of monarchies, than this spontaneous adoption of great public measures
which simply commend themselves to good sense and a sound judgment.

Correspondence: . . . "Females Not Suitable for Nurses."
[To the Editor of the *American Medical Times*.]

Our women appear to have become almost wild on the subject of hospital
nursing. We honor them for their sympathy and humanity. Nevertheless,
a man who has had experience with women nurses among male surgical
cases, cannot shut his eyes to the fact that they, with the best intentions in
the world, are frequently a useless annoyance. Cases are continually occurring
in male surgical wards of such a character as require strong arms, and
attentions which any reasonable medical man is loth to exact from female
nurses. Imagine a delicate refined woman assisting a rough soldier to the
close-stool, or supplying him with a bed-pan, or adjusting the knots on a

T-bandage employed in retaining a catheter in position, or a dozen offices of a like character which one would hesitate long before asking a female nurse to perform, but which are frequently and continually necessary in a military hospital. Besides this, women, as a rule, have not the physical strength necessary. For example—a man having gunshot wounds of grave severity affecting the lower extremities, with perhaps incontinence of urine, or diarrhoea, would not improbably be attacked with bed-sores if not kept scrupulously clean. Should the soft parts of the back begin to ulcerate, local attention becomes doubly necessary. The patient, under these circumstances, requires often to be lifted up carefully, and bodily, so as not to alter the comparative position of his limbs to his body. To do this properly, at least *four* strong men are required, who, stationed two at the shoulders and two at the hips (one hand from each lower assistant steadying the thigh and leg of that side), can thus raise the man steadily and carefully. A fifth would not be out of place in supporting the feet, while the medical attendant washes the excoriated parts, applies the needed dressings, and throws upon the surface of the bed a clean sheet.

Women, in our humble opinion, are utterly and decidedly unfit for such service. They can be used, however, as the regular administrators of the prescribed medicines, and in delicate, soothing attentions which are always so grateful to the sick, and which at the same time none know so well how to give as do noble, sensible, tenderhearted women.

But as hospital nurses for wounded men, they are by nature, education, and strength totally unfitted, i. e. when we consider *all the duties* surgical nurses are called upon to perform. In conclusion, it may be well to state that a surgeon on duty with troops, by showing proper interest in the men, without allowing himself to be humbugged by them, will gain their affection as well as respect.

S. G.

300. *The Medical and Surgical Reporter*, November 8, 1862, p. 160

[Miss Dorothea Dix was appointed superintendent of Army nurses early in the Civil War. Below are the qualifications which she formulated for nurses for the hospitals of the Sanitary Commission.]

Editorial

Women Nurses for the Army.—We have had several inquiries in regard to women nurses for the military hospitals. Many are still wanted. Miss D. L. Dix is the superintendent of the Women Nurses, and the following are her amended rules:

No candidate for service in the Women's Department for nursing in the military hospitals of the United States, will be received below the age of (35) thirty-five, nor above fifty.

Only women of strong health, not subject of chronic disease, nor liable to sudden illness, need apply. The duties of the station make large and continued demands on strength.

Matronly persons of experience, good conduct, or superior education and serious disposition, will always have preference; habits of neatness, order, sobriety and industry are prerequisites.

All applicants must present certificates of qualification and good character from at least two persons of trust, testifying to morality, integrity, seriousness, and capacity for the care of the sick.

Obedience to rules of the service, and conformity to special regulations, will be required and enforced.

Compensation, as regulated by act of Congress, forty cents a day and subsistence. Transportation furnished to and from the place of service, over military routes only.

Amount of luggage limited within small compass. Dress plain, (colors, brown, grey or black): and, while connected with the service, without ornaments of any sort.

No applicants accepted for less than six months' service, or for the war; for longer periods always have preference.

D. L. Dix.

Approved—Wm. A. Hammond, Surgeon-General.

301. The *Medical and Surgical Reporter*, September 10, 1864, p. 32

[The following circular letter, published in this medical periodical, is of interest as indicating the relative pay of women nurses and women cooks.]

Pay of Female Nurses

Surgeon-General's Office,
Washington, D. C., August 27, 1864.

[Circular Letter.]

So much of Circular Letter dated Surgeon-General's Office, Washington, June 15th, 1864, granting increased pay to female nurses is hereby revoked, as the Act of Congress of August 3, 1861, fixes the pay of female nurses in general or permanent hospitals at forty cents a day, and one ration in kind, or by commutation, in lieu of all emoluments except transportation in kind.

Female cooks will continue to receive sixty cents a day and one ration.

By order of the Acting Surgeon-General,

C. H. Crane, Surgeon, U. S. Army.

302. *Letters of a Family during the War for the Union 1861–1865*

[Several members of the Woolsey family, socially minded residents of New York, participated in one capacity or another in the Civil War. Abby Howland Woolsey, one of the sisters, was a worker on the State Charities Aid Association of New York and a member of the special committee which planned the Bellevue School of Nursing in 1873. She later visited hospitals in Europe and reported her findings in *A Century of Nursing*.[38] Jane Stuart Woolsey, another sister, wrote of her war ex-

388

perience in *Hospital Days.*[39] The brief account, *Three Weeks at Gettysburg,* was written by another member of the family, Georgeanna Muirson Woolsey Bacon.[40] The selection of letters is from the correspondence of the family during the war. In addition to the books and letters written by the sisters, their brother, Charles William Woolsey, also contributed to the literature of the war.[41]]

[Written by GMW (Georgeanna Muirson Woolsey)]

It was hard work getting myself acceptable and—accepted. What with people at home, saying "Goodness me! a nurse!" "All nonsense!" "Such a fly-away!" and what with the requisites insisted upon by the grave committee, I came near losing my opportunity.

First, one must be just so old, and no older; have eyes and a nose and a mouth expressing just such traits, and no others; must be willing to scrub floors, if necessary, etc., etc. Finally, however, by dint of taking the flowers out of my bonnet and the flounce off my dress; by toning down, or toning up, according to the emergency, I succeeded in getting myself looked upon with mitigated disapprobation, and was at last sat upon by the committee and passed over by the Examining Board. The Board was good to me. It had to decide upon my physical qualifications; and so, having asked me who my grandfather was, and whether I had had the measles, it blandly put my name down, leaving a blank, inadvertently, where the age should have been, and I was launched, with about twenty other neophytes, into a career of philanthropy more or less confused.

Then began serious business. Armed with a blue ticket, I presented myself with the others at the door of a hospital and was admitted for instruction. "Follow me," said our guide, and we followed in procession. "This will be your ward; you will remain here under so and so, and learn what you can; and this, yours; and this, *yours.*" That was mine! I shall never forget the hopeless state of my mind at this exact point. To be left standing in the middle of a long ward, full of beds, full of sick men—it was appalling! I seized another nurse, and refused to be abandoned. So they took pity, and we two remained, to use our eyes and time to the advantage of the Army of the Potomac which was-to-be. We took off our bonnets and went to work. Such a month we had of it, walking from room to room, learning what we could—really learning something in the end, till finally, what with writing down everything we saw, and making elaborate sketches of all kinds of bandages and the ways of applying them, and what with bandaging everybody we met, for practice, we at last made our "reverses" without a wrinkle; and at the end of the month were competent to any very small emergency, or very simple fracture.

. . . .

[GMW to EWH (Eliza Woolsey Howland)]

May 15, 1861.

I supposed you would go to Albany; I am sure I should, and I hope you will take into serious consideration the small plan I suggested to you about

being a nurse—at any rate about fitting yourself as far as you can for looking after the sick. If you go, as I suppose you will want to, to Washington in
the fall with Joe [Eliza's husband] I invite you to join me. Mrs. Trotter and
I were yesterday examined by the Medical Committee, Drs. Delafield, Wood
and Harris, and with ten other women admitted to the course of instruction
at the New York Hospital. We are to learn how to make beds for the
wounded, cook food properly for the sick, wash and dress wounds, and
other things as they come along in the proper care of the wards—fresh air,
etc. Not that we have any idea of really going south now, no one will till
the fall, and two or three companies of ten each who are fitting themselves
at Bellevue Hospital will at any rate go first. Then if there is really a necessity for more nurses we shall send substitutes agreeing to pay their expenses,
—unless the opposition in the family has come to an end, in which case,
having tested our strength and endurance a little in this training, we shall
be very glad to carry out our plan and go. We three might very usefully
employ ourselves in Washington if we went no further south, and I shall
not be satisfied at all to stay at home while Joe is down there. So, my dear,
be keeping the little plan in view in making your arrangements, and don't
say a word to anybody about our being at the Hospital; I don't want to
have to fight my way all through the course, and be badgered by the connection generally, besides giving a strict account of myself at home. We all
mean to be very brave about Joe, and I am sure you will be;—it's a way you
have; especially as you and I, and perhaps Mrs. Trotter, will be near him
in Washington at one of the hotels or hospitals.

.   .   .   .

[AHW (Abby Howland Woolsey) to the Sisters still abroad]
We are gradually growing accustomed to things that a few weeks ago
would have appalled us, or which we would have received as horrid jokes—
such, for instance as Georgy's training at the hospital. She comes home
fagged-looking but determined to "stick it out." Did you know, Carry
[Caroline Carson Woolsey], that Miss Bessie and Miss Mattie Parsons are
walking the hospitals in Boston? Some of the ladies there fainted every day
for a week, when Dr. Bigelow made them mad by telling them "They had
tried it long enough; they were unfit for it and must go home." It will not
surprise us if by and by Georgy starts for the wars. *Nothing* astonishes us
nowadays; we are *blasées* in revolutions and topsy-turvyings; or, as Joe
elegantly expresses it: "How many exciting things we have had this winter!
First, parlor skates, and now, civil war! . . ."

.   .   .   .

[Dr. Eliz. Blackwell to GMW]

New York, July 30 [1861]
My dear Miss Woolsey: I was extremely glad to receive your excellent
letter yesterday. Had I known that you were residing in Washington, I should
have requested you some time before to collect information for our society.

We had become extremely anxious about these women; we could not learn who had safely arrived, where they were, what they were doing, nor how they fared in any respect; and a check of considerable amount, sent to one of them, was unacknowledged. As we pledged ourselves to protect these women, pay their expenses, their wages, etc., you may imagine that we felt extremely uneasy about them . . .

I will ask you now, to find out for us where Miss E. H. and Mrs. N. S. are placed. They were sent from New York by night train, July 25, direct to Miss Dix, and should have reached Washington last Friday morning.

Will you also visit the Georgetown Hospital and report on two nurses whom we sent on last Saturday. We should like some unprejudiced account of this Hospital . . .

I will see that any nurse going to Alexandria in future is furnished with a certificate signed by some proper authority here. We feel much obliged to you for all the trouble you have taken in this matter . . .

As the government payment commences Aug. 5th, from that time our society hands the nurses over to the government.

I remain very truly yours,
E. Blackwell.

[The following account of the "Patent Office" Hospital is taken from G.'s letter to the Sanitary Commission Fair's paper.]

One of the first extemporized hospitals of the war was in the top story of the Patent office, where the 19th Indiana regiment was brought, nearly every man of them. The great, unfinished lumber room was set aside for their use, and rough tables—I can't call them beds—were knocked together from pieces of the scaffolding. These beds were so high that it was impossible to reach them, and we had to make them up with brooms, sweeping off the mattresses, and jerking the sheets as smooth as we could. About six men could be accommodated on one table. These ran the whole length of the long room, while on the stacks of marble slabs, which were some day to be the floor, we spread mattresses, and put the sickest men. As the number increased, camp-beds were set up between the glass cases in the outer room, and we alternated—typhoid fever, cog-wheels and patent churns—typhoid fever, balloons and mouse-traps (how *many* ways of catching mice there are!)— typhoid fever, locomotives, water-wheels, clocks,—and a general nightmare of machinery.

Here, for weeks, went on a sort of hospital pic-nic. We scrambled through with what we had to do. The floors were covered with lime dust, shavings, nails, and carpenter's scraps. We had the rubbish taken up with shovels, and stacked in barrels at one end of the ward. The men were crowded in upon us; the whole regiment soaked with a malignant, malarial fever, from exposure, night after night, to drenching rains, without tents. There was so much of this murderous, blundering want of prevision and provision, in the first few months of the war—and is *now,* for that matter.

391

Gradually, out of the confusion came some system and order. Climbing up to the top of the Patent office with each loaf of bread was found not to be an amusing occupation, and an arrangement of pulleys was made out of one of the windows, and any time through the day, barrels of water, baskets of vegetables and great pieces of army beef, might be seen crawling slowly up the marble face of the building.

Here, for weeks, we worked among these men, cooking for them, feeding them, washing them, sliding them along their tables, while we climbed up on something to make up their beds with brooms, putting the same powders down their throats with the same spoon, all up and down what seemed half a mile of uneven floor;—coaxing back to life some of the most unpromising, watching the youngest and best die.

I remember rushing about from apothecary to apothecary, in the lower part of the city, one Sunday afternoon, to get, in a great hurry, mustard to help bring life into a poor Irishman, who called me Betty in his delirium, and, to our surprise, got well, went home, and at once married the Betty we had saved him for.

By-and-by the regiment got through with the fever, improvements came into the long ward, cots took the place of the tables, and matting covered the little hills on the floor. The hospital for the 19th Indiana became the "U. S. General Hospital at the Patent Office," and the "volunteers for emergencies" took up their saucepans and retired.

[G. to Mother]

May 1, '61.

We are in sight of the abandoned rebel quarters at Ship Point, now used as a hospital on low, filthy ground surrounded by earth-works, rained on half the time and fiercely shone on the other half, a death place for scores of our men, who are piled in there covered with vermin, dying with their uniforms on and collars up, dying of fever. Of course there is that vitally important thing, medical etiquette, to contend with here as elsewhere, and so it is:— "Suppose you go ashore and ask whether it would be agreeable to have the ladies come over, just to walk through the hospital and talk to the men?" So the ladies have gone to talk to the men with spirit lamps and farina and lemons and brandy and clean clothes, and expect to have an improving conversation! . . .

[EWH to JH (Joseph Howland)]

May 7th, '62.

My dear Joe: Down in the depths of the Ocean Queen, with a pail of freshly-made milk punch alongside of me, a jug of brandy at my feet, beef tea on the right flank, and untold stores of other things scattered about, I write a hurried note on my lap, just to tell you that we keep well, but have been so busy the last 48 hours that I have lost all track of time. You had scarcely left us the other day when our first installment of sick men came aboard—150 men—before anything whatever was ready for them. We had only just taken possession of the ship, as you saw, and not an article had been unpacked or a bed made. With two spoons, and ten pounds of Indian meal (the only food on board) made into gruel, G. and I managed, however, to feed them all and got them to bed. They have come in the same way ever since, crowded upon us unprepared, and with so few to do for them; and we have now nearly 600, and more coming tonight. . . . Until today we have had only our small force who were detached from the Webster, and I may say without vanity that G. and I, and the two young doctors, Wheelock and Haight, have done *everything*. We women have attended to the feeding of the 400 or 500, and those two young fellows have had the responsibility of their medical care! Last night, however, a large party of surgeons, dressers, and nurses arrived from New York, and though today things have been frightfully chaotic, they will settle down soon and each one will have his own work to do . . .

G. and I look after the special diet and the ordering of all the food. Beef tea is made by the ten gallons and punch by the pail. I was so busy yesterday morning that I didn't know when you left, and only saw the last of the fleet far up York River.

.   .   .   .

[E. to J. H.]

Floating Hospital, Spaulding,
Off White House, May 22, [1862].

We are going on shore presently to see what we can do for the large field hospital there. Two of our doctors, Ware and Draper of New York, spent the day yesterday trying to organize it and make the men tolerably comfortable. They furnished from the Commission nearly a thousand mattresses, secured them fresh water in hogsheads (which they were entirely without) and saw that all who needed medicine got it. System and food seem to be the great wants, and today we ladies will attend to the latter, take them supplies and show the hospital cooks how to prepare them. There are 1,200 or more sick men there, and until the Commission took hold they were in a most wretched plight, lying on the damp ground without beds, without food or water, and with little or no care. . . . I hope *you* take all necessary precautions in this wretched climate. Don't give up your quinine . . .

Later.—Directly after I wrote you this morning Georgy and I went to the shore to breakfast the men we had dinnered and teaed yesterday, and there we had a little house nearby which Dr. Ware had found, nicely cleaned out for a hospital or resting place for the sick when the other overflows. The floor of one of the rooms upstairs is six inches deep in beans. That makes a good bed for them. . . . Meantime Mrs. Griffin and the others got this boat in order for sick, and this afternoon fifty odd have been brought on board. Tomorrow it will fill up and leave for New York.[42]

393

303. Jane Stuart Woolsey. *Hospital Days*

[Jane Stuart Woolsey, one of the Woolsey sisters of New York, served in the hospitals until the end of the war. Following the service there, she worked among the freedmen at Richmond, Virginia.[43]]

First Days

On a blue-and-gold day in the edge of November, a hundred years ago, two ladies, with their luggage, were carefully packed into an ambulance, the conveyance of the period, at the door of a great city hotel. They were setting out—with an easy and cheerful-minded confidence in the unknown, which seems strange to them as they look back at it, but which must have been part of the spirit of the time—for a lonely outpost hospital to which they had been invited by the officer in charge, as supervisors of the nursing and cooking department.

. . . .

Special Diets

On the morning after their arrival, the newcomers, who had already been formally mustered into the service of the United States, were put on duty in published orders, and were waited on in the store-room by women-nurses in a body, somewhat prepared to resent if occasion offered, but soon melting and smiling on observing the unformidable aspect of the new authority. "Them dear lambs!" said old Mrs. B., afterwards, "What I was afraid of was caps . . ."

An exploration was then made of every nook and corner of the Hospital. A little ripple of smiles followed the Surgeon in Charge up and down the wards, and the men to whom he spoke or whom he touched, loosening or righting strap or bandage, looking proud and pleased.

In the course of this tour of inspection the Superintendent received a few words of instruction as to her position and its duties. She might visit in the wards, distribute little extra comforts, talk with the men, write letters and "sympathize as much as she had time and inclination for," but her serious business was to see that the women-nurses did their duty, and that the Special Diet was everything that it ought to be. She was required to know what quantity and quality of raw material was furnished by the commissary steward; to see that this was properly çooked, properly distributed from the diet kitchen, received in good order in the wards, carefully divided there; that each patient got, without unlawful leakage, the exact articles ordered for him by the ward medical officer; in short, she was expected to follow the food from the commissary storehouse down the sick man's throat. . . . "Observe, observe continually; your observation is worth more than my theory." [said the Surgeon in Charge].

. . . .

The Superintendent has in her possession many original orders on the diet kitchen, of which the following are specimens:

Private H. (Inflammation of stomach) Hot cakes, cheese and molasses candy.

Private C. (Chronic diarrhoea.) Graded flour porridge, lemonade, oyster soup, oatmeal gruel and peppermint tea.

Private J. (Chronic diarrhoea.)

Breakfast.	Dinner.	Supper.
Coffee.	Roast Beef.	Oyster Soup.
Steak.	Fish.	Raw Cabbage.
Eggs.	Boiled Cabbage.	Cheese.
Bread.	Radishes.	Bread.
Butter.	Bread.	Butter.
Milk-punch.	Tea.	Coffee.

Private K. (Typhoid fever.)

Breakfast.	Dinner.	Supper.
Mutton Chops.	Beefsteak.	Milk.
Potatoes.	Potatoes.	Tea.
Bread.	Tea.	Arrowroot.
Coffee.	Coffee.	Cake.
Doughnuts.	Butter.	Butter.
Butter.	Plum Pudding.	Pudding.

The woman-nurse in each little ward receives her tray or trays, having her china plates and cups, her knives and forks and tumblers, set out in order beforehand; divides the food according to a duplicate of the ward return hanging over her table, and the men-nurses carry it about. She follows immediately down the ward, helps and feeds those who are unable to help themselves, and sees that all have enough. If anything goes wrong, she is directed to send word at once to the superintendent. She has means of heating over any simple thing if the patient does not incline to it at the fixed hour. A sick man will often take his food nicely if he may have his own time about it, and does not feel himself under observation. In critical cases a fresh ration is prepared instead of the *rechauffe*.

Take a page at random from the Superintendent's shabby, little yellow note-book. What hospital nurse doesn't know the sort. "Cushing complains of the steak; it is too rare."—The Superintendent observes with pain that the Defenders all prefer their steaks cut thin and *fried*.—Jeffries wants more seasoning in his soup; it is "too fresh," he says, and Brooks must have his tomatoes raw, with vinegar. Thompson says the men-nurses are too slow;

he says he "wants particular attention paid to him;" he "can't eat fish-hash," and he "can't eat soup." Bates wants "crust coffee," and explains to me how it should be made. No. 35 hasn't touched his breakfast. "If he could only have some Boston brown bread." Mem.: to try and get him some. Eustace is tired of all his drinks; try mulled sherry. Cocoa in F poor and washy today. More small cans wanted for gruels. Ward return wrong—explain to woman-nurse. Quinn running down; try champagne in a long-spouted feeding cup. Mem.: to show nurse in K how to get more dish-towels and hot-water cans for cold feet. Scott says he can't get along without "jel" for his tea every night. Cut up No. 802's chicken and feed him with it, on his intimation that he will eat it if I do; he admits that it is not as bad as he expected.

·   ·   ·   ·   ·   ·   ·

Women-Nurses

Was the system of women-nurses in hospitals a failure? There never was any system. That the presence of hundreds of individual women as nurses in hospitals was neither an intrusion nor a blunder, let the multitude of their—unsystematized—labors and achievements testify. So far as I know, the experiment of a compact, general organization was never fairly tried. Hospital nurses were of all sorts, and came from various sources of supply; volunteers paid or unpaid; soldiers' wives and sisters who had come to see their friends, and remained without any clear commission or duties; women sent by State agencies and aid societies; women assigned by the General Superintendent of Nurses; sometimes, as in a case I knew of, the wife or daughter of a medical officer drawing the rations, but certainly not doing the work of a "Laundress." These women were set adrift in a hospital, eight to twenty of them, for the most part slightly educated, without training or discipline, without company organization or officers, so to speak, of their own, "reporting" to the surgeons, or in the case of persons assigned by her, to the General Superintendent, which is very much, in a small way, as if Private Robinson should "report" to General Grant.

There was a standing misunderstanding on the question, for instance, who was authorized to supply women-nurses. An attempt was made, late in 1863, ostensibly to clear up this question. In order No. 351 of the War Department, clause Two says: Women-nurses will be assigned only on application to the General Superintendent, unless, adds clause Three, they are specifically appointed by the Surgeon General. Of course, surgeons in charge wishing to retain or employ nurses without the "certificate" of the General Superintendent, applied for their "special appointment" by the Surgeon General, which was promptly obtained. This, with the other provisions of the order, practically abolished the office of General Superintendent of Nurses, and threw the selection into the hands of surgeons in charge, which, where the surgeon in charge was an "honest gentleman" and a faithful and efficient officer, was a wise enough measure.[44]

304. Katharine Prescott Wormeley. *The Cruel Side of the War, With the Army of the Potomac*

[Katharine Prescott Wormeley (1830–1908), author and philanthropist, was born in England. Her father was a rear admiral in the British Navy. Miss Wormeley took an active part in public affairs, especially those relating to sanitation and work with women and girls. She was an accomplished French scholar and was best known for her translations of works of French writers. During the Civil War she participated in relief measures for Union soldiers and was superintendent of a hospital for convalescent soldiers at Portsmouth, Rhode Island.[45] The book quoted below was issued previously under the title, *The Other Side of the War.* It consists of letters from the headquarters of the United States Sanitary Commission during the Peninsular Campaign in Virginia in 1862.]

> Headquarters U. S. Sanitary Commission,
> Steamer "Wilson Small,"
> Off Yorktown, May 12 [1862].

Dear A.,—Transferred to this boat. Mr. Olmsted came on board at twelve o'clock last night and ordered Mrs. Griffin and me off the "Daniel Webster." We had just received, stowed, and fed two hundred and forty-five men, most of them very ill with typhoid fever. The ship sailed at eight o'clock this morning, and will be in New York tomorrow night. Mrs. Trotter went back in charge of our department, and Mrs. Bellows (wife of the president of the Sanitary Commission) accompanied her.

The "Webster" could not get up to the wharf, so the sick men were brought off to us in tug boats. As each man came on board (raised from one vessel and lowered to the second deck of ours in cradles), he was registered and "bunked." In my ward, as each man was laid in his berth, I gave him brandy and water, and after all were placed, tea and bread and butter, if they could take it, or more brandy or beef-tea if they were sinking. Of course it was painful; but there was so much to be done, and done quietly and quickly, that there was no time to be conscious of pain. But fever patients *are* very dreadful, and their moans distressing. The men were all patient and grateful . . .

We did not get them all settled and the watches set until 1 A. M.; after which Mrs. Griffin and I packed up, to leave the ship at daybreak. Oh! if I had it to do over again, I'd have an organized Carpet-bag, with compartments for everything. As it was, all was poked and stamped upon.

This is a little boat, headquarters of the Sanitary Commission, Mr. Olmsted, the General Secretary, in charge of the whole transport service, and Mr. Knapp, his second in command living on board. At present she is filled in every available corner by severely wounded men brought from the battlefield of Williamsburg,—wounded chiefly in the legs and thighs. Today Mrs.

Griffin and I are supernumeraries, the ladies on board being sufficient for all purposes. They are, so far as I have yet ascertained, Miss Mary Gardiner, of New York, Mrs. Joseph Howland [Eliza Woolsey], wife of the colonel of a regiment in the advance, a tall symmetrical Miss Whetten, and a pretty little creature, half nun, half soubrette, whose name I don't know. They all seem easy and at home in their work, as if they had been at it all their lives. I use my eyes and learn, and have taken a hand here and there as occasion offered. Terrible things happened yesterday. Many of the wounded of the Williamsburg battle were found lying in the woods with their wounds not dressed, and they starving. Mrs. Strong saw them, and says it was like going over a battle-field.

There is a general cry throughout the female department for "Georgy." "Where is Georgy?" "Oh, if Georgy were here!" Georgy is on board a hospital boat called the "Knickerbocker," which appears to be missing. As I have nothing to do, I speculate a good deal as to who and what "Georgy" may be.[46]

"Wilson Small."
May 13 [1862].

Dear Mother,—Yours of the ninth received. The mails come with sufficient regularity . . .

I took my first actual watch last night; and this morning I feel the same ease about the work which yesterday I was surprised to see in others. We begin the day by getting them all washed; and freshened up, and breakfasted. Then the surgeons and dressers make their rounds, open the wounds, apply the remedies, and replace the bandages. This is an awful hour; I sat with my fingers in my ears this morning. When it is over, we go back to the men and put the ward in order once more; remaking several of the beds, and giving clean handkerchiefs with a little cologne or bay-water on them,— so prized in the sickening atmosphere of wounds. We sponge the bandages over the wounds constantly,—which alone carries us round from cot to cot almost without stopping, except to talk to some, read to others, or with letters for them; occasionally giving medicine or brandy, etc., according to order. Then comes dinner, which we serve out ourselves. After that we go off duty, and get first washed and then fed ourselves; our dinner-table being the top of an old stove, with slices of bread for places, fingers for knives and forks, and carpet-bags for chairs,—all this because everything available is being used for our poor fellows. After dinner other ladies keep the same sort of watch through the afternoon and evening, while we sit on the floor of our staterooms resting, and perhaps writing letters, as I am doing now . . .

"Knickerbocker," May 26 [1862]

Dear Mother,—I believe my last words on Saturday were that I was "called off,"—and so effectually called that this is my first quiet moment

398

since then. We were called to go on board the "Wissahickon," from thence to the "Sea-Shore," and run down in the latter to West Point, to bring off twenty-five men said to be lying there sick and destitute. Two doctors went with us. After hunting an hour through the fleet for the "Sea-Shore" in vain, and having got as low as Cumberland, we decided (*we* being Mrs. Howland and I; for the doctors were new to the work, and glad to leave the responsibility upon us women) to push on in the tug, rather than to leave the men another night on the ground, for a heavy storm of wind and rain had been going on all day. The pilot remonstrated, but the captain approved; and if the fireman had not suddenly let out the fires and detained us two hours, we might have got our men on board and returned comfortably soon after dark. But the delay cost us the precious daylight. It was night before the last man was got on board. There were fifty-six of them,—ten very sick ones.

The boat had a little shelter-cabin. As we were laying the mattresses on the floor, while the doctors were finding the men, the captain stopped us, refusing to let us put typhoid fever cases below the deck,—on account of the crew, he said,—and threatening to push off at once from the shore. Mrs. Howland and I looked at him. I did the terrible, and she the pathetic; and he abandoned the contest. The return passage was rather an anxious one. The river is much obstructed with sunken ships and trees, and we had to feel our way, slackening speed every ten minutes. If we had been alone, it would not have mattered; but to have fifty men upon our hands unable to move was too heavy a responsibility not to make us anxious. The captain and the pilot said the boat was leaking (we heard the water gurgling under our feet), and they remarked casually that the river was "four fathoms deep about there;" but we saw their motive and were not scared. We were safe alongside the "Spaulding" by midnight; but Mr. Olmsted's tone of voice as he said, "You don't know how glad I am to see you," showed how much he had been worried . . .[47]

305. *Life, Letters and Journals of Louisa May Alcott*

[Louisa May Alcott (1832–1888), American novelist and writer of children's books, served as a nurse at the Union Hospital at Georgetown, D.C., for six weeks in 1862–63. She is best known for her books, *Little Women* and *Little Men*. Some of her poems and short stories were published in the *Atlantic Monthly*. Her letters from Georgetown (excerpts from which follow) were first published in the *Boston Commonwealth*. Miss Alcott also wrote of her war experiences in a book for children called *Hospital Sketches and Companion Fireside Stories*.[48] A quotation from this book is given in Reading No. 306.]

Journal kept at the Hospital, Georgetown, D.C.

1862

November—Thirty years old. Decided to go to Washington as nurse if I could find a place. Help needed, and I love nursing, and must let out my pent-up energy in some new way. Winter is always a hard and a dull time and if I am away there is one less to feed and warm and worry over.

I want new experiences, and am sure to get 'em if I go. So I've sent in my name, and bide my time writing tales, to leave all snug behind me, and mending up my old clothes,—for nurses don't need nice things, thank Heaven!

1863

Monday [January] 4th—I shall record the events of a day as a sample of the days I spend:—

Up at six, dress by gaslight, run through my ward and throw up the windows, though the men grumble and shiver; but the air is bad enough to breed a pestilence; and as no notice is taken of our frequent appeals for better ventilation, I must do what I can. Poke up the fire, add blankets, joke, coax, and command; but continue to open doors and windows as if life depended upon it. Mine does, and doubtless many another, for a more perfect pestilence-box than this house I never saw,—cold, damp, dirty, full of vile odors from wounds, kitchens, washrooms, and stables. No competent head, male or female, to right matters, and a jumble of good, bad, and indifferent nurses, surgeons, and attendants, to complicate the chaos still more.

After this unwelcome progress through my stifling ward, I go to breakfast with what appetite I may; find the uninvitable fried beef, salt butter, husky bread, and washy coffee; listen to the clack of eight women and a dozen men,—the first silly, stupid, or possessed of one idea; the last absorbed with their breakfast and themselves to a degree that is both ludicrous and provoking, for all the dishes are ordered down the table full and returned empty; the conversation is entirely among themselves, and each announces his opinion with an air of importance that frequently causes me to choke in my cup, or bolt my meals with undignified speed lest a laugh betray to these famous beings that a "chiel's amang them takin' notes."

Till noon I trot, trot, giving out rations, cutting up food for helpless "boys," washing faces, teaching my attendants how beds are made or floors are swept, dressing wounds, taking Dr. F. P.'s orders (privately wishing all the time that he would be more gentle with my big babies), dusting tables, sewing bandages, keeping my tray tidy, rushing up and down after pillows, bed-linen, sponges, books, and directions, till it seems as if I would joyfully pay down all I possess for fifteen minutes' rest. At twelve the big bell rings, and up comes dinner for the boys, who are always ready for it, and never entirely satisfied. Soup, meat, potatoes, and bread is the bill of fare. Charley Thayer, the attendant, travels up and down the room serving out the rations, saving little for himself, yet always thoughtful for his mates, and patient as a woman with their helplessness. When dinner is over, some sleep, many read, and others want letters written. This I like to do, for they put in such odd things, and express their ideas so comically, I have great fun interiorally, while as grave as possible exteriorly. A few of the men word their para-graphs well and make excellent letters. John's was the best of all I wrote. The answering of letters from friends after some one has died is the saddest and hardest duty a nurse has to do.

Supper at five sets everyone to running that can run; and when that flurry is over, all settle down for the evening amusements, which consist of newspapers, gossip, the doctor's last round, and, for such as need them, the final doses for the night. At nine the bell rings, gas is turned down, and day nurses go to bed. Night nurses go on duty, and sleep and death have the house to themselves.

My work is changed to night watching, or half night and half day,—from twelve to twelve. I like it, as it leaves me time for a morning run, which is what I need to keep well, for bad air, food, and water, working and watching, are getting to be too much for me. I trot up and down the streets in all directions, sometimes to the Heights, then half way to Washington, again to the hill, over which the long trains of army wagons are constantly vanishing and ambulances appearing. That way the fighting lies, and I long to follow.

Ordered to keep my room, being threatened with pneumonia. Sharp pain in the side, cough, fever, and dizziness. A pleasant prospect for a lonely soul five hundred miles from home! Sit and sew on the boys' clothes, write letters, sleep, and read, try to talk and keep merry, but fail decidedly, as day after day goes, and I feel no better. Dream awfully, and wake unre-freshed, think of home, and wonder if I am to die here, as Mrs. R., the matron is likely to do. Feel too miserable to care much what becomes of me. Dr. S. creaks up twice a day to feel my pulse, give me doses, and asks if I am at all consumptive or some other cheering question. Dr. O. examines my lungs and looks sober. Dr. J. haunts the room, coming by day and night with wood, cologne, books, and messes, like a motherly little man as he is. Nurses, fussy and anxious, matron dying, and everything very gloomy. They want me to go home, but I *won't* yet.

January 16th—Was amazed to see Father enter the room that morning, having been telegraphed to by order of Mrs. R. without asking leave. I was very angry at first, though glad to see him, because I knew I should have to go. Mrs. D. and Miss Dix came, and pretty Miss W., to take me to Willard's to be cared for by them. I wouldn't go, preferring to keep still, being pretty ill by that time.

On the 21st I suddenly decided to go home, feeling very strangely, and dreading to be worse. Mrs. R. died, and that frightened the doctors about me; for my trouble was the same,—typhoid pneumonia. Father, Miss K., and Lizzie T. went with me. Miss Dix brought a basket of bottles of wine, tea, medicine, and cologne, besides a little blanket and pillow, a fan, and a testament. She is a kind old soul, but very queer and arbitrary.

Was very sorry to go, and "my boys" seemed sorry to have me. Quite a flock came to see me off; but I was too sick to have but a dim idea of what was going on . . .[49]

306. Louisa May Alcott. *Hospital Sketches and Companion Fireside Stories*

[In this account, written for children, Miss Alcott named herself "Nurse Periwinkle." In a postscript the date and place are given as, "Concord, April, 1863."]

[Washington]
"They've come! they've come! hurry up, ladies—You're wanted."
"Who have come? The rebels?"
This sudden summons in the gray dawn was somewhat startling to a three days' nurse like myself, and, as the thundering knock came at our door, I sprang up in my bed, prepared
                    "To gird my woman's form,
                    And on the ramparts die,"
if necessary; but my room-mate took it more coolly, and, as she began a rapid toilet, answered my bewildered question,—
"Bless you, no child; it's the wounded from Fredericksburg; forty ambulances are at the door, and we shall have our hands full in fifteen minutes."
"What shall we have to do?"
"Wash, dress, feed, warm and nurse them for the next three months, I dare say. Eighty beds are ready, and we were getting impatient for the men to come. Now you will begin to see hospital life in earnest, for you won't probably find time to sit down all day, and may think yourself fortunate if you get to bed by midnight. Come to me in the ball-room when you are ready; the worst cases are always carried there, and I shall need your help . . ."
Having a taste for "ghastliness," I had rather longed for the wounded to arrive, for rheumatism wasn't heroic, neither was liver complaint, or measles . . .
A second bang at the door . . . and Joey (a six years' old contraband,) announced—
"Miss Blank is jes' wild fer ye, and says fly around right away. They's comin' in, I tell yer, heaps on 'em—one was took out dead, and I see him,—hi! warn't he a goner!"

.   .   .   .   .   .

The sight of several stretchers, each with its legless, armless, or desperately wounded occupant, entering my ward, admonished me that I was there to work, not to wonder or weep; so I corked up my feelings, and returned to the path of duty, which was rather "a hard road to travel" just then. . . . Presently, Miss Blank tore me from my refuge behind piles of one-sleeved shirts, odd socks, bandages and lint; put basin, sponge, towels, and a block of brown soap into my hands, with these appalling directions:
"Come, my dear, begin to wash as fast as you can. Tell them to take off

socks, coats and shirts. Scrub them well, put on clean shirts, and the attendants will finish them off, and lay them in bed."

If she had requested me to shave them all, or dance a hornpipe on the stove funnel, I should have been less staggered; but to scrub some dozen lords of creation at a moment's notice, was really—really—. However, there was no time for nonsense, and having resolved when I came to do everything I was bid, I drowned my scruples in my wash-bowl, clutched my soap manfully, and assuming a business-like air, made a dab at the first dirty speciman I saw, bent on performing my task *vi et armis* if necessary . . .

Having done up our human wash, and laid it out to dry, the second syllable of our version of the word War-fare was enacted with much success. Great trays of bread, meat, soup and coffee appeared; and both nurses and attendants turned waiters, serving bountiful rations to all who could eat. . . . It was a lively scene; the long room lined with rows of beds, each filled by an occupant, whom water, shears, and clean raiment had transformed from a dismal ragamuffin into a recumbent hero, with a cropped head. To and fro rushed matrons, maids, and convalescent "boys" skirmishing with knives and forks; retreating with empty plates; marching and counter-marching, with unvaried success; while the clash of busy spoons made most inspiring music for the charge of our Light Brigade . . .

All having eaten, drank, and rested, the surgeons began their rounds; and I took my first lesson in the art of dressing wounds.

. . . .

It was long past noon before these repairs were even partially made; and, having got the bodies of my boys into something like order, the next task was to minister to their minds, by writing letters to anxious souls at home; answering questions, reading papers, taking possession of money and valuables; for the eighth commandment was reduced to a very fragmentary condition, both by the blacks and whites, who ornamented our hospital with their presence . . .

At five o'clock a great bell rang, and the attendants flew, not to arms, but to their trays, to bring supper, when a second uproar announced that it was ready . . .

Then came the doctor's evening visit; the administration of medicines; washing feverish faces; smoothing tumbled beds; wetting wounds; singing lullabies; and preparations for the night. By twelve, the last labor of love was done; the last "good night" spoken; and, if any needed a reward for that day's work, they surely received it, in the silent eloquence of those long lines of faces, showing pale and peaceful in the shaded rooms, as we quitted them followed by grateful glances that lighted us to bed, where rest, the sweetest, made our pillows soft, while Night and Nature took our places, filling that great house of pain with the healing miracles of Sleep, and his diviner brother, Death.[50]

307. *Crusader and Feminist: Letters of Jane Grey Swisshelm*

[Jane Grey (Cannon) Swisshelm (1815–1884) was born in Pittsburgh of Scotch-Irish parents. At the age of nineteen she married James Swisshelm. In 1842, under a pen name, she began her writing career with stories and poems for the *Dollar Newspaper* and *Neal's Saturday Gazette* of Philadelphia. A few years later she became the editor of the *Pittsburgh Saturday Visiter,* a leading liberal newspaper. Separated from her husband, she moved to St. Cloud, Minnesota, in 1857, where she again edited a newspaper. She was a leader in the fight against slavery and in the movement to improve the legal status of women. She was opposed by Sylvanus B. Lowrey, political dictator of northern Minnesota. During a brief period of inactivity, while waiting for her next work as clerk in the War Department to begin, she offered her services as nurse in the Campbell Hospital near Washington, D.C. She nursed the wounded throughout the war, following which she resumed her duties in the War Department.[51] Her letters, quoted here, appeared first in the *St. Cloud Democrat.* In 1934 they were collected in one volume with the above title, by the Minnesota Historical Commission.]

[*St. Cloud Democrat,* June 18, 1863]
Campbell Hospital, Washington,
May 19 [1863]

I have been here in the hospital ten days, dressing wounds, wetting wounds, giving drinks and stimulants, comforting the dying, trying to save the living. The heroic fortitude of the sufferers is sublime, yet I have held the hands of brave, strong men while shaking in a paroxysm of weeping. The doctors have committed to my special care wounded feet and ankles, and I kneel reverently by the mangled limbs of these heroes, and thank God and man for the privilege of washing them. I want whiskey—barrels of whiskey— to wash feet, and thus keep up circulation in wounded knees, legs, thighs, hips. I want lots of pickles, pickles, pickles, lemons, lemons, lemons, oranges. No well man or woman has a right to a glass of lemonade. We want it all in the hospitals to prevent gangrene. I will get lady volunteers to go through the wards of as many hospitals as I can supply with drinks. My business is dressing wounds where amputation may be avoided by special care.

Oh, God! there is plenty of work; with the great advantages of the most skillful physicians, the utmost cleanliness, and best ventilation, the exceeding and beautiful tenderness of ward masters and nurses, there is much to do, if the right persons appeared to do it. Dr. Baxter, physician in charge, will not permit female nurses here, and from the manner in which he cares for his patients, and the reasons he gives for his decision I have no disposition to quarrel with it . . .

. . . .

[*St. Cloud Democrat,* September 17, 1863]

I have many letters from ladies asking how they may be able to devote themselves to the care of the sick and wounded soldiers; and many more asking questions about the management of hospitals. For answer, I can only "tell my experience."

I had my appointment and was receiving my salary; but for want of rooms, the Government was not ready for me to go to work. When room was ready I was to be notified.

About the first of May, when the rumors first reached the city that the army of the Potomac had crossed the Rappahannock and that a battle was in progress, I went to Miss [Dorothea L.] Dix and tendered my gratuitous services in helping to take care of the wounded either here or at the front. I had previously visited her to call her attention to the dirt and destitution of the regimental hospital of the 2d Vermont artillery, and then, as now, found her very urbane and anxious to do, and have done, all in her power to mitigate the suffering of the sick and wounded; but she informed me that their arrangements were complete and there was nothing I could do.— The points were all supplied with efficient experienced nurses; and the diet list, supplied by Government, gave the patients everything the surgeons deemed proper and anything more was not permitted.—The sending of supplies she looked upon as a mistake and as likely if not certain to be resented by surgeons as an impertinent interference. I had and have no doubt she said what circumstances justified her in believing to be strictly true; and felt that there was nothing for me to do; but, to make assurance doubly sure, I went to the Sanitary Commission and tendered my service. Here too I was assured that all arrangements were complete in as far as laborers were concerned. They would receive any amount of contributions in stores and money, but their officers, agents and distributors of every class are employed at liberal salaries and gratuitous services are not in the programme. So I settled down to *wait,* as *labor* was not supplied.[52]

308. Jane Grey Swisshelm. *Half a Century*

[This is the autobiography of Mrs. Swisshelm, published in 1880.]

Next morning while we were attending to a Colonel, and Lieutenant Colonel, both of the same regiment, and both badly wounded and just brought in, one said to the other: "My God, if our men in Fredericksburg could have a little of this care!" "Why?" said I, "I have heard that everything possible was being done for them?"

"Everything possible!" exclaimed one, and both together began the most terrible recital of the neglect and abuse of the wounded in that horrible place— . . . We set down our basins; Georgie [Willets] started in one direction and I in another to find transportation . . .

An hour after I was on the way, and Georgie a few moments in advance . . .

It was raining when we reached Fredericksburg, at four o'clock on Sabbath, and I went to the surgeon in command, reported, and asked him to send me to the worst place—the place where there was most need.

"Then I had better send you to the Old Theatre, for I can get no one to stay there!"

He gave me my appointment, and I went to a Corps Surgeon, who signed it, and advised me not to go to the theater—I could do nothing, as the place was in such dreadful condition, while I could be useful in many other places.

   .   .   .   .

The second morning of my work in the old theater, Miss Hancock came to see how I got along. She was thoroughly practical, and a most efficient laborer in the hospital field, and soon thought of something to better the condition of the man minus clothes, who lay quite near my desk and the front door, and caught my dress whenever he could to plead for a blanket. She could get no blanket; but was stationed in the Methodist Church, where there was a surgeon in charge, and everything running in regular order. In a tent adjoining, this man could be laid out of the draught and chill of that basement, and she would do her best to get some clothing for him. She sent two men with a stretcher, who took him to the church tent, where I fear he was not much better provided for than in the place he left.

   .   .   .   .   .

From the engine house I went to the Methodist church. Miss Hancock had been detailed to the General Hospital, just being established, and I found a house full of men in a sad condition. Nine o'clock, on a hot morning, and no wounds dressed; bandages dry and hard, men thirsty and feverish, nurses out watching that stream pouring through the city, and patients helpless and despondent.

I got a basin of water and a clean rag, never cared for sponges, and went from one to another, dripping water in behind those bandages to ease the torment of lint splints, brought drinks and talked to call their attention from the indefinite dread which filled the air, and got up considerable interest in— I do not remember what—but something which set them to talking.

Some wounds I dressed, and while engaged on one, a man called from the other side of the house to know what the fun was all about, when the man whose wound I was attending placed a hand on each of his sides, screamed with laughter, and replied:

"Oh, Jim! do get her to dress your wound, for I swear, she'd make a dead man laugh!"

I found some of the nurses; a surgeon came in who would, I thought, attend to them, and I went back to my post to find every man on duty.[53]

309. *South After Gettysburg Letters of Cornelia Hancock from the Army of the Potomac 1863–1865*

[These letters were written by Cornelia Hancock to various members of her family while she was serving as volunteer nurse. Miss Hancock (1839–1926) was born in southern New Jersey. After the war ended, she turned her attention to various other fields of usefulness, such as educational assistance to those unable to obtain schooling, social work in Philadelphia, and activity in housing for the underpriviledged.[54]]

The summons came on the morning of July fifth, 1863. . . . In an hour's time I was off for Philadelphia. . . . It was late in the afternoon when we reached Philadelphia. . . . Dr. Child with a number of other physicians, had determined to leave that night by the eleven o'clock train for Gettysburg. I was to accompany him.

He and the Hon. Judge Kelly had aided Miss Eliza Farnham, a well-known public-spirited woman, with a number of others of "suitable age" to get passes as volunteer nurses. The ladies in the party were many years older than myself, and I was under the especial care of Miss Farnham. . . . The morning found us in Baltimore where there was stir and some knowledge of events. Here Dorothea Dix appeared on the scene. She looked the nurses over and pronounced them all suitable except me. She immediately objected to my going farther on the score of my youth and rosy cheeks. I was then just twenty-three years of age. In those days it was considered indecorous for angels of mercy to appear otherwise than gray-haired and spectacled. Such a thing as a hospital corps of comely young maiden nurses, possessing grace and good looks was then unknown. Miss Farnham explained that she was under obligation to my friends who had helped her get proper credentials. The discussion waxed warm and I have no idea what conclusion they came to, for I settled the question myself by getting on the car and staying in my seat until the train pulled out of the city of Baltimore. They had not forcibly taken me from the train, so I got into Gettysburg the night of July sixth—where the need was so great that there was no further cavil about age.

. . . . . .

General Hospital Gettysburg, Pa.
Aug. 6th, 1863.

My dear Sister

We have all our men moved now to General Hospital. I am there, too, but the order in regard to women nurses has not yet been issued, and I do not know what my fate will be; I only know that the boys want me to stay very much, and I have been assigned to ward E. It is a great deal nicer here except that I have but fourteen of my old boys which is very trying—it is just like parting with one's family. I go to see the boys and some of them cry that I cannot stay. I have the first four tents abreast of the cook house, the handiest tents in the whole hospital. I have Steward Olmstead for my *headquarter influence,* and we have an elderly doctor for our ward. I have a large hospital tent and sleep with three other ladies, so unless I struggle very hard to find it my friends need fear no harm for me. I am better than I am at home. I feel so good when I wake up in the morning. I received a letter announcing Sallie S's death. It does not appear to me as if one death is anything to me now. I do want my watch very much indeed, if you can get any show of a safe way of sending it—do so; I want my own gold one. I expect I shall be able to draw twelve dollars from the government now, but if thee can draw any money for hospital purposes or for me, send it along, for it is a poor place to be without money. If there should be an opportunity to send my purple dress, best bonnet and mantilla, I should like to have them; this hospital will not stay here more than three weeks and nobody knows what I may want to do by that time. I may come home if there is no other battle. Dr. Dwinelle gave me a splendid recommendation to Dr. Chamberlain, Surgeon in charge here. I am good friends with Sanitary, Christian, and all here, if it only lasts. One of the boys died yesterday, and one had his leg amputated fresh. Cadet Brown I sent to your house to tell you I was well. Col. Colville is getting some better; he expects Dr. Child here.

No citizens are allowed in Camp without a pass only after four o'clock. The militia go around after dark and pick up stragglers to take them out of camp. The other night they asked me if I was a detailed nurse. As it was before I was sworn in, I had to say "No." They said their orders were peremptory, so I would have to go, but Steward Olmstead appeared and told them that I was all right, so they went away. I expect I shall be in the guard house!—but that is only a part of soldiering if I am. I do not meddle or make up with any one here but the ward master, doctor of our ward and Steward Olmstead. We have twenty women here about, some of them are excellent, but a more willful, determined set you never saw. Send this letter to mother for I hate to take the time to write often.

C. Hancock

Fredericksburg, Va.
[1864]

My dear Mother

I was the first and only Union woman in the city. I believe today there were some of Miss Dix' nurses came thru. I have good quarters. We calculated there are 14,000 wounded in the town; the Secesh help none, so you may know there is suffering equal to any thing anyone ever saw, almost as bad as Gettysburg, only we have houses, and churches for the men. I am well, have worked harder than I ever did in my life; there was no food but hard tack to give the men so I turned in and dressed their wounds. It was all that could be done. I hear from my friends at the front one by one. Almost every one I knew was shot dead except the Doctor. Some of them are taken prisoners, Dr. Aiken for one; Dr. Dudley was safe last night. Lieut. Fogg was shot dead, so was Capt. Madison—this battle is still raging. I am glad I am here but I really thought my heart would break as one after another they told me was dead. If they only accomplish getting to Richmond. If not, it is a dear battle. There is very heavy firing today. I hope Dr. Dudley will get· thru safe. He sent a Doctor to see me, told him he knew I would get thru. He is out on the front with his Regt . . .

I am going out on the front to our new div. hospit. in a few days but you need not be concerned . . .

Thine in haste
Cornelia Hancock [55]

310. Mary Livermore. *My Story of the War: A Woman's Narrative of Four Years' Personal Experience*

[Mary Ashton (Rice) Livermore (1820–1905), American reformer and ardent advocate of woman suffrage, temperance, and higher education for women, served with the United States Sanitary Commission during the Civil War. She later edited and contributed to the *Agitator,* a suffrage paper. The wife of a Universalist minister, she assisted her husband in editing a religious weekly, *The New Covenant,* from 1857 to 1869. With Frances E. Willard she edited *A Woman of the Century: Biographical Sketches of Leading American Women,* published in 1893.[56]]

My second visit to the Cairo hospitals, was made in company with Miss Mary Safford, then a resident of Cairo. She commenced her labors immediately when Cairo was occupied by our troops. If she was not the first woman in the country to enter upon hospital and camp relief, she was certainly the first in the west. There was no system, no organization, no knowledge of what to do, and no means with which to work. As far as possible she brought order out of chaos, systematized the first rude hospitals, and with her own means, aided by a wealthy brother, furnished necessaries, when they could be obtained in no other way.

Surgeons and officers everywhere opposed her; but she disarmed them by the sweetness of her manner and her speech; and she did what she pleased. . . . She threw herself into hospital work with such energy, and forgetfulness of self, that she broke down utterly before the end of the second year of the war.

.   .   .   .

The hospital at Mound City occupied a block of brick stores, built before the war, to accomodate the prospective commerce of the town. . . . A Shaker-like cleanliness and sweetness of atmosphere pervaded the various wards, the sheets and pillows were of immaculate whiteness, and the patients who were convalescing were cheerful and contented. The "Sisters of the Holy Cross" were employed as nurses, and by their skill, quietness, gentleness, and tenderness, were invaluable in the sick-wards. Every patient gave hearty testimony to the kindness and skill of the "Sisters." [57]

"Mother Angela" was the matron, the "Superieure," of these "Sisters"— a gifted lady, of rare cultivation and executive ability, with winning sweetness of manner. . . . The "Sisters" had nearly broken up their famous schools at South Bend, Ind., to answer the demand for nurses . . .

After the battle of Belmont she [Mother Bickerdyke] was appointed matron of the large post hospital at Cairo, which was filled with the wounded. She found time, however, to work for, and to visit daily, every other hospital in the town.

Rested and recuperated, and having placed her two sons at boarding-school where she could feel easy about them, she reported to the medical director at Memphis, as she had been ordered, in January, 1863. Immense hospitals were being organized in that city, which was also being made a base of military and medical supplies. She was first set to organizing the Adams Block Hospital, and, that completed, she was sent to Fort Pickering, to reorganize the "Smallpox Hospital." There had been great neglect here; and the loathsome place had been left uncared for until it was fouler and more noisome than an Augean stable. But Mother Bickerdyke was just the Hercules to cleanse it. She raised such a hurricane about the ears of the officials whose neglect had caused its terrible condition, as took the heads from some of them, and sent back to their regiments several private soldiers who had been detailed as nurses.[58]

311. *Personal Memoirs of John H. Brinton, Major and Surgeon, U.S.V., 1861–1865*

[Dr. John H. Brinton (1832–1907) graduated from the University of Pennsylvania (LL.D.) and received his medical degree from Jefferson College.[59] As will be seen from the following, Dr. Brinton did not favor the use of lay women as nurses in the Army hospitals.]

Mound City Hospital

But if the men were bad, the women were worse. Just at this period the craze spread among our good people that the women of the country could make themselves useful by acting as nurses for the sick and wounded. So out they came, these patriotic women of the North. The Secretary of War, the generals commanding departments, divisions or military posts, were besieged by them. By strained construction of certain paragraphs in the army regulations, and of acts of Congress, positions, paid positions, were devised for them. They besieged all officers and persons high in authority, and these, on the general military principle of sending a disagreeable person as far away as possible, sent the fair petitioners to as far away positions as they could. And the women went, and on the arrival of certain trains would stalk into the office of district commanders, and establish themselves solemnly against the walls, entrenched behind their bags and parcels. They defied all military law. There they were, and there they would stay, until some accommodation might be found for them. In self-defence the adjutant general would send them to the medical director, and he, gallantly or not, as might be his nature, would forward them to the surgeon in charge of hospitals. To him at last these wretched females would come. "They did not wish much," not they, "simply a room, a bed, a looking glass, someone to get their meals and do little things for them," and they would nurse the "sick boys of our gallant Union Army." "Simply a room." Can you fancy half a dozen or a dozen old hags, for *that* is what they were (our modern efficient trained nurses were unknown), surrounding a bewildered hospital surgeon, each one clamorous for her little wants? And rooms so scarce and looking glasses so few! And then, when you had done your best, and had often sacrificed the accomodations for the sick to their benefit, how little gratitude did one receive! Usually nothing but complaints, fault-finding as to yourself, and backbiting as to companions of their own sex. In short this female nurse business was a great trial to all the men concerned, and to me at Mound City became intolerable.

I determined, therefore, to try to get rid of them from the Mound City Hospital. In answer to my request to the Catholic authorities of, I think, North and South Bend, Indiana, a number of sisters were sent down to act as nurses in the hospital. Those sent were from a teaching and not from a nursing order, but in a short time they adapted themselves admirably to their new duties. I have forgotten the exact title of the order to which they belonged,—I think they were sisters of Notre Dame. I remember their black and white dresses, and I remember also, that when I asked the Mother who accompanied them, what accomodations they required, the answer was, "One room, Doctor," and there were in all, I think, fourteen or fifteen of them. So I procured good nurses for my sick and the whole tribe of sanitary "Mrs. Brundages" passed away. The sick patients gained by the change, but for a few days I was the most abused man in that department, for the newspapers gave me no mercy.

. . . .

Whenever we were badly beaten and when popular feeling was dissatisfied, Stanton was in the habit, at his own instance, of issuing or peremptorily directing the issuing of, an appeal to the North, in the first place for lint and bandages, and secondly, for surgeons and nurses. As a natural result, the Surgeon-General's office would be flooded with boxes of linen scrappings and home-made bandages, which would be piled away in the stables and yards, or sent off where really not wanted, inasmuch as the articles themselves were usually not in shape or condition for issuance to hospitals, already usually fully stocked. Then, too, both doctors and nurses were most often of little use. Most were not competent; they were untrained, did not know what to do, or how to take care of soldiers,—still less could they take care of themselves. As for the women, sanitarians or nurse corps, they were terrible,—helpless, irritable and unhappy; each one thinking herself of much importance, and acting under the direct orders of the Secretary of War, and very often indeed they had seen him before starting. What to do with these poor women was indeed a problem. They would sit in your office, if you happened to be a Medical Director, by the hour at the time, each one with an enamelled leather bag between her feet waiting to be sent somewhere, anywhere.[60]

312. Walt Whitman's Articles in the *New York Leader*, 1862

[Walt Whitman (1819–1892), American poet, served as an errand boy in a lawyer's office, was a country schoolteacher, and edited several newspapers. In 1855, *Leaves of Grass* was published, but it was not successful until Emerson wrote a letter commending it.[61] In 1862 Whitman went to Virginia to care for his brother who was wounded, and remained as unofficial nurse in the hospitals. Much of his record of the Civil War is contained in *Specimen Days and Collect* (1882–1883), *The Wound Dresser* (1898), and *Sequel to Drum-Taps* (1866). In his later life Whitman was a clerk in the Indian Bureau and was employed in the Attorney General's office.[62]

Before going to the front in 1862, he contributed a series of articles dealing with the Broadway Hospital, to the *New York Leader*. At this time he was visiting the sick and wounded in this hospital. The articles are signed "Velsor Brush." [63]]

[City Photographs II The Broadway Hospital]

.   .   .   .   .   .

The Nurses

Some of the nurses are real characters, and favorable specimens, at that. I saw a vigorous-looking women a Swedess by birth, Mrs. Jackson, who has been a nurse here for thirty years. I saw another nurse among the soldiers in the North Building, Mrs. Mack, whose good size and healthy and handsome appearance, I thought ought to do good, salutary service, even just to see her moving around among the sick.

Aunty Robinson

But by what I hear from the doctors in the Hospital, no sketch of that establishment could be fair unless it put in a word about Aunty Robinson, a colored nurse, who has officiated there in that capacity for over twenty years. This good creature has all the appearance of one of the most favorable samples of the Southern *mammy,* or house nurse, in the families of the high old Carolina and Virginia planters. She has big old-fashioned gold ear-rings in her ears, and wears a clean, bright red and yellow blue handkerchief around her head, and such an expression on her face, that I at once made up my mind, if ever I should be unfortunate enough to go to the Hospital as a patient, I should want to be nursed by Aunty Robinson.[64]

313. Walt Whitman. *Specimen Days and Collect.*

[Although *Specimen Days* was published in 1882–1883, most of it was probably written twenty years before. The most useful part of it for nursing history is concerned with Whitman's hospital experiences in Washington during the Civil War. It had been published in 1875 as *Memoranda During the War.*[65]]

Wednesday, February *4th* [1863]. Visited Armory Square hospital, went pretty thoroughly through wards E and D. Supplied paper and envelopes to all who wish'd—as usual, found plenty of men who needed those articles. Wrote letters. Saw and talked with two or three members of the Brooklyn 14th regt. A poor fellow in Ward D, with a fearful wound in a fearful condition, was having some loose splinters of bone taken from the neighborhood of the wound. The operation was long, and one of great pain—yet, after it was well commenced, the soldier bore it in silence. He sat up, propp'd—was much wasted—had lain a long time quiet in one position (not for days only but weeks,) a bloodless, brown-skinn'd face, with eyes full of determination—belonged to a New York regiment. There was an unusual cluster of surgeons, medical Cadets, nurses, etc. around his bed—I thought the whole thing was done with tenderness, and done well. . . . I liked the woman nurse in Ward E—I noticed how she sat a long time by a poor fellow who just had, that morning, in addition to his other sickness, bad hemorrhage—she gently assisted him, reliev'd him of the blood, holding a cloth to his mouth, as he coughed it up—he was so weak he could only just turn his head over on the pillow.

.   .   .   .

June 18 [1863]
Bed 3, Ward E, Armory, has a great hankering for pickles, something pungent. After consulting the doctor, I gave him a small bottle of horseradish; also some apples; also a book. Some of the nurses are excellent. The woman nurse in this ward I like very much. (Mrs. Wright—a year afterwards I found her in Mansion house hospital, Alexandria—she is a perfect nurse.)

.   .   .   .

I have noticed through most of the hospitals that as long as there is any chance for a man, no matter how bad he may be, the surgeon and nurses work hard, sometimes with curious tenacity, for his life, doing everything, and keeping somebody by him to execute the doctor's orders, and minister to him every minute night and day. See that screen there. As you advance through the dusk of early candlelight, a nurse will step forth on tiptoe, and silently but imperiously forbid you to make any noise, or perhaps to come near at all.

. . . . . .

Female Nurses for Soldiers

There are many women in one position or another, among the hospitals, mostly as nurses here in Washington, and among the military stations; quite a number of them young ladies acting as volunteers. They are a help in certain ways, and deserve to be mention'd with respect. Then it remains to be distinctly said that few or no young ladies, under the irresistible conventions of society, answer the practical requirements of nurses for soldiers. Middle-aged or healthy and good condition'd elderly women, mothers of children, are always best. Many of the wounded must be handled. A hundred things which cannot be gainsay'd must occur and must be done. The presence of a good middle-aged or elderly woman, the magnetic touch of hands, the expressive features of the mother, the silent soothing of her presence, her words, her knowledge and privileges arrived at only through having had children, are precious and final qualifications. It is a natural faculty that is required; it is not merely having a genteel young woman at a table in a ward. One of the finest nurses I met was a red-faced illiterate old Irish woman; I have seen her take the poor wasted naked boys so tenderly up in her arms. There are plenty of excellent clean old black women that would make tip-top nurses.[66]

314. Walt Whitman's Articles in the *New York Times*

[The two brief quotations below are from letters which Walt Whitman wrote to his mother during the war. A number of these were published in the *New York Times,* and later included in the volume entitled *The Wound Dresser.*[67]]

The military hospitals, convalescent camps, etc., in Washington and its neighborhood, sometimes contain over fifty thousand sick and wounded men. . . . Upon a few of these hospitals I have been almost daily calling as a missionary, on my own account, for the sustenance and consolation of some of the most needy cases of sick and dying men, for the last two months . . .

Every ward has a ward-master, and generally a nurse for every ten or twelve men. A ward surgeon has generally, two wards—although this varies. Some of the wards have a woman nurse; the Armory-square wards have some very good ones. The one in Ward E is one of the best.

W. W.

New York Times, Dec. 11, 1864.

. . . For nurses, middle-aged women and mothers of families are best. I am compelled to say young ladies, however refined, educated, and benevolent, do not succeed as army nurses, though their motives are noble; neither

414

do the Catholic nuns, among these home-born American young men, mothers full of motherly feelings, and however illiterate, but bringing reminiscences of home, and with the magnetic touch of hands, are the true women nurses. Many of the wounded are between fifteen and twenty years of age.

I should say that the Government, from my observation, is always full of anxiety and liberality toward the sick and wounded. The system in operation in the permanent hospitals is good, and the money flows without stint. But the details have to be left to hundreds and thousands of subordinates and officials. Among these, laziness, heartlessness, gouging, and incompetency are more or less prevalent. Still I consider the permanent hospitals, generally, well conducted.

W. W.

315. Correspondence of Pastor Passavant

[Pastor William A. Passavant,[68] Lutheran pastor of Pittsburgh, had sent some of the deaconesses from his institution to participate, under the direction of Miss Dix, in the nursing in the war hospitals.]

From *The Missionary* (date not given), by Pastor Passavant.

The first night of the Sisters among the sick was that of Thursday, the twenty-third, a memorable day in the future of our nation. A soldier of one of the Brooklyn regiments had accidentally shot himself that morning, and life seemed to be fast ebbing away. One of the Sisters was watching by his bedside and a second was ministering to the other poor sufferers who filled the hall . . .

From letters to Pastor Passavant's mother (date not given).

Our Sisters write often from Washington and speak very encouragingly. Miss Dix appears to be much pleased with them and is determined to carry out some necessary reforms through their aid. I cannot enter into particulars of the nursing work in Washington. It would take me hours to talk all over. Several of the papers speak very honorably of our Sisters in the hospital in the Capitol building . . .

The Sisters are doing good work in Washington, and, I presume, went down to Fort Monroe with Miss Dix on the news of the late sad battle. They greatly desire me to be in Washington to aid Miss Dix, as they fear she cannot endure the great fatigue and exertion of her position.

Letters from Dorothea L. Dix to Pastor Passavant

Dear Sir, I may not have the evidence to go by to show the value I have placed on the services rendered by Sister Elizabeth and by other Sisters in this beloved Christian duty. Although we would like to see the end of this

415

unhappy war, it is my purpose to have a substantial evidence made of my appreciation of our friends and their toil in the cause of humanity.

Yours cordially,

D. L. Dix.

Dec. 26, 1861, Washington.

Washington, Oct. 5, 1862.

Dear Sir, Probably no request was ever more reluctantly complied with by any person more or less concerned in the affairs of a hospital than is your recalling Sister Barbara, from the Military Hospital service to a more limited and remote field of action. I have still to say if it be at all possible to construct other plans for another point that we all should most gratefully receive and welcome our precious friend and nurse again to this field of labor.

Yours with esteem,

D. L. Dix.[69]

316. The Diary of Sister Anthony O'Connell

[Sister Anthony O'Connell, who came to be known as the "Angel of the Battlefield" because of her work in the Civil War, was a member of the Sisters of Charity of Cincinnati. The excerpt from her diary, quoted below, is undated, but would have been written between May 1 and August 15, 1861.[70] The Tenth Regiment Hospital, with an encampment of 12,000 men, was located at Camp Dennison, about fifteen miles from Cincinnati on the Little Miami Railroad.[71] The Sisters were also at Cumberland, New Creek, and Shiloh, and, after their return to Cincinnati, cared for the soldiers sent up the river to them.[72]]

The Most Rev. Archbishop Purcell and Mayor Hatch called upon us at the desire of Gov. Dennison, May 1, 1861 and requested that a colony of Sisters of Charity be sent to Camp Dennison to attend the sick soldiers, the worst form of measles had broken out among them and they needed immediate attention.

Sisters Anthony and Sophia were the first Sisters sent to Camp Dennison, but Sisters Bernadine, Alphonsa, Lawrence and Magdalen followed soon after.[73]

317. *Baltimore Catholic Mirror*, February 25, 1862

[The following letter to the editors, signed simply "E," is in the Archives of the Sisters of Charity at Mount St. Joseph, Ohio.]

Messrs. Editors: It is with great pleasure I tell you that eight Sisters of Charity have recently arrived in our Mountain City from Cincinnati. They have come to take charge of the military hospitals here. A considerable number of soldiers from General Lauder's division have fallen sick, in consequence of the inclemency of the weather, to which they were more or less exposed, while encamped on the banks of the Potomac and Patterson's Creek. . . . Our Community was much gratified and delighted at the unexpected appearance in their midst, of these estimable and most praiseworthy ladies, who have so devotedly received the appellation of "Angels of Mercy". . . .

Already, I have been informed, the good fruits of the Sisters' labors are manifest with regard to the patients confined in the two hospitals under their charge. The sick men seem astonished and cannot comprehend the devotedness, the zeal and unwearying patience of the Sisters. Some declared that had the Sisters been here from the beginning, not a man would have died. The cleanliness of these two hospitals, the improvement in the patients, the great change for the better in the cooking and preparation of food suitable for the delicate constitutions of the sick, are subjects of grateful remarks by the patients, who all combine to sound the praises of their inestimable nurses.

E.

318. Oscar L. Jackson. *The Colonel's Diary* . . .

[Colonel Jackson (1840–1920) commanded the 63rd Regiment during the Civil War. At the end of the war he practiced law and helped to codify the laws of Pennsylvania.[74]]

[Mar. 14, 1861—June 16, 1863].

October 4th to November 20th. During this time I remained in hospital on Seminary Hill at Corinth and, after three weeks, gradually improved. My colored woman, Jane, waited on me with as much care as if I had been a brother. Night and day she bathed my wound. Frequently I begged in vain for her to go to her own quarters and take some rest, as other nurses would tend me. She would say, "Oh, Captain, they will forget, and you know how soon the fever rises when I quit bathing your brow." . . . I am much indebted to her for her care. In fact, the surgeon says I never would have got well if I had not been carefully watched.[75]

319. Kate Cumming. *A Journal of Hospital Life in the Confederate Army of Tennessee from the Battle of Shiloh to the End of the War*

[The writer, a Southern woman, gives a firsthand account of the care of the sick in the Confederate Army of Tennessee. The *Journal,* probably written with no thought of publication, is given as it was written. It is on the whole, accurate as to dates.[76] The narrative was rewritten and published in 1895 as *Gleanings from Southland.* It is evident from it that some of the surgeons in the Confederate Army shared the prejudice of their Northern brethren against women nurses in the hospitals.]

April 7, 1862.

After we returned to Mrs. Haughton's, I was quite amused in listening to her granddaughter's account of a visit which they had just made to the hospital. It seems that the surgeons entertain great prejudice against admitting ladies into the hospital in the capacity of nurses. . . . Is the noble example of Miss Nightingale to pass for nothing? I trust not.

April 12 [1862], Corinth.

I sat up all night, bathing the men's wounds and giving them water. Every one attending to them seemed completely worn out. Some of the doctors told me that they had scarcely slept since the battle. As far as I have seen, the surgeons are very kind to the wounded, and nurse as well as doctor them.

The men are lying all over the house, on their blankets, just as they were brought from the battle-field. They are in the hall, on the gallery, and crowded into very small rooms. The foul air from this mass of human beings at first made me giddy and sick, but I soon got over it. We have to walk, and when we give the men any thing kneel, in blood and water; but we think nothing of it at all. There was much suffering among the patients last night; one old man groaned all the time. He was about sixty years of age, and had lost a leg. He lived near Corinth, and had come there the morning of the battle to see his two sons, who were in the army, and he could not resist shouldering his musket and going into the fight. I comforted him as well as I could. He is a religious man and prayed nearly all night.

Another, a very young man, was wounded in the leg and through the lungs, had a most excruciating cough, and seemed to suffer awfully. One fine-looking man had a dreadful wound in the shoulder. Every time I bathed it he thanked me, and seemed grateful. He died this morning before breakfast. Men who were in the room with him told me that he prayed all night. I trust that he is now at rest, far from this dreary world of strife and bloodshed. I could fill whole pages with descriptions of the scenes before me.

Other ladies have their special patients, whom they never leave. One of them, from Natchez, Miss., has been constantly by a young man, badly wounded, ever since she came here, and the doctors say that she has been the means of saving his life. Many of the others are doing the same. Mrs. Ogden and the Mobile ladies are below stairs. I have not even time to speak to them. Mr. Miller is doing much good; he is comforting the suffering and dying, and has already baptised some.

This morning, when passing the front door, a man asked me if I had any thing to eat, which I could give to some men at the depot awaiting transportation on the cars. He said they had eaten nothing for some days. Some of the ladies assisting me, we took them hot coffee, bread, and meat. The poor fellows ate eagerly, and seemed so thankful. One of the men, who was taking care of them, asked me where I was from. When I replied Mobile, he said that Mobile was the best place in the Confederacy. He was a member of the Twenty-first Alabama Regiment; I have forgotten his name. I have been busy all day, and can scarcely tell what I have been doing; I have not taken time even to eat, and certainly not time to sit down. There seems to be no order. All do as they please. We have men for nurses, and the doctors complain very much, at the manner in which they are appointed; they are detailed from the different regiments, like guards. We have a new set every few hours. I can not see how it is possible for them to take proper care of the men, as nursing is a thing that has to be learned, and we should select our best men for it—the best, not physically, but morally—as I am certain that none but good, conscientious persons will ever do justice to the patients.

January 16 [1863].
[Chattanooga]

I have just returned from another horseback ride with Mrs. N[Newsome]; we visited the small-pox hospital, but were not allowed to go in; about six of Mrs. N.'s nurses were there as patients. She inquired how they were, and if they needed any thing. They have very nice quarters, and one of our ablest army surgeons—Dr. Kratz—to attend them. The mortality from this loathsome disease is little or nothing.

[Mobile], Feb. 10 [1863].

I found few of the patients whom I had left here; some have died, and others have gone to other hospitals. Mr. Noland and Mr. Kelly, two of our best nurses, are not expected to live.

[Mobile], [Feb. 23, '63].

The doctors do not like the wives of the men to come and nurse them; they say they invariably kill them with kindness. There are some ladies who come to take care of their relatives, who seem to understand nursing, and are a great help, not only to their own folks, but to others around them; these the doctors do not object to.

September 28, [1863].—Last evening, Rev. Dr. Husten made a speech at the depot, calling on the people to send up provisions and nurses to Chickamauga, for the purpose of feeding and nursing the wounded, as General Bragg has gone with his whole army to take Chattanooga, and requires the services of every man who is able to travel, and there are not enough left to take care of the sufferers. Our cooks have been up all night long, cooking food to send up. The same has been done in all the other hospitals.

This morning Mrs. Johnston called, and I went with her to a meeting, which was held in town, about the wounded.

419

Dr. Heustis addressed us, and presented a picture of suffering that would have wrung the heart of the most hardened, and said he had only told us about our own men; that if they were in such distress we could guess in what state the prisoners were.

He told us the principal thing needed was something to eat, and he believed that in one place where the men were lying, that if a basket full of biscuits was put down in the midst of them, they would let out a shout of joy that would rend the air. He had worked day and night while there, dressing wounds and giving the men water to drink, and said he believed many persons could be kept busy doing nothing but the latter. He urged all the men to go that could possibly do so; said that ladies could not go yet, as there was no place for them to stay. The enemy had destroyed a portion of the railroad, and the wounded had to be taken to a place called the "Burnt Shed," some twenty miles distant from the battlefield, there to await transportation on the cars.

Colonel Colyer of Tennessee made a very stirring speech, and was ready himself to go. A collection was then taken up, and many hundreds of dollars given. Mrs. J. introduced me to Dr. Heustis. I told him I was very anxious to go; I knew I could get some place to stay, as I was well acquainted in that neighborhood; the Burnt Shed being only a short distance from Cherokee Springs. He tried to persuade me not to think of it. On my way home I met our chaplain, Mr. Green, who told me he was going, and that if I wished I could go with him, and stay with a very nice lady, a friend of his. I intend leaving this afternoon, and am busy collecting what I can take with me. Dr. Devine has just received a box full of delicacies from Mississippi, for troops from that state. It is impossible to send any thing to the army at present. He has given me some nice wine and other things. —

Some of the ladies of the place intend going up in a few days, but none are ready to go at present. Mrs. Colonel Griffin gave me a black man for a servant.

February 20, [1865].

Since my return I have visited three of the hospitals; they have very few patients. The Levert (so called in honor of the late Dr. L. of this place) is set apart for officers. Our old patient, Captain Curran, is in it, and, much to my astonishment, is recovering.

This hospital is a small one, but seems perfect in every department. The surgeon—Dr. Redwood—was captured at Shiloh, and was for some time practicing in prisons in the North, and has his hospital arranged as they have them there. A hospital like his is all very well in a place like Mobile; but I am afraid, if he had a few runs like we have had, it would not be quite so nice. Captain C. asked me if I would like to be in such a one. I answered him no; for then I might forget we had a war on hand, with all these nice things around me. There is one room trimmed with blue, another with

420

yellow, etc. The whole hospital is not as large as one of our wards. I asked Captain C. what he thought would become of all these "pretty things," if some few hundreds of wounded were brought in from the field, as we have had them many a time. I think the blue and yellow spreads would be *slightly soiled.*

On one of my visits there, Captain Curran informed me that the day previous his surgeon had neglected to state what was to be his diet, and he had to fast all day, as the matron could not give him any thing not prescribed. To think of a wounded man, who is convalescing, fasting a whole day! I think I should have broken the rules that day. I believe in discipline, but, as I heard a friend say, we need not break the rules, just bend them a little . . .

The other hospital (the Canty, so called in honor of General C.) is a very handsome building. It was a city hospital, and part of it is still reserved for the use of the sick citizens. The Sisters of Charity are its matrons, and we all know what they are in hospitals. And, by the way, why can we not imitate them in this respect, during these war times? Here one of them is a druggist; another acts the part of steward; and, in fact, they could take charge of the whole hospital, with the exception of the medical department . . .

The Ross Hospital, so called in honor of Dr. R. of this place, is, like the others, *parfait* in every respect. Dr. Needlet of Missouri is surgeon, and Mrs. Crocker matron . . .

While visiting the Ross Hospital, Mrs. C. showed me a book large enough to keep all of the records of the Confederacy, in which she has to note every mouthful eaten by the patients, and every drop of whisky that they drank. According to the rules in this book, she will be compelled to keep some half dozen of assistants. On looking at its size, I could not but think that paper must be more plentiful than we thought for. The diet-lists are amusing to read. We know there are such articles as those named in them, from having seen them in good old peace times, but that is about all we know of them. The lists always put me in mind of the receipt, "First catch your hare, and then make your pie." [77]

320. Susan Leigh Blackford. *Letters from Lee's Army*

[Although the Confederacy had no organization comparable to the United States Sanitary Commission, its Women's Relief Society devoted its energies to collecting money for assistance to the sick and wounded, and in general, relieving their suffering. In addition, thousands of Southern women volunteered for nursing. The Blackford family was one of the "first families of Virginia." The letters comprise the correspondence of the distinguished Charles Blackford, judge advocate under General Longstreet, and his wife. The letters were privately printed in 1894. The present edition was compiled by Susan Leigh Blackford, granddaughter of the correspondents.[78]]

A letter from Mrs. Blackford.

Lynchburg, July 8th, 1861.

I did not write you this morning as I usually do, because I have been at father's all day sewing for the soldiers. While I was there I was sent for to see old Mrs. John M. Otey, who was at Mrs. Spence's making arrangements to establish a Ladies' Hospital for the soldiers in opposition to Dr. Owen's. You know perhaps, that he will not allow the ladies to enter his hospital, or do anything for the patients. Mrs. Otey proposes to have a house and matron and a staff of hired nurses, all under the supervision of the ladies, with a change every day of those who are to stay in the hospital and directing the cooking and general service. If the scheme can be carried through it will be a good one and the poor men will be more comfortable than they are now. I promised Mrs. Otey I would co-operate with her as far as it was in my power but I did not think I could do any nursing. I think you would not like me to do that. Mrs. Otey said she was very glad to have her son associated with you and that he sounded your praises very loudly.

From Mrs. Blackford.

May 7th [1864]

Yesterday was my regular time for writing you, but I really did not have time to do so. The wounded soldiers commenced arriving on Saturday, and just as soon as I heard of it, which was before breakfast, I went to see Mrs. Spence to know what I could do for them. She said the ladies had been so shamefully treated by the surgeons that she was afraid to take any move in the matter. I told her I would go and see Dr. Randolph and ask him if we could not do something. I went down and did so at once and asked him what we could do. He said we might do anything we pleased in the way of attention to them; send or carry anything to them we wished and he would be glad of our help. As soon as I reported to Mrs. Spence what he said she started messengers in every direction to let it be known and I went to eleven places myself. We then determined to divide our provisions into two divisions: the bread, meat and coffee to be sent to the depot, the delicacies to the hospitals. The reception of wounded soldiers here has been most hospitable. You would not believe there were so many provisions in town as have been sent to them.

On Saturday evening I went up to Burton's factory, where most of the wounded were taken, and found the committee of ladies who had been selected, of whom I was one, just going in with the supper. I went in with them. We had bountiful supplies of soup, buttermilk, tea, coffee and loaf bread, biscuits, crackers and wafers. It did my heart good to see how the poor men enjoyed such things. I went around and talked to them all. One man had his arm taken off just below the elbow and he was also wounded through the body, and his drawers were saturated with blood. I fixed his pillow comfortably and stroked his poor swelled and burning arm. Another

I found with his hand wounded and his nose bleeding. I poured water over his face and neck, and after the blood ceased to flow wiped his pale face and wounded hand which was black from blood and powder. They were very grateful and urged us to come and see them again.

On Sunday evening news came that six hundred more would arrive and Mrs. Spence sent me word to try and do something. The servants were away and I went into the kitchen and made four quarts of flour into biscuits and two gallons of coffee, and Mrs. Spence gave me as much more barley, so I made by mixing them, a great deal of coffee. I am very tired.

May 12th.

My writing desk has been open all day, yet I have just found time to write you. Mrs. Spence came after me just as I was about to begin this morning and said she had just heard that the Taliaferro's factory [tobacco warehouse] was full of soldiers in a deplorable condition. I went down there with a bucket of rice milk, a basin, towel, soap, etc. to see what I could do. I found the house filled with wounded men and not one thing provided for them. They were lying about the floor on a little straw. Some had been there since Tuesday and had not seen a surgeon. I washed and dressed the wounds of about fifty and poured water over the wounds of many more. The town is crowded with the poor creatures, and there is really no preparations for such a number. If it had not been for the ladies many of them would have starved to death. The poor creatures are very grateful, and it is a great pleasure to us to help them in any way. I have been hard at work ever since the wounded commenced coming. I went to the depot twice to see what I could do. I have had the cutting and distribution of twelve hundred yards of cotton cloth for bandages, and sent over three bushels of rolls of bandages, and as many more yesterday. I have never worked so hard in all my life and I would rather do that than anything else in the world. I hope no more wounded are sent here as I really do not think they could be sheltered. The doctors, of course, are doing much, and some are doing their full duty, but the majority are not. They have free access to the hospital stores and deem their own health demands that they drink up most of the brandy and whiskey in stock, and, being fired up most of the time, display a cruel and brutal indifference to the needs of the suffering which is a disgrace to their profession and to humanity.

Next morning.

It is now but a little after five o'clock, and as I go to the hospitals directly after breakfast I have arisen early to finish my letter. Almost all the men at Taliaferro's are Longstreet's men and express the greatest desire to see the General. When I told the men I had been in East Tennessee with them they seemed most pleased. Your mother is much interested in the soldiers. They seem to arouse her more than anything else. She does a great deal for them.

Evening.

I have been in the hospital nearly all day dressing wounds and nursing. I went to enquire about General Longstreet and saw Captain Gorse and was glad to hear that the general was better and that he rested well last night.

May 18th.

I have been constantly engaged with wounded soldiers. My work, however, is much reduced, as the men have been scattered about to the different hospitals and are better cared for. I shall not undertake so much again. I was nearly broken down by my efforts and could not perform any other duties. I went up yesterday evening to see Eliza Gordon, not expecting to see General Longstreet. I had been there but a short time when he sent for me and insisted I should come up and see him which, of course, I did. He is very feeble and nervous and suffers much from his wound. He sheds tears on the slightest provocation and apologizes for it. He says he does not see why a bullet going through a man's shoulder should make a baby of him.

I stopped just here on yesterday to go to church and thence in pursuit of little Spratt. Mary and I found him,—a most forlorn looking person with a wound in his face and most miserably clad. He was very gentlemanly, but the saddest person I ever saw. He did not have the ghost of a smile about his face while I was talking to him. I promised to send him down some soup and rice milk, for the hospital rations are very indifferent for the men, and most uninviting. From Miller's we went to the college, where all the patients have been put into tents. Some of my patients have been placed in the Langhorne Hospital, so I can see and attend them every day. There are three wounded yankees there, one of them a splendid looking man from Ohio. I talked with him a good deal and found him very intelligent and very sick of the war. He says he has been kindly treated ever since he has been here, and does not intend to fight any more. The yankees are mixed up with our men and are treated exactly alike. They seem well contented. The hospital fare is very bad. I broke open a corn pone prepared for one of the sick and found it full of dry meal; no pains had been taken in making it up, though water was the only ingredient, enough was not supplied.[79]

321. *Diary of a Southern Refugee During the War*

[The writer of this diary, Judith Brockenbrough McGuire, was the wife of Reverend John P. McGuire, Principal of the Episcopal High School, near Alexandria. The diary, which was not intended for publication, opens on May 4, 1861, and closes on May 4, 1865.[80]]

The Briars, June 12 [1861].

Winchester is filled with hospitals, and the ladies are devoting their energies to nursing the soldiers. The sick from the camp at Harper's Ferry are brought there. Our climate seems not to suit the men from the far South. I hope they will soon become acclimated. It rejoices my heart to see how much everybody is willing to do for the poor fellows. The ladies there think no effort, however self-sacrificing, is too great to be made for the soldiers. Nice food for the sick is constantly being prepared by old and young. Those who are very sick are taken to private houses, and the best chambers in town are occupied by them.

.   .   .   .

August 20 [1862]

Lynchburg is full of hospitals, to which the ladies are very attentive; and they are said to be well kept. I have been to a very large one today, in which our old home friends, Mrs. R. [Mrs. Rowland], and Miss E. M. [Emily Mason], are matrons. Everything looked beautifully neat and comfortable.[81]

322. Letter of Ella Newsome Trader

[Ella Newsome Trader was the daughter of Rev. T. S. N. King, a Baptist clergyman. She was born at Brandon, Mississippi. When the war came, Mrs. Newsome, as she was then, volunteered her services in the cause of the Confederacy. Having unusual executive ability, she organized hospitals in Memphis, Bowling Green, Nashville, Chattanooga, Corinth, Marietta, and Atlanta.[82]]

The scenes in The Tishomingo Hotel Hospital after the battle of Shiloh beggar description. Every yard of space on the floors, as well as all the beds, bunks, and cots were covered with the mangled forms of badly wounded soldiers.

.   .   .   .

Every morning at daylight we went to the Hospital, remaining there until eleven or twelve every night that we did not stay all through the night to sit up with some poor fellow shot in the lungs and who had to be fanned every moment to enable him to breathe at all.[83]

323. Louise Wigfall Wright. *A Southern Girl in '61* *

[Mrs. Wright was the daughter of a Southern senator.[84]]

Macon, July 11, 1864.

... You see by the heading of my letter that already we have been forced to leave Atlanta—not that it has fallen, but Mrs. Johnston received a letter from the General in which he advised her to send us off at once—to remain until the fate of the city was decided either one way or the other ...

I shall never forget the horrors of that journey from Atlanta to Macon. We left in a hospital train, filled with wounded, sick and dying soldiers, in all imaginable stages of disease and suffering. My little sister and myself and one other lady were the only other passengers on the train, except the officer put in charge of us to see us safe to our journey's end. I never imagined what a hideous, cruel thing war was until I was brought into direct contact with these poor victims of "Man's inhumanity to man." For this was no modern hospital train with arrangements for hygiene and the relief of suffering. There was scant supply of the common comforts, and even decencies of life—no cushions nor air pillows for weary heads; no ice to cool the fevered thirst; no diet kitchen for broths and delicate food for these half starved sufferers; no wine or brandy to revive the failing pulse and stimulate the weakened vitality; not even medicine enough to check the ravages of disease; no anaesthetics nor anodynes to ease their agonies—for the supply of medicines and anodynes was daily diminishing, and they could not be replaced, as our foes had declared them "contraband of war." There was not even a place in that crowded car where the sick could lie down, but, packed in as close as possible on the hard uncomfortable seats, they made that journey, as best they might, in uncomplaining martyrdom. I reached Macon sick at heart over the suffering I had witnessed and was so powerless to avert . . .[85]

324. Annie K. Kyle's Account of Nursing at a Hospital in Fayetteville

[Mrs. Kyle of North Carolina, a "frail woman on crutches," cared for the sick as head nurse in the hospital at Fayetteville, after her husband had been under fire at Morris Island.[86]]

[Date not given]

They were bringing the wounded from Fort Fisher, Wilmington and other points. We already had one hospital and were establishing another. I shall never forget the doctor's look of amazement when I applied for the situation. My reply was: "Doctor I don't want any pay, but I must have constant occupation or I will lose my mind." I went every morning at nine o'clock and stayed until one, and I always went late in the afternoon to see that the wants of the patients were attended during the night. I always dressed all the wounds every morning, and I soon found that my grief and sorrow were forgotten in administering to the wants of the sick. Such patience and fortitude I have never seen. Not one murmur did I ever hear escape the lips. My Prayer Book was my constant companion. I carried it in my pocket and many poor soldiers have I soothed and comforted with Holy prayers. One day as I entered the hospital I noticed a new face, I made my way to him as I was struck by his gray hair, and said: "You are too old to be here." He smiled and his answer was quite a rebuke: "One never gets too old to fight for ones home and fireside. I had no sons so I came myself." [87]

CONCLUDING STATEMENT

The documentation of nursing in the wars in which the United States engaged in its early history indicates that, before the Civil War, sick and

426

wounded soldiers were cared for mainly by individuals, although some provision was made for hospitals at the time of the Revolutionary War. Interesting evidence of care by individuals in the French and Indian Wars are the bills rendered for nursing the soldiers.

In the Revolutionary War, this method continued to be employed, but in addition, as has been said, provision was made by Congress for a Medical Department of the Army. In these plans, nurses were provided for as part of the necessary personnel. Among the many problems facing George Washington as Commander-in-Chief of the Continental Army was the welfare of sick and wounded soldiers, and the difficulty of obtaining nurses, partly because of the low payment allowed them. The official records of certain states and of Congress mention payment of nurses for attendance on the sick and wounded. Personal memoirs indicate that individuals in the vicinity of battles being waged cared for the wounded.

From the numerous documents resulting from the Civil War, it is clear that early in the war the United States Sanitary Commission provided for a corps of volunteer women nurses, under a superintendent, Miss Dorothea L. Dix, who outlined the qualifications necessary for this service. Among the qualifications mentioned were suitable age, between thirty-five and fifty, good health, and good character, as well as plainness in appearance and dress. Several personal accounts indicate that the sick were cared for chiefly in hospitals behind the battle lines and on hospital transports. In addition to these nurses employed by the government, various other women and men participated in one way or another in the nursing of the wounded.

Although the Confederacy did not have an organization comparable to the Sanitary Commission, the Women's Relief Society performed many functions of caring for the sick and wounded. Many thousands of Southern women devoted their entire time, energies, and money in this cause also, and participated in the nursing of the patients.

It is assumed that the experiences of the Civil War emphasized the lack of proper preparation for their functions of most of the nurses who participated. At about this time public interest in nursing, and preparation for it, became intensified. The Appendix, which follows this chapter, presents two documents: one was prepared by a committee of physicians, making certain recommendations relative to the education of nurses; the other indicates the growing interest on the part of women in the opportunities in the emerging profession of nursing, and was published as an editorial in a prominent women's magazine.

427

Appendix

TWO DOCUMENTS INDICATING THE RISING INTEREST IN THE UNITED STATES IN THE EDUCATION OF NURSES

A. "Report of Committee on the Training of Nurses," *Transactions of the American Medical Association,* 1869, pp. 161–174

[The chairman of this committee, Dr. Samuel D. Gross (1805–1884), secured his medical degree at Jefferson Medical College, Philadelphia, in 1828. He taught at several medical colleges and at Jefferson Medical College from 1858. He contributed outstandingly to his profession as a teacher, an inventor of surgical instruments and techniques, and a founder of the American Medical Association.*]

Good nursing, as has very justly been observed by an intelligent writer, is half the battle in disease; if the other half be as well managed, the result can hardly fail to be all that the nature of the case demands. It is often incomparably more valuable to a sick man than the most skilled medication. It is the right hand of the medical practitioner. Thousands of human beings are daily lost by bad nursing.

Nursing, in its more exalted sense, is as much of an art and a science as medicine. The educated physician is sought for far and wide; his skill is in constant requisition; day and night he is at the bedside of the sick and the dying; at every visit he makes his prescription and leaves his instruction; he literally wars with disease and death; he necessarily from causes which no human agency can control, loses many patients; and many also who could be saved if his efforts were properly seconded by efficient nursing. The commander of an army cannot be victorious if he is not properly aided by his subordinates, the lieutenants, whose duty it is to carry out his orders and the minor details of the campaign. In private life there is hardly one really

* *Columbia Encyclopedia,* 2nd ed., article on "Samuel David Gross."

good, intelligent, or accomplished nurse in a hundred who exercise the functions of that office, one who is perfectly familiar with all the duties and requirements of the sick-room; and what is true of private society is still more true of the hospitals, almshouses, infirmaries, asylums, jails, work-houses, and similar institutions in the United States. It is a mistake to suppose, as is so often done, that any and every individual, whether male or female, is fitted for such an occupation, as if nursing, like poetry, were a gift of nature. Many persons are utterly incapacitated by their constitution and habits for such a task, and yet, as society is now constituted, there is hardly one who may not, sooner or later, be compelled to exercise it.

To afford the proper facilities for carrying out this grand design [of providing adequate nursing service for all], the Committee are of the opinion: 1st. That every large and well-organized hospital should have a school for the training of nurses, not only for the supply of its own necessities, but for private families, the teaching to be furnished by its own medical staff, assisted by the resident physicians.

2dly. That, while it is not at all essential to combine religious exercises with nursing, it is believed that such a union would be eminently conducive to the welfare of the sick in all public institutions; and the Committee therefore earnestly recommend the establishment of nurses' homes, to be placed under the immediate supervision and direction of deaconesses, or lady superintendents, an arrangement which works so well in the nurses' homes at London, Liverpool, Dublin, and other cities in Europe, and at the Bishop Potter Memorial House in Philadelphia.

3dly. That in order to give thorough scope and efficiency to this scheme, district schools should be formed, and placed under the guardianship of the county medical societies in every State and Territory in the Union, the members of which should make it their business to impart, at such time and place as may be most convenient, instruction in the art and science of nursing, including the elements of hygiene, and every other species of information necessary to qualify the student for the important, onerous, and responsible duties of the sick-room.

The Committee would further suggest the importance of forming in every convenient place nurses' societies, the regular members of which should, in all cases, other things being equal, have the preference, as it respects the recommendation of the practitioner over the ordinary ignorant or uneducated nurse. In this manner an *esprit de corps* could be established which could not fail to be highly advantageous to the public as well as to the medical profession.

The Committee, in view of the importance of the subject discussed in this report, beg leave to offer the following resolution: *Resolved,* that a copy of this Report, authenticated by the signatures of the President and Secretary of this Association, be sent to the State Medical Societies of the different States of the Union, inviting their cooperation in the establishment of schools for the training of nurses for hospitals and private families, in accordance with the principles therein advocated.

S. D. Gross, M.D. LL.D.,
Chairman.

B. "Lady Nurses," *Godey's Lady's Book and Magazine,* Vol. LXXXII (January to June, 1871), pp. 188–189

[The founder and publisher of this successful woman's magazine was Louis A. Godey (1804–1878). In 1837 Mr. Godey appointed Mrs. Sarah J. Hale as editor, a position she held for forty years. Mrs. Hale (1788–1879) had been editor of the *Ladies Magazine* of Boston before coming to Philadelphia to become editor of *Godey's Lady's Book.* The latter magazine strongly influenced women's fashions and manners. Mrs. Hale was an advocate of education of women, as well as many other causes. Her interest in professional education of nurses is illustrated by the following editorial.*]

Much has been lately said of the benefits that would follow if the calling of sick nurse were elevated to a profession which an educated lady might adopt without a sense of derogation, either on her own part or in the estimation of others. A writer in an English periodical suggests that this result could be brought about by raising the scale of remuneration in the case of ¯lady nurses. He adduces the instance of the surgeon, who was formerly a mere mechanical assistant to the physician, and frequently combined the office with that of barber, but who is now a gentleman, receiving as high fees and held in the same estimation as other members of the medical profession. It appears evident, however, that the writer mistakes the effect for the cause. The surgeon of the present day is not respected because he receives high fees; but he obtains these fees because he is a well-educated and thoroughly-trained professional man ...

There can be no doubt that the duties of sick nurse, to be properly performed, require an education and training little, if at all, inferior to those possessed by members of the medical profession. To leave these duties to untaught and ill-trained persons is as great a mistake as it was to allow the office of surgeon to be held by one whose proper calling was that of a mechanic of the humblest class. The manner in which a reform may be effected is easily pointed out. Every medical college should have a course of study and training especially adapted for ladies who desire to qualify themselves for the profession of nurse; and those who had gone through the course, and passed the requisite examination, should receive a degree and

* *Columbia Encyclopedia,* 2nd ed., articles on "Louis Antoine Godey," and "Sarah Josepha (Buell) Hale"; and Ruth Finley, *The Lady of Godey's* (Philadelphia: Lippincott, 1931).

diploma, which would at once establish their position in society. The "graduate nurse" would in general estimation be as much above the ordinary nurse of the present day as the professional surgeon of our times is above the barber-surgeon of the last century.

It would not, however, be necessary that the professional nurse should be educated in a medical institution, although the degree or diploma should in all cases proceed from one. In this respect the example of the English universities might be followed, in awarding degrees to out-students who are found qualified to pass the requisite examination. Physicians (either doctors or *doctresses*) might receive pupils desirous of qualifying themselves for the profession of nurse. If the pupil had already a good general education (which would be absolutely essential), a year devoted to the special studies of medicine and science, and another year of reading and practice combined, would probably be sufficient for this object. It must be borne in mind, however, that in this profession, as in all others, there would be no short road to proficiency, and that the higher the qualifications the better, as a general rule, would be the remuneration.

When once the value of the "graduate nurses" became known, there is no doubt that the demand for them would be very great. Every village of a thousand inhabitants would, with the country about it, give occupation for two or three, at least. In any case of severe and protracted illness, their services would be called for as a matter of course, when the circumstances of the family allowed it. Every physician would be glad to recommend an assistant, on whose intelligent cooperation he could rely, and who would be too well informed to interfere with the treatment, as uneducated nurses are apt to do. There are many diseases in which the patient must owe his recovery chiefly to the diet, regimen, and careful attendance. In all such cases the graduate nurse would be invaluable. In committing the control of the sick-room into her hands, the family would feel the same sense of relief and security as is felt by the passengers in a ship, when in stormy weather off a dangerous coast, an experienced pilot comes on board to take charge of the vessel.

There would be the further advantage that the nurse would not be an ignorant and unrefined person, with whom association would be unpleasant, but an educated lady, who would form an acceptable addition to the family circle during a period of anxiety and trouble—one who could give useful counsel on many subjects besides those of the sick chamber, and who would know how to economize not only her own health and strength, but the health and strength of the household, which are apt to be taxed too severely, when any member of it is ill for a long period. In short, whenever such a profession is once established, it will soon be deemed as useful and respectable as any other; and to revert to our former comparison, we shall wonder as much that we could have done without its members as we now wonder that our ancestors were content to allow the operations of surgery to be performed by a hair-cutter.

Notes

In the notes which follow, symbols have been used for brevity to indicate general reference works and works appearing frequently. Complete citations of the references will be found in the bibliography.

BT = *Babylonian Talmud*
CaE = *Catholic Encyclopedia*
CE = *Columbia Encyclopedia*, 2nd edition
DAB = *Dictionary of American Biography*
DAH = *Dictionary of American History*
DNB = *Dictionary of National Biography*
EAH = *Encyclopedia of American History*
EB = *Encyclopaedia Britannica*, 11th edition
NPNF = *Select Library of Nicene and Post-Nicene Fathers of the Christian Church*
PPTS = *Palestine Pilgrims' Text Society*
SAC = *Sussex Archeological Collections*
WWA = *Who's Who in America*
WWW = *Who Was Who 1897–1916*

CHAPTER 1

The Nurse in the Literature of Early Civilizations

(Pp. 23–37 of text)

1. Heidel, *Babylonian Genesis,* 4.
2. *Ibid.,* 11.
3. *EB,* "Talmud."
4. *BT,* vol. 3, Part 1, 287.
5. Sarma, "Hindu Medicine and Its Antiquity," *Annals of Medical History,* May, 1931, 318–324.
6. *EB,* "Surgery."
7. *Charaka-Samhita,* 102–103, 168–169.
8. *English Translation of the Sushruta-Samhita,* I, 176–179, 305–307.

9. *CE,* "Homer."
10. *Complete Works of Homer. Iliad,* 111–114.
11. *Ibid. Odyssey,* Bk. I, 13; Bk. XIX, 303.
12. *EB,* "Theocritus."
13. *Idylls of Theocritus,* II, 125.
14. *EB,* "Plutarch;" *CE, idem.*
15. *Plutarch's Lives: Alcibiades,* IV, 3.
16. *Ibid.: Lycurgus,* I, 83.
17. *EB,* "Plato;" *CE, idem.*
18. Plato, *Laws,* II, 7–8.
19. *EB,* "Xenophon."
20. Xenophon, *Memorabilia and Oeconomicus,* 425.
21. *EB,* "Hippocrates."
22. *Genuine Works of Hippocrates,* I, 240, 252; II, 10–11.
23. Hippocrates, *Decorum,* II, 299.
24. *CE,* "Vitruvius."
25. Vitruvius, *On Architecture,* I, 209.
26. *CE,* "Pliny the Elder," and "Pliny the Younger."
27. *Pliny's Letters,* I, 449.
28. *EB,* "Anatomy."
29. *CE,* "Aulus Cornelius Celsus."
30. Celsus, *De Medicina,* I, 165.
31. *EB,* "Brehon Laws."
32. Translator's note: "The man who acts as his nurse-tender—That is the man who is employed to lift him up and lay him down."
33. Translator's note: "For concealment from the physician—What was the nature of the concealment or fraud attempted to be practised on the physician it is impossible to define."
34. I.e., "a heifer in her third year, not yet bulled."
35. *Ancient Laws of Ireland,* III, 475.

CHAPTER 2

Some Sources for the Study of Nursing in the Early Christian Era

(Pp. 38–64 of text)

1. Quoted in Robinson, *Ministry of Deaconesses,* 10.
2. Quoted in *ibid.*
3. *Ibid.*
4. Hefele, *History of the Councils of the Church From the Original Documents.*
5. "On the Early History and Modern Revival of Deaconesses," *Church Quarterly Review,* xlvii (1899), 302–341.
6. St. Basil, *Letters,* I, 199.

7. *NPNF,* 2nd ser., III, 256, 286.

8. Robinson, *op. cit.,* 91.

9. *Ibid.,* 10.

10. A question has arisen among scholars concerning the word "wives" in this passage. The word "their" is not present in the Greek. The opinion expressed by some is that "deaconess" is meant rather than "wives," because of the context. See Henry Wheeler, *Deaconesses, Ancient and Modern* (New York: Hunt and Eaton, 1889), pp. 89–90.

11. *EB,* "Apostolical Constitutions."

12. *Didascalia Apostolorum,* 11–17, 70–79.

13. *Apostolical Constitutions,* 93, 104, 230, 241.

14. *CE,* "Canon;" *EB,* "Council of Trent."

15. *NPNF,* 2nd ser., XIV, 40.

16. Hefele, *op. cit.,* II, 412, 418; III, 163, 401; IV, 80.

17. "Votum castitis," i.e., "That blessing by which the grade of penitence was conveyed to anyone, and [which] was always available if penitent was not condemned to public penitence."

18. Hefele, *op. cit.,* IV, 187, 369, 429, 440, 456, 474, 480; V, 226.

19. *Rule of St. Benedict,* xiii, xxvii.

20. *Ibid.,* 68–69.

21. *Letters of Abelard and Heloise,* 211–212.

22. *Ibid.*

23. Clarke, *Saint Gregory of Nyssa: The Life of Saint Macrina,* 7, 10; *EB,* "Basilian Monks."

24. Clarke, *op. cit.,* 58–60.

25. Palladius, *Paradise of the Holy Fathers,* I, xxv.

26. *Ibid.,* 164, 183.

27. *CE,* "Saint John Chrysostom."

28. *NPNF,* 1st ser., X, ix, 407.

29. *Ibid.,* 407.

30. *EB,* "Saint Gregory of Nazianzen."

31. *NPNF,* 2nd ser., VII, 395.

32. *Ibid.,* 416.

33. *Dialogues of St. Gregory, Surnamed the Great,* 163.

34. *EB,* "Gregory."

35. *Dialogues of St. Gregory,* 163.

36. *EB,* "Pliny the Younger."

37. See *Pliny's Letters,* Bk. X, Letter XCVII.

38. *Ibid.,* Bk. X, Letter XCVI, Vol. II, 403.

39. *Select Letters of St. Jerome,* xiii.

40. *NPNF,* 2nd ser., VI, 158–160, 197, 202, 206.

41. *EB,* "Basil."

42. *NPNF,* 2nd ser., VIII, 179–180, 205, 208.

43. *Ibid.,* I, 45.

44. *CE,* "Eusebius of Caesarea;" *EB, idem.*

45. *NPNF,* 2nd ser., I, 307.

46. *EB,* "Sozomen," and "Socrates [Scolasticus];" *CE, idem.*
47. *NPNF,* 2nd ser., II, 296, 414.
48. *CE,* "Theodoret;" *EB, idem.*
49. *NPNF,* 2nd ser., III, 145.
50. *CE,* "Procopius;" *EB, idem.*
51. *Procopius,* VII, 173, 329, 347.
52. *CE,* "William of Tyre."
53. William Archbishop of Tyre, *History of Deeds Done Beyond the Sea,* II, 241–245.
54. Beazley, *Dawn of Modern Geography,* I, 110–111.
55. *PPTS. Of the Holy Places Visited by Antoninus Martyr,* II, 11, 19, 28.
56. Muratori, *Antiquitates Italicae,* V, 572.
57. *Melanges d'Archeologie,* 245. Quoted in Robinson, *op. cit.,* 91.
58. Thorp, *Charles Kingsley,* 111.
59. Kingsley, *Hypatia,* 88.

CHAPTER 3

Nursing in the Literature of the Middle Ages

(Pp. 65–106 of text)

1. Sabatier, *Life of St. Francis of Assisi,* 147.
2. *EB,* "Thomas Fuller."
3. Fuller, *Historie of the Holy Warre,* 47.
4. *CE,* "Anna Comnena;" *EB,* "Crusades."
5. Comnena, *Alexiad,* 408.
6. *CE,* "Jean Sire de Joinville;" *EB, idem,* and "Crusades."
7. Villehardouin and de Joinville, *Memoirs of the Crusades,* 162.
8. Quoted in King, *Knights Hospitallers in the Holy Land,* 26, 278–279.
9. Quoted in Schermerhorn, *On the Trail of the Eight-Pointed Cross,* 21.
10. Some authorities state that a Master, Roger by name, intervened between Gerard and Raymond. This is considered by others to be unlikely.
11. *EB,* "Crusades," and "Knights of the Order of the Hospital of St. John of Jerusalem."
12. Quoted in King, *op. cit.,* 324–326.
13. Porter, *History of the Knights of Malta,* I, 94–97.
14. Vertot, *History of the Knights of Malta,* I, 73.
15. Translator's note: "Servants, not necessarily of noble birth."
16. Quoted in Hume, "Medical Work of the Knights Hospitallers of St. John of Jerusalem," *Bulletin of the Institute of the History of Medicine,* June, 1938, 426–428.
17. Vertot, *op. cit.,* I, 167.
18. Quoted in King, *Rule Statutes and Customs of the Hospitallers,* 80.
19. Quoted in Hume, *op. cit.,* 561–581.
20. Quoted in Vertot, *op. cit.,* II, 1–27 at end of book.
21. Beazley, *Dawn of Modern Geography,* II, 139.

22. Quoted in *Early Travels in Palestine,* 39.

23. Beazley, *op. cit.,* II, 186.

24. *PPTS, Fetullus,* V, vi.

25. *Ibid.,* 39.

26. Beazley, *op. cit.,* II, 190, 196.

27. *PPTS. Description of the Holy Land by John of Wurzburg,* V, 44–45.

28. Beazley, *op. cit.,* II, 196.

29. *PPTS. Theodorich's Description of the Holy Places,* V, 23, 43, 46.

30. Beazley, *op. cit.,* III, 399–401.

31. *PPTS. Ludolph von Suchem's Description of the Holy Land,* XII, 106–107.

32. *CE,* "John Howard;" *EB, idem.*

33. Howard, *Account of the Principal Lazarettos in Europe,* 58–60.

34. *DNB,* "Sir Richard Colt Hoare."

35. "And where there is a decline in the vigor of ancient truth, it is closely followed by inertia and soon (unless I prophesy falsely) by defection." Translation by Irwin Stein.

36. Hoare, *Recollections Abroad During the Year 1790,* 184.

37. *EB,* "Francois Emmanuel Guignard Saint Priest."

38. Quoted in Hume, *op. cit.,* 531. Translation by Henriette Callot.

39. Moorman, *Sources for the Life of St. Francis of Assisi,* 13, 23–24, 33, 37.

40. Quoted in Englebert, *Saint Francis of Assisi,* 225.

41. Bullarium Romanum, iii. Quoted in *Select Historical Documents of the Middle Ages,* p. 346.

42. Various writers give different dates for these.

43. Moorman, *op. cit.,* 61–66.

44. Thomas of Celano, *Lives of St. Francis of Assisi,* 17, 38–40, 81, 305.

45. Holzapfel, *History of the Franciscan Order,* 553.

46. Moorman, *op. cit.,* 141.

47. St. Bonaventura, *Life of St. Francis,* Ch. II, 6.

48. Moorman, *op. cit.,* 68–69.

49. *Legend of S. Francis by the Three Companions,* 24.

50. Moorman, *op. cit.,* 131–133.

51. *Mirror of Perfection of St. Francis of Assisi,* 71, 96, 162.

52. Moorman, *op. cit.,* 159–169.

53. *"Little Flowers" and Life of St. Francis with "Mirror of Perfection,"* 44–45.

54. See also Ch. XC, *Mirror of Perfection,* p. 81.

55. Moorman, *op. cit.,* 13–15.

56. Thomas of Celano, *Life of St. Clare,* 113–114.

57. *Life and Works of Charles Kingsley,* XVI, 3–4.

58. Theodoric of Thuringen, *Vita Sancte Elisabethae,* Vol. IV, Bk. III, Ch. VI, 129; Bk. VI, Ch. IV, 140; Bk. VII, Ch. V, 144. Quoted in Hughes, *Women Healers in Medieval Life and Literature,* 133–134.

59. *CE,* "Charles Forbes René de Tryon, Comte de Montalembert."

60. Montalembert, *Life of Saint Elizabeth*, 12, 423.

61. *EB*, "Charles Forbes René de Montalembert."

62. Montalembert, *op. cit.*, 152–158, 195, 274, 276.

63. Pope-Hennessy, *Canon Charles Kingsley, A Biography*, 8.

64. *Charles Kingsley: His Letters and Memories of His Life*, I, 45.

65. Thorp, *Charles Kingsley 1819–1875*, 41.

66. Kingsley, *Poems*, 152–154.

67. Raymond of Capua, *Life of Saint Catherine of Sienna*, vii–lx, 14–17, 22, 25, 275.

68. *Ibid.*, 93–95, 101–102.

69. *CaE*, "Augusta Theodosia Drane."

70. Drane, *History of St. Catherine of Siena*, I, viii–xi.

71. *Ibid.*, 221–223.

72. *EB*, "Beguines."

73. *Ibid.*, "Robert Southey;" *CE, idem.*

74. *Life and Correspondence of the Late Robert Southey*, IV, 127–132.

75. Southey, *Journal of a Tour in the Netherlands in the Autumn of 1815*, 50–54.

76. *DNB*, "Robert Gooch, M.D."

77. De Bunsen, *Elizabeth Fry's Journeys on the Continent, 1840–1841*, 8.

78. *EB*, "Bridgittines."

79. Aungier, *History and Antiquities of Syon Monastery*, xi.

80. *Ibid.*, 395–396.

81. *Fifty Earliest Wills in the Court of Probate, London*, 52.

82. Quoted in Child, *English and Scottish Popular Ballads*, III, 105–106.

83. Quoted in Hughes, *op. cit.*, 147.

84. Quoted in Clay, *Mediaeval Hospitals of England*, 5, 33, 78, 86.

85. Moore, *Past and Present State of St. Bartholomew's Hospital*, I, 381–382.

86. Quoted in *ibid.*, 384–385.

87. *EB*, "Bedlam."

88. Gregory, *Historical Collections of a Citizen of London in the Fifteenth Century*, xliii.

CHAPTER 4

Some References to European Nursing, Sixteenth to Eighteenth Centuries

(Pp. 107–147 of text)

1. *EB*, "Sir Thomas More."

2. More, *Utopia*, 89.

3. Stow, *Survay of London*, 9–11.

4. *CE*, "John Stow."

5. Stow, *op. cit.*, 9–11.

6. ———, *Annales*, 940.

7. ———, *Survay*, 434–435.

8. *Ibid.*, I, 42, 57–58. This is a longer edition of the *Survay*. Quoted in Clark, *Working Life of Women in the Seventeenth Century*, 244–246.

9. Nichols and Wray, *History of the Foundlings' Hospital*, 7, 13, 19.

10. Quoted in *ibid.*, 41, 167.

11. Morris, *History of the London Hospital*, 26, 56.

12. Quoted in *ibid.*, 57.

13. *Memoranda, References, and Documents Relating to the Royal Hospitals of the City of London*, 17.

14. *Ibid.*, 9–21.

15. *Ibid.*, 83–103.

16. *EB*, "Lambeth."

17. Parsons, *History of St. Thomas's Hospital*, II, 124.

18. Quoted in *ibid.*, I, 232.

19. *DNB*, "Thomas Fuller."

20. Fuller, *Exanthematologia*, 208–209.

21. Nolan, *Essay on Humanity*, iii, 48.

22. *Ibid.*, 11–15, 33–35.

23. See pp. 81–82.

24. *CE*, "John Howard."

25. Howard, *Account of the Principal Lazarettos in Europe*, 86, 93, 180–182.

26. Hodges, *Loimologia*, title page.

27. *Ibid.*, 8–9, 25–26.

28. *Shutting Up of Infected Houses Soberly Debated*. Quoted in Nicholson, *Historical Sources of Defoe's Journal of the Plague Year*, 36.

29. Austin, *Anatomy of the Pestilence*, 25–27.

30. Vincent, *God's Terrible Voice in the City*, title page.

31. *Ibid.*, 34.

32. *DNB*, "Daniel Defoe."

33. Defoe, *Due Preparations for the Plague*, xxi.

34. ———, *Journal of the Plague Year*, 95–96, 112.

35. *CE*, "Samuel Pepys;" *EB*, idem.

36. Nicholson, *op. cit.*, 44.

37. *Diary and Correspondence of Samuel Pepys*, II, 276.

38. *Diary of Lady Margaret Hoby*, ix–x, 47.

39. *Ibid.*, 63, 86, 100–101, 169–171, 184–186, 191–195.

40. Weigall, "An Elizabethan Lady," *Quarterly Review*, July, 1911, 119–138.

41. Quoted in *ibid.*, 125.

42. *DNB*, "Lucius Cary."

43. Marriott, *Life and Times of Lucius Cary*, 67–71, 331.

44. Duncon, *Holy Life and Death of the Lady Letice*, 14, 40.

45. *EB*, "Lewes."

46. *SAC*, Ross, *Hastings Documents*, XXIII, 90.

47. *Ibid., Extracts from the Journal and Account Book of the Rev. Giles Moore,* I, 65.

48. Mat seems to have been his niece or his goddaughter or both.

49. *SAC, Extracts from the Journal of the Rev. Giles Moore,* I, 2, 100, 119.

50. *Ibid.,* Turner, *Ancient Parochial Account Book of Cowden,* XX, 91.

51. *Ibid.,* 117–118.

52. Packard, *Life and Times of Ambroise Paré,* 10–20.

53. *Workes of that Famous Chirurgion Ambroise Parey,* 1168–1171.

54. *CE,* "John Robinson."

55. *EB,* "John Robinson."

56. *Works of John Robinson,* III, 421.

57. *Ibid.,* 429.

58. Young, *Chronicles of the Pilgrim Fathers,* vii, ix, 4, 412–414.

59. Willison, *Saints and Strangers,* 60–62, 72–79.

60. Quoted in Young, *op. cit.,* 455.

61. *EB,* "Saint Vincent de Paul;" *CE, idem.*

62. Emanuel, *Charities of St. Vincent de Paul,* 103.

63. Coste, *Life and Works of Saint Vincent de Paul,* I, 83.

64. Abelly, *Saint Vincent de Paul,* I, xxiii. Quoted in Adderley, *Monsieur Vincent,* 52–56.

65. *Regles Communes,* Ch. vii, Art. 1 and 3; Ch. iv, Art. 4. Quoted in Emanuel, *op. cit.,* 149, 167.

66. *Regles Particulieres aux Soeurs de Paroisses,* Ch. ix, xi, xiii, xiv, xvlii, Art. 4; Art. 16, 1–4. Quoted in Emanuel, *op. cit.,* 148, 150–151, 180–181.

67. These rules seem to refer also to the hospital at Angers.

68. Coste, *op. cit.,* I, 237, 283.

69. Quoted in Emanuel, *op. cit.,* 187–189.

70. *Conferences aux Filles de la Charite,* I, 76. Quoted in Bougaud, *History of St. Vincent de Paul,* I, 277, 283–284.

71. *Ibid.,* I, 5–6, No. 1, July 31, 1634; 30, No. 4, Aug. 12, 1640; 56, No. 8, July 14, 1642; II, 319, No. 79, Nov. 11, 1657; 614, Aug. 24, 1659. Quoted in Emanuel, *op. cit.,* 147–150.

72. *Lettres et Conferences de S. Vincent de Paul (Suppl.),* 167–168. Quoted in Coste, *op. cit.,* I, 395.

73. Abelly, *op. cit.,* I, 371, 491. Quoted in Coste, *op. cit.,* I, 283–284.

74. Translator's note: "Henrietta Gesseaume was a most intelligent, resourceful, but rather independent Daughter of Charity. As she was a clever pharmacist, she was of great service to the hospital at Nantes, where she served from 1646 to 1655."

75. Translator's note: "Isabella, or Elizabeth, Martin, was one of the most accomplished of the first Daughters of Charity. She was sister-servant of the hospital at Angers in 1640, of the house at Richelieu in 1641, of the hospital at Nantes in 1646."

76. Letters 224, 354. Quoted in *Letters of St. Vincent de Paul,* 73, 78.

77. *Lettres et Conferences (Suppl.)*, 314–315. Quoted in Emanuel, *op. cit.*, 141.

78. *Memoire addresse a l'archeveque de Paris*, 498. Quoted in Emanuel, *op. cit.*, 141.

79. *Lettres et Conferences (Suppl.)*, 167–168, 452. Quoted in Emanuel, *op. cit.*, 150, 180.

80. Abelly, *op. cit.*, X, 661. Quoted in Coste, *op. cit.*, I, 345.

81. Quoted in Adderley, *op. cit.*, 116.

82. Abelly, *op. cit.*, 323. Quoted in Coste, *op. cit.*, I, 355.

CHAPTER 5

Some References to Nursing Reforms in Europe in the First Half of the Nineteenth Century

(Pp. 148–210 of text)

1. See also pp. 170–176.

2. See also pp. 96–98.

3. See pp. 62, 135–137.

4. *DNB*, "John Flint South."

5. South, *Facts Relating to Hospital Nurses*, 21, 25, 28.

6. *Ibid.*, 9–16, 25–29.

7. *WWW*, "Frances Power Cobbe."

8. *EB*, "Ernest Abraham Hart."

9. Quoted in Twining, *Workhouses and Pauperism and Women's Work in the Administration of the Poor Law*, 29.

10. Forster, *Life of Charles Dickens*, II, 30.

11. Dickens, *Martin Chuzzlewit*, Ch. XIX, XXIX. See also Ch. XXV.

12. *EB*, "Sir Henry Wentworth Acland."

13. This was Felicia Skene.

14. Acland, *Memoir of the Cholera at Oxford in the Year 1854*, 98–99, 139.

15. See pp. 250–251.

16. See pp. 156–157.

17. See pp. 160–162.

18. Rickards, *Felicia Skene of Oxford A Memoir*, 1–2, 21, 71, 93, 110–111.

19. Miss Hughes, the sister of Rev. Thomas Chamberlain of St. Thomas-the-Martyr, Oxford, was head of a sisterhood in Oxford.

20. See Reading No. 145.

21. Rickards, *op. cit.*, 100–105.

22. Goodman, *Experiences of an English Sister of Mercy*, 1, 32, 55.

23. *Ibid.*, 32–33.

24. *EB*, "Sir James Paget;" *CE, idem.*

25. *Memoirs and Letters of Sir James Paget*, 353.

26. *EB*, "William Augustus Muhlenberg;" *CE, idem.*

27. [Keller], *History of the St. Luke's Hospital Training School for Nurses,* 9–12.

28. Letter of Pastor Muhlenberg, dated 1855. Quoted in Ayres, *Life and Work of William Augustus Muhlenberg,* 282.

29. *CE,* "Joseph Lister, 1st Baron Lister;" *EB, idem.*

30. Godlee, *Life of Lord Lister,* vii.

31. Quoted in *ibid.,* 254–255.

32. *WWW,* "John Beddoe;" *DNB, 2nd suppl., idem.*

33. Beddoe, *Memories of Eighty Years,* 56–57.

34. *CE,* "William Ernest Henley."

35. Godlee, *op. cit.,* 256.

36. Henley, *In Hospital,* 12.

37. See p. 174.

38. *DNB, Suppl.,* "Sir Edward Henry Sieveking."

39. Pöel, *Life of Amelia Wilhelmina Sieveking,* 5, 23, 282–284. See also pp. 187–188.

40. Quoted in *ibid.,* 246–249, 263.

41. *EB,* "Newspapers;" and "Medicine."

42. *The Lancet,* July 15, 1865; July 29, 1865; Aug. 12, 1865; Aug. 26, 1865; Nov. 18, 1865; April 7, 1866.

43. Tooley, *History of Nursing in the British Empire,* 218–219.

44. *WWW,* "Louisa Twining."

45. Twining, *op. cit.,* 61, 68, 76, 133, 138, 150, 156, 187.

46. *DNB,* "Robert Gooch, M.D."

47. See pp. 96–98.

48. See pp. 98–99.

49. Southey, *Sir Thomas More; or Colloquies on the Progress and Prospects of Society,* II, 318.

50. *Life and Correspondence of Robert Southey,* IV, 156; V, 25, 237; VI, 52, 71–72.

51. Liddon, *Life of Edward Bouverie Pusey,* III, 1; *EB,* "Edward Bouverie Pusey."

52. Quoted in Liddon, *op. cit.,* III, 6.

53. [Stanley], *Hospitals and Sisterhoods,* 38.

54. Quoted in *ibid.,* 38–41.

55. *Sisterhoods; Schools for Nurses,* 3, 6, 12, 16–18; *Saturday Review,* 1866.

56. *EB,* "Archibald Campbell Tait."

57. Quoted in Davidson and Benham, *Life of Archibald Campbell Tait,* I, 457.

58. *DNB,* "John William Ogle."

59. Pöel, *op. cit.,* 322.

60. Adams, *Good Samaritans,* 362.

61. *Memorial of Two Sisters: Susanna and Catherine Winkworth,* 235.

62. Quoted in Pöel, *op. cit.,* 282–285.

63. Howson, "Deaconesses; or the Official Help of Women in Parochial Work and in Charitable Institutions," *Quarterly Review,* September, 1860, 342–387.

64. *EB,* "Theodor Fliedner."

65. Fliedner, *Kurzer Abriss Seines Lebens,* 60. Quoted in *Life of Pastor Fliedner,* 58–68.

66. Disselhoff, "The Deaconesses of Kaiserswerth: A Hundred Years' Work." *International Nursing Review,* Vol. IX, Nos. 1–4 (1934), 22.

67. *Der Armen-und Kranken-Freund,* No. 5, 142, 157. Quoted in Disselhoff, *op. cit.,* 22–24.

68. Cook, *Life of Florence Nightingale,* II, 437.

69. [Nightingale], *Institution of Kaiserswerth on the Rhine,* 16–23.

70. Cook, *op. cit.,* I, 92–93. See Reading No. 168.

71. See also second part of Reading No. 189.

72. Quoted in Tooley, *Life of Florence Nightingale,* 69. Portions of the letter are quoted in Cook, *op. cit.,* I, 112–113; and in Matheson, *Florence Nightingale A Biography,* 99–100.

73. Quoted in Cook, *op. cit.,* I, 112.

74. *Ibid.,* II, 126–130; *CE,* "John Lair Mair Lawrence, 1st Baron Lawrence."

75. *"Una and Her Paupers,"* 36–37, 122–123.

76. *Ibid.,* 120, 171, 175, 182.

77. De Bunsen, *Elizabeth Fry's Journeys on the Continent 1840–1841,* 100–101.

78. Quoted in *Memoirs of the Life of Elizabeth Fry,* II, 357–358.

79. Gerberding, *Life and Letters of W. A. Passavant,* 140–154.

80. *Ibid.,* 145–146.

81. Liddon, *op. cit.,* III, 14, 17.

82. Quoted in *ibid.,* 27.

83. Beale, "Nursing the Sick in Hospitals, Private Families, and Among the Poor," *Medical Times and Gazette,* Mar. 15, 1875, 270–271; Apr. 26, 1873, 438–439.

84. See pp. 198–200.

85. *Memoirs of the Life of Elizabeth Fry,* II, 373.

86. Archives of the Nursing Sisters. Quoted in Tooley, *History of Nursing in the British Empire,* 29.

87. Quoted in Ryder, *Elizabeth Fry Life and Labors,* 316.

88. Archives of the Nursing Sisters. Quoted in Tooley, *History of Nursing in the British Empire,* 29.

89. *Memoirs of the Life of Elizabeth Fry,* II, 373.

90. *Ibid.,* 373–375.

91. Archives of the Nursing Sisters. Quoted in Tooley, *History of Nursing in the British Empire,* 41.

92. Morris, *History of the London Hospital,* 26; Ives, *British Hospitals,* 19–22.

93. Quoted in Haldane, *British Nurse in Peace and War,* 51.

94. Cooke, *Mildmay*, 6, 9–14, 39–43.
95. *Life and Letters of Rev. William Pennefather*, 409.
96. Lonsdale, *Sister Dora*, 13, 37, 222.
97. *EB*, "Mark Pattison."
98. Quoted in Lonsdale, *op. cit.*, 38–39, 168–169, 175–176.
99. *Ibid.*, 131.
100. Quoted in *ibid.*, 131–135.
101. Ludlow, *Woman's Work in the Church*, 249.
102. Quoted in *ibid.*
103. [Atkinson], *Life and Work of Mary Aikenhead*, 1, 25, 44.
104. Quoted in *ibid.*, 133.

CHAPTER 6

Some References to the Life of Florence Nightingale
Before 1860

(Pp. 213–256 of text)

1. *EB*, "Julia Ward Howe;" *CE, idem.*
2. Howe, *Reminiscences, 1819–1899*, 138–139.
3. *CE*, "Laura Elizabeth (Howe) Richards."
4. Richards, "Letters of Florence Nightingale," *Yale Review*, Winter, 1935, 326–347.
5. *EB*, "Lucy Stone;" *CE, idem*, and "Elizabeth Blackwell."
6. Quoted in Blackwell, *Pioneer Work in Opening the Medical Profession to Women*, 150.
7. *EB*, "Elizabeth Cleghorn Gaskell."
8. *DNB*, "Catherine Winkworth." See pp. 187, 460, 463.
9. Quoted in Haldane, *Mrs. Gaskell and Her Friends*, 98–101.
10. Darwin, *Century of Family Letters*, I, xxviii–xxxiii.
11. *Ibid.*, II, 155, 159–160.
12. See pp. 160–164.
13. Rickards, *Felicia Skene of Oxford A Memoir*, 109–111.
14. Ramsey, *Thomas Grant, First Bishop of Southwark*, 1–8, 37, 135.
15. The number was later increased to five.
16. Quoted in Ramsey, *op. cit.*, 136–139.
17. Note by author: "No payment was ever made to the Sisters from Bermondsey, and they never claimed any. Miss Nightingale knew they were acting from a higher motive, and in this respect distinguished them from all her other helpmates."
18. Quoted in Ramsey, *op. cit.*, 139–143, 170.
19. Cook, *Life of Florence Nightingale*, I, 163, 173, 197, 441; II, 236, 305.
20. *EB*, "Sidney Herbert."
21. Quoted in Stanmore, *Sidney Herbert*, I, 343–345.
22. Reid, *Richard Monckton Milnes*, I, 63, 404, 425–429.

23. Pope-Hennessy, *Monckton Milnes,* 307.

24. Quoted in Reid, *op. cit.,* I, 505.

25. *EB,* "International Arbitration," and "Shanghai."

26. Hornby, *Constantinople During the Crimean War,* 152–161.

27. *DNB,* "Lord Sydney Godolphin Osborne."

28. Osborne, *Scutari and Its Hospitals,* 23–37.

29. Pincoffs, *Experiences of a Civilian in Eastern Military Hospitals,* title page.

30. *Ibid.,* 69–70, 78–80, 178.

31. Dunne, *Trip to Constantinople,* title page.

32. *Ibid.,* 146–152.

33. Cook, *op. cit.,* I, 188–194.

34. Quoted in Stanmore, *op. cit.,* I, 412–414.

35. *Catholic World,* April, 1880, 55–63.

36. Cook, *op. cit.,* I, 79.

37. Quoted in Stanmore, *op. cit.,* I, 373, 375, 406–408.

38. [Taylor], *Eastern Hospitals and English Nurses,* 39, 94.

39. *Ibid.,* 39–40, 94–95.

40. Cook, *op. cit.,* II, 464.

41. Aloysius, *Memories of the Crimea,* 6–9, 34–37, 53–54, 65–67.

42. See p. 164.

43. Goodman, *Experiences of an English Sister of Mercy,* 1.

44. *Ibid.,* 55–65, 101–105.

45. *DNB,* "Anna Maria Hall," and "Samuel Carter Hall." For note about Mrs. Herbert, see p. 239.

46. Quoted in Tooley, *Life of Florence Nightingale,* 92.

47. Martineau, *Biographical Sketches,* 360–365.

48. Cook, *op. cit.,* I, 176.

49. Quoted in Tooley, *op. cit.,* 100.

50. *EB,* "Stratford Canning, Stratford de Redcliffe."

51. Cook, *op. cit.,* I, 206.

52. See pp. 160–164.

53. Rickards, *op. cit.,* 29.

54. Skene, *With Lord Stratford in the Crimean War,* 37–38.

55. Cook, *op. cit.,* I, 257, 456–457; II, 55, 157; *DNB,* "Sir John McNeill."

56. *Memoir of the Rt. Hon. Sir John McNeill,* 403–404.

57. *WWW,* "General Sir George Wentworth Alexander Higginson."

58. Higginson, *Seventy-one Years of a Guardsman's Life,* 318–319.

59. *Life of Henry Wadsworth Longfellow,* II, 332.

60. Jameson, *Sacred and Legendary Art,* II, 658.

61. *Poetical Works of Henry Wadsworth Longfellow,* 511–512.

62. See pp. 195–196.

CHAPTER 7

Selections from the Literature of the New Profession of Nursing

(Pp. 257–300 of text)

1. See p. 378.

2. Quoted in Blackwell, *Pioneer Work in Opening the Medical Profession to Women*, 175.

3. See pp. 196–198.

4. *"Una and Her Paupers,"* ix.

5. *Ibid.*, 253–256, 317, 321–323, 328.

6. Lees, *Handbook for Hospital Sisters*, xvi.

7. Note by Miss Lees: "This was the custom at St. Thomas's Hospital when I was there as a 'Nightingale probationer;' and I have not seen a better method in any other English hospital or infirmary. All these things were hemmed and made in the female wards, where also old linen was repaired."

8. Cook, *op. cit.*, I, 458–459.

9. Richards, *Reminiscences of Linda Richards*, 33.

10. Nightingale, "Reform of Sick Nursing and the Late Mrs. Wardroper," *British Medical Journal*, Dec. 31, 1892, 1448, note.

11. See pp. 196–198.

12. Cook, *op. cit.*, II, 446.

13. Quoted in Dunbar, *Origin and Early Development of Two English Training Schools for Nurses*, 20, 34–37, 52.

14. See pp. 216–217, 263–268.

15. See preceding note.

16. Cook, *op. cit.*, I, 383, 417; II, 439.

17. Nightingale, *Notes on Hospitals*, iii, 181, Appendix.

18. Cook, *op. cit.*, I, 408–409; II, 442.

19. Nightingale, *Army Sanitary Administration and Its Reform*, 3.

20. Cook, *op. cit.*, II, 163–164.

21. *Ibid.*, 452.

22. *Ibid.*, 124–126. See p. 262.

23. Rathbone, *Sketch of the History and Progress of District Nursing*, x–xxi.

24. Nightingale, "Sick-Nursing and Health-Nursing," *Woman's Mission*, 184–198.

25. Cook, *op. cit.*, II, 438.

26. [Nightingale], *Subsidiary Notes as to the Introduction of Female Nursing into Military Hospitals*, 1–3.

27. See pp. 183–185.

28. *Sisterhoods; Schools for Nurses*, 18–19.

29. *EB*, "Medicine."

30. Chavasse, *Advice to a Wife on the Management of Her Own Health*, title page.

31. *Ibid.,* 167–171.

32. *EB.,* "James Hinton."

33. *DNB,* "Jane Ellice Hopkins."

34. *Life and Letters of James Hinton,* 255.

35. See pp. 174–176.

36. Twining, *Workhouses and Pauperism and Women's Work in the Administration of the Poor Law,* 108, 207, 262–264.

37. See pp. 275–276.

38. See p. 262.

39. Rathbone, *op. cit.,* 1–3, 14–16, 21–28, 37–53, 79–82, 109–112.

40. Rathbone, *William Rathbone,* 156, 174–179, 182.

41. See p. 262. See also Reading No. 236.

42. Platt, *Story of the Ranyard Mission,* 11–13, 20–21.

43. "Pioneers . . . were women of more education than most of the Bible-women." Platt, *op cit.,* 50.

44. *Ibid.,* 61–70.

CHAPTER 8

Some References to Early American Nursing in Homes and Hospitals

(Pp. 303–363 of text)

1. Hume, "El Hospital de Jesus Nazareno," *Gaceta Medica de Mexico,* Vol. LVIII, Suppl. No. 4 (August, 1938), p. 10.

2. Atherton, *Saintly Life of Jeanne Mance,* 27.

3. *CE,* "Virginia."

4. Willison, *Saints and Strangers,* 105, 145–146.

5. *Historic New York: Half Moon Papers,* II, 297.

6. O'Connor, "Charity Hospital of Louisiana at New Orleans," *Louisiana Historical Quarterly,* XXXI (1948), 1–109.

7. *Autobiography of Benjamin Franklin,* 281–282.

8. *CE,* "Elizabeth Ann (Bayley) Seton."

9. *EB,* "William Augustus Muhlenberg."

10. Gerberding, *Life and Letters of W. A. Passavant,* 188.

11. *EB,* "Hernan or Hernando Cortes;" *CE, idem.*

12. MacNutt, *Letters of Cortes,* I, 77–98.

13. Quoted in Hume, *op. cit.,* 9.

14. Nasatir, "Royal Hospitals in Colonial Spanish America," *Annals of Medical History,* November, 1942, 481–503.

15. Quoted in *ibid.,* 493–496.

16. *CE,* "Jesuit Relations."

17. *Jesuit Relations,* XVI, 9, 19, 21–23; XIX, 9, 11, 23–25; XXIV, 23, 113, 159, 263; XXV, 121, 127, 195; XXVI, 201; XXVII, 77, 193; XXVIII, 241, 277; XXIX, 81–83.

18. Dollier de Casson, *History of Montreal,* 5–8, 46–49.

19. *Ibid.,* 89, 97, 107, 125, 245.

20. Charlevoix, *Letters to the Dutchess of Lesdiguieres,* newspaper clipping on inside front cover. See Reading No. 251, last paragraph of journal, 1645.

21. *Ibid.,* 24.

22. Simcoe, *Diary of Mrs. John Graves Simcoe,* ix, 1, 9.

23. *Ibid.,* 66–67.

24. *EB,* "François Alexandre Frédéric, duc de La Rochefoucauld-Liancourt;" *CE, idem.*

25. La Rochefoucauld-Liancourt, *Travels Through the United States of North America and Upper Canada,* I, 317, 320.

26. J. C. B., *Travels in New France,* xi–xii.

27. "Quebec became a bishopric in 1674, but M. de St. Valier did not succeed M. de Laval until 1688." (Footnote, p. 13.)

28. J. C. B. *op. cit.,* 12, 20–22.

29. Knox, *Historical Journal of the Campaign in North America,* I, xviii, xix.

30. *Ibid.,* 460; II, 108, 212–214.

31. Wakefield, *Excursions in North America,* title page, 1.

32. *Ibid.,* 302–303.

33. Hall, *Travels in Canada and the United States in 1816 and 1817,* 1.

34. *Ibid.,* 61–62.

35. Hall, *Travels in North America in the Years 1827 and 1828,* I, 1.

36. *Ibid.,* II, 133.

37. *CE,* "William Bradford."

38. *EB,* "William Bradford."

39. *Bradford's History of Plimoth Plantation,* 2 Booke, 111–112, 387–389.

40. *CE,* "Moravia."

41. *Records of the Moravians in North Carolina 1758–1783,* I, 73.

42. *Ibid.,* I, 122, 133; II, 680, 715, 723; III, 1138; IV, 1717; V, 2301, 2330; VII, 3178, 3343, 3378, 3414, 3449.

43. *CE,* "Benjamin Rush;" *EB, idem.*

44. *Autobiography of Benjamin Rush,* 201.

45. *Ibid.,* 201–202.

46. *Baltimore. Series of Letters and Other Documents Relating to the Late Epidemic of Yellow Fever,* title page.

47. *Ibid.,* 35, 51, 153.

48. Warrington, *Nurse's Guide,* title page.

49. *Ibid.,* iii, 13–15.

50. Longshore, *Principles and Practice of Nursing,* title page.

51. *Ibid.,* 2.

52. Unpublished paper by Mary B. Poppenheim for *The Southern Magazine.*

53. *Year Book 1941 City of Charleston South Carolina,* 217.

54. Poppenheim, *op. cit.*

55. Photostatic copy of report in Library, School of Nursing, Western Reserve University.

56. *Directory Cleveland and Ohio City for the Years 1837–38.*

57. *Cleveland Directory, 1850–51,* 184.

58. *Ibid., 1856,* 7.

59. *Ibid., 1857,* 274.

60. *Apron Full of Gold,* v.

61. *Ibid.,* 22–23.

62. *WWA, 1942–43,* "Alfred Worcester."

63. Worcester, *Nurses and Nursing,* 45–46.

64. *CE,* "Peter Stuyvesant."

65. *Documents Relative to the Colonial History of the State of New York,* I, title page.

66. *Ibid.,* 300, 425.

67. *CE,* "Henry Hudson;" *EB, idem.*

68. *Historic New York: Half Moon Papers,* II, 296.

69. *Ibid.,* 296–297.

70. Wiley, *Cyclopedia of Delaware County, Pennsylvania,* 37.

71. Smith, *History of Delaware County, Pennsylvania,* 96–139.

72. *Rec. Upland Court,* 102. Quoted in *ibid.,* 116.

73. *Public Records of the Colony of Connecticut from October, 1706, to October, 1716,* 231.

74. Cruzat, "Ursulines of Louisiana," *Louisiana Historical Quarterly,* Vol. II, No. 1 (January, 1919), 5–7. Treaty in Vol. 2, Register of the Accounts of the Indies, Depot of Charts and Archives of the Marines.

75. *Ibid.,* 5–23.

76. "Cabildo Archives, French Period," *ibid.,* III (1920), 555–556.

77. *Ibid.*

78. "Sidelights on Louisiana History," *ibid.,* I (1917–1919), 110; III (1920), 551–552; IV (1921), 366–367; *EB,* "Louisiana."

79. Translation of handwritten transcript of extract of despatch of May 20, 1737, from Bienville and Salmon to the Count de Maurepas. In Collection of French Reproductions, Library of Congress.

80. Packard, *History of Medicine in the United States,* 181–182.

81. Quoted in *ibid.*

82. *CE,* "Benjamin Franklin;" *EB, idem.*

83. Franklin, *Some Account of the Pennsylvania Hospital,* 30–45.

84. *CE,* "John Bigelow;" *EB, idem.*

85. *Autobiography of Benjamin Franklin,* 281–282.

86. Morton and Woodbury, *History of the Pennsylvania Hospital,* 544.

87. Original in Library of Pennsylvania Hospital.

88. The inscription on the building as given by Benjamin Franklin in *Some Account of the Pennsylvania Hospital,* p. 83, and by Francis R. Packard, M.D., in *Some Account of the Pennsylvania Hospital* (Philadelphia: Engle Press, 1938), p. 15, differs in some small details from this account of it.

89. Watson, *Annals of Philadelphia,* 399–400.

90. Packard, *Some Account of the Pennsylvania Hospital,* 3–5.

91. *EB,* "Henry Wadsworth Longfellow;" *CE, idem.*

92. Longfellow, *Evangeline,* 142–146.

93. *Statutes at Large of Virginia,* VIII, 21, 378–379; XI, 47, 167, 384; XII, 272–274.

94. *Account of the New York Hospital,* 1820 ed., 3.

95. Quoted in *ibid.,* 3, 15.

96. *Account of the New York Hospital,* 1811 ed., 29, 47–49.

97. See pp. 336–337.

98. *Longworth's American Almanack* (1805), 83, 148.

99. Archives of the Sisters of Charity, Mount St. Joseph, Ohio.

100. *Ibid.*

101. *Ibid.*

102. *Ibid.*

103. Robinson, *Ministry of Deaconesses,* 118.

104. [Keller], *History of the St. Luke's Training School for Nurses,* 9–12.

105. *EB,* "Henry Codman Potter;" *CE, idem.*

106. Potter, *Sisterhoods and Deaconesses,* 98–105.

107. Gerberding, *op. cit.,* 24, 113, 145, 188.

108. *Ibid.,* 147, 176, 184, 188, 259, 264.

109. Florence Nightingale and Annie M. Andrews.

CHAPTER 9

Selected Documents of Early War Nursing in the United States

(Pp. 364–427 of text)

1. See pp. 321–322.

2. *CE,* "French and Indian Wars."

3. Latin, *Scilicet;* suggested meaning here: "specifically," "to wit," "namely."

4. Quoted in Sheldon, *History of Deerfield, Massachusetts,* I, 568–569.

5. Original in Armed Forces Medical Library, History of Medicine Division, Cleveland, Ohio.

6. *Journals of American Congress, 1774–1788,* I, 124–125, 325, 342, 382, 383, 389, 419, 424, 500, 546, 549; II, 40, 79.

7. *DAB,* "William Shippen;" *CE, idem.*

8. *Journals of American Congress, 1774–1788,* II, 87.

9. "Text of William Shippen's First Draft of a Plan for the Organization of the Military Hospital," *Annals of Medical History,* Vol. 1, No. 2 (Summer, 1917), 174–176.

10. See p. 370, and March 29, 1777. It is stated there that the number of patients to nurses should be 10 to 1.

11. "Text of William Shippen's First Draft . . . ," 174.

12. *Official Letters to the American Congress,* I, title page.

13. *Ibid.,* 212.

14. *Orderly Book of George Washington.*

15. *Ibid.,* 24.

16. *DAH,* I, 437.

17. *Calendar of Virginia State Papers,* VIII, 83, 161, 185, 195, 227.

18. Ellet, *Women of the American Revolution,* I, 319; *EAH,* 102–105.

19. Quoted in Ellet, *op. cit.,* I, 319–320.

20. *Ibid.,* I, 119; de Riedesel, *Letters and Memoirs Relating to the War of American Independence,* 5–6.

21. de Riedesel, *op. cit.,* 184–185.

22. *Documents of the United States Sanitary Commission,* Doc. No. 2, 4–6.

23. *Ibid.*

24. *CE,* "Henry Whitney Bellows;" *EB, idem.*

25. Bellows, *Report Concerning the Woman's Central Association of Relief,* 2–3, 8.

26. *CE,* "Frederick Law Olmsted;" *EB, idem.*

27. *Report of Committee Appointed to Visit Military Hospitals,* 5–6.

28. Forman, *Western Sanitary Commission,* 16.

29. *Ibid.,* 5–7, 20–21.

30. *CE,* "John Strong Newberry;" *EB, idem.*

31. Newberry, *United States Sanitary Commission in Valley of Mississippi,* 488–490.

32. See Reading No. 296.

33. See pp. 377–378.

34. Newberry, *Visit to Fort Donelson, Tenn.,* 7.

35. See p. 378.

36. *CE,* "Frederick Law Olmsted;" *EB, idem.*

37. *Hospital Transports,* 17, 25, 84, 143, 147.

38. Woolsey, *Century of Nursing,* iii.

39. See pp. 394–396.

40. [Bacon], *Three Weeks at Gettysburg.*

41. *Letters of a Family During the War for the Union,* II, 396–404, 668–688.

42. *Ibid.,* I, 79–80, 85–86, 89, 151, 189–190, 338–339; II, 365.

43. Brockett, *Woman's Work in the Civil War,* 342.

44. Woolsey, *Hospital Days,* 9, 15–18, 30–32, 41–42.

45. *DAB,* "Katherine Prescott Wormeley."

46. The evidence indicates that "Georgy" was Georgeanna Woolsey. See Reading No. 302 for other references to Mrs. Howland (Eliza Woolsey).

47. Wormeley, *Cruel Side of the War,* 20–27, 74–75.

48. *CE,* "Louisa May Alcott;" *EB, idem.*

49. Life, *Letters and Journals of Louisa May Alcott,* 115–119.

50. Alcott, *Hospital Sketches,* 25–29, 36–37.

51. *Crusader and Feminist,* 1–30.

52. *Ibid.,* 233, 255–256.

53. Swisshelm, *Half a Century,* 304–306, 317–318, 334.

54. *South After Gettysburg,* vii–ix.

55. *Ibid.,* 15–16, 86.

56. *EB,* "Mary Ashton (Rice) Livermore;" *CE, idem.*

57. See Reading No. 309.

58. Livermore, *My Story of the War,* 206, 217, 480, 502.

59. *Personal Memoirs of John H. Brinton,* 10.

60. *Ibid.,* 43–44, 199.

61. *EB,* "Walt Whitman."

62. *CE,* "Walt Whitman."

63. *Walt Whitman and the Civil War,* 17.

64. Quoted in *ibid.,* 33.

65. *Walt Whitman,* 473.

66. *Ibid.,* 508–509, 521, 533, 557.

67. Whitman, *Wound Dresser,* title page.

68. See introductory note to Reading No. 282.

69. Gerberding, *Life and Letters of W. A. Passavant,* 308, 310, 317–318.

70. Sister Rosarita, letter dated July 30, 1954.

71. Archives of Sisters of Charity, Mount St. Joseph, Ohio.

72. Sister Rosarita, letter dated July 30, 1954.

73. Archives of Sisters of Charity, Mount St. Joseph, Ohio.

74. Jackson, *Colonel's Diary,* 1, 234, 239.

75. *Ibid.,* 88.

76. Cumming, *Journal of Hospital Life in Confederate Army of Tennessee* (5).

77. *Ibid.,* 11, 13, 57, 60, 94, 164–165.

78. Blackford, *Letters from Lee's Army,* vi–viii.

79. *Ibid.,* 22, 259–262.

80. *Women of the South in War Times,* 71.

81. *Diary of a Southern Refugee During the War,* 29, 132.

82. *Women of the South in War Times,* 132.

83. Quoted in *ibid.,* 135–136.

84. Wright, *Southern Girl in '61,* title page.

85. *Ibid.,* 178–180.

86. Anderson, *North Carolina Women of the Confederacy,* 40.

87. *Ibid.*

Bibliography

With Acknowledgments to Publishers

A complete bibliography on the subject of this source book would be very extensive and has not been attempted here. Besides the works to which reference has been made in the text, the writer inevitably examined innumerable other source materials. The bibliography which follows includes only those items which were used in the preparation of the manuscript.

MANUSCRIPTS

Annual Report of the Board of Managers to the Ladies Benevolent Society, September 15th, 1824, 2 pp. (By permission of Board of Managers, Ladies Benevolent Society, Charleston, S. C.)

Archives of Sisters of Charity, Mount St. Joseph, Ohio. (By permission of Sisters of Charity of Cincinnati.)

Bill rendered by David Field to the Province of Massachusetts Bay, for services during the French and Indian Wars, Deerfield, November, 1775, 2 pp. (By permission of Armed Forces Medical Library, History of Medicine Division, Cleveland, Ohio.)

Letter of Florence Nightingale, May 6, 1881, to the Nurses at St. Thomas's Hospital, 16 pp. (By permission of School of Nursing, Western Reserve University, Cleveland, Ohio.)

Note of Benjamin Franklin to Sister Elizabeth, June 4, 1753, 1 p. (By permission of Pennsylvania Hospital.)

Transcript of Extract of Despatch of 20 May 1737 from Bienville and Salmon to the Comte de Maurepas. (By courtesy of Library of Congress.)

PRINTED DOCUMENTS AND BOOKS

Abelly, Louis. *Saint Vincent de Paul*. Paris, 1664, 14 vols.

An Account of the New York Hospital. New York: Printed by Collins, 1811, 74 pp.

Bibliography

An Account of the New York Hospital. New York: Mahlon Day, 1820, 62 pp.

Acland, Henry Wentworth. *Memoir of the Cholera at Oxford in the Year 1854.* London: Churchill, 1856, 172 pp.

Adams, W. H. Davenport. *Good Samaritans; or Biographical Illustrations of the Law of Human Kindness.* London: Sonnenschein, 1883, 403 pp.

Adderley, James Granville. *Monsieur Vincent.* London: Arnold, 1902, 169 pp. (By permission of Edward Arnold [publishers] Ltd.)

Alcott, Louisa May. *Hospital Sketches and Companion Fireside Stories.* Boston: Little, Brown, 1916, 379 pp.

Aloysius, Sister Mary. *Memories of the Crimea.* London: Burns, 1897, 128 pp. (By permission of Burns, Oates & Washburne, Ltd.)

Ancient Laws of Ireland. Dublin: Thom, 1865, 6 vols.

Anderson, Lucy (Worth) London. *North Carolina Women of the Confederacy.* Fayetteville, N. C.: Cumberland Printing Co., 1926, 141 pp.

Apostolical Constitutions: Constitutions of the Holy Apostles by Clement, Bishop and Citizen of Rome. Edited by James Donaldson. Edinburgh: Clark, 1870, 280 pp.

Apron Full of Gold The Letters of Mary Jane Megquier from San Francisco, 1849–1856. Edited by Robert Glass Cleland. San Marino, Calif.: Huntington Library, 1949, 99 pp. (By permission of the Huntington Library.)

Atherton, William Henry. *The Saintly Life of Jeanne Mance First Lay Nurse in North America.* St. Louis: Catholic Hospital Association, 1945, 95 pp. Reprinted from *Hospital Progress,* June, July, August, 1945, as *Bulletin 282.*

[Atkinson, Sarah]. S. A. *The Life and Work of Mary Aikenhead.* New York: Longmans, 1924, 476 pp. (By permission of Longmans, Green & Co., Inc.)

Aungier, George James. *The History and Antiquities of Syon Monastery.* London: Nichols, 1840, 567 pp.

Austin, William. *The Anatomy of the Pestilence, in the Year of Our Lord, 1665, A Poem in Three Parts.* London: Brooke, 1666, 109 pp.

Autobiography of Benjamin Franklin. Edited by John Bigelow. Philadelphia: Lippincott, 1868, 399 pp.

The Autobiography of Benjamin Rush; His "Travels Through Life," together with his Commonplace Book for 1789–1813. Edited by George W. Corner. Princeton, N. J.: Princeton University Press, 1948, 399 pp. (By permission of Princeton University Press.)

Autobiography of Samuel D. Gross, M.D. with Sketches of His Contemporaries. Philadelphia: Barrie, 1887, 2 vols.

Ayres, Sister Anne. *The Life and Work of William Augustus Muhlenberg.* New York: Randolph, 1880, 524 pp.

B., J. C. *Travels in New France.* Edited by Sylvester K. Stevens, Donald H. Kent, and Emma Edith Woods. Harrisburg: Pennsylvania Historical Commission, 1941, 167 pp. (By permission of the Pennsylvania Historical and Museum Commission.)

Bibliography

The Babylonian Talmud. Translated by Rabbi Dr. I. Epstein. London: Soncino Press, 1938, 32 vols.

[Bacon, Georgeanna Muirson (Woolsey)]. *Three Weeks at Gettysburg.* New York: Randolph, 1863, 24 pp.

Baltimore. A Series of Letters and Other Documents Relating to the Late Epidemic of Yellow Fever. Baltimore: Warner, 1820, 211 pp.

Beazley, C. Raymond. *Dawn of Modern Geography.* New York: Peter Smith, 1949, 3 vols.

Beddoe, John. *Memories of Eighty Years.* Bristol: Arrowsmith, 1910, 321 pp. (By permission of J. W. Arrowsmith, Ltd.)

Bellows, Henry Whitney. *Report Concerning the Woman's Central Association of Relief at New York to the United States Sanitary Commission at Washington.* New York: Bryant, 1861, 31 pp. Document No. 32, *The Documents of the United States Sanitary Commission.* New York: 1866–71, 2 vols.

Blackford, Susan Leigh. *Letters from Lee's Army.* Edited by Charles Minor Blackford, III. New York: Scribners, 1947, 312 pp. (By permission of Charles Scribner's Sons.)

Blackwell, Elizabeth. *Pioneer Work in Opening the Medical Profession to Women, and Autobiographical Sketches.* London: Longmans, 1895, 236 pp.

Boghurst, William. *Loimographia: An Account of the Great Plague of London in the Year 1665.* Edited by Joseph Frank Payne. London: Shaw, 1894, 99 pp.

Bougaud, Mon. *History of St. Vincent de Paul, Founder of the Congregation of the Mission and of the Sisters of Charity.* London: Longmans, 1899, 2 vols.

Bradford's History of Plimoth Plantation. Boston: Wright and Potter, 1901, 555 pp.

Brockett, Linus Pierpont. *Woman's Work in the Civil War.* Philadelphia: Zeigler, McCurdy, 1867, 799 pp.

Buckler, Georgina Grenfell. *Anna Comnena: A Study.* London: Oxford University Press, 1929, 558 pp.

Calendar of Virginia State Papers. Richmond, 1875, 11 vols.

Celsus. *De Medicina.* Translated by W. G. Spencer. Cambridge, Mass.: Harvard University Press, 1935, 3 vols. (Reprinted by permission of Harvard University Press.)

Charaka-Samhita. Translated by Kaviraj Avinash Chandra Kaviratna. Calcutta: Published by the translator, 1890–1925, 4 vols.

Charles Kingsley: His Letters and Memories of his Life. Edited by His Wife. London: Paul, 1888, 2 vols.

Charlevoix, Father [Pierre François Xavier de]. *Letters to the Dutchess of Lesdiguieres.* London: Goadby, 1763, 384 pp.

Chavasse, Pye Henry. *Advice to a Wife on the Management of Her Own Health and on the Treatment of Some of the Complaints Incident to Pregnancy, Labor, and Suckling.* New York: Routledge, 1873, 273 pp.

Child, Francis James. *The English and Scottish Popular Ballads.* Boston: Houghton Mifflin, 1882, 5 vols.

Chronicles of the Pilgrim Fathers of the Colony of Plymouth from 1602 to 1625. Compiled by Alexander Young. Boston: Little, Brown, 1884, 502 pp.

Clark, Alice. *Working Life of Women in the Seventeenth Century.* New York: Dutton, 1919, 332 pp.

Clarke, W. K. Lowther. *Saint Gregory of Nyssa: The Life of Saint Macrina.* London: Society for Promoting Christian Knowledge, 1916, 79 pp. (By permission of The Society for Promoting Christian Knowledge and The Macmillan Company.)

Clay, Mary Rotha. *Mediaeval Hospitals of England.* London: Methuen, 1909, 357 pp. (By permission of Methuen & Co., Ltd.)

Cleveland Directory, 1850–51; 1856; 1857.

Comnena, Anna. *The Alexiad.* Translated by Elizabeth A. S. Dawes. London: Paul, Trench, Trubner, 1928, 439 pp. (By permission of Routledge and Kegan Paul, Ltd.)

The Complete Works of Homer. The Iliad and the Odyssey. The Iliad. Translated by Andrew Lang, Walter Leaf, and Ernest Myers, 463 pp. *The Odyssey.* Translated by S. H. Butcher and Andrew Lang, 383 pp. Modern Library, n. d.

Conferences de S. Vincent de Paul aux Filles de la Charité. Paris, 1881, 2 vols.

Cook, Sir Edward. *The Life of Florence Nightingale.* London: Macmillan, 1913, 2 vols. (By permission of St. Martin's Press, Inc.)

Cooke, Harriette J. *Mildmay: or The Story of the First Deaconess Institution.* London: Stock, 1893, 214 pp.

Coste, Pierre. *The Life and Works of Saint Vincent de Paul.* London: Burns, 1934, 3 vols. (By permission of Burns, Oates & Washburne, Ltd.)

Crusader and Feminist: Letters of Jane Grey Swisshelm. Edited by Arthur J. Larsen. Saint Paul: Historical Society, 1934, 327 pp. (By permission of Minnesota Historical Association.)

Cumming, Kate. *A Journal of Hospital Life in the Confederate Army of Tennessee from the Battle of Shiloh to the End of the War.* Louisville, Ky.: Morton, 1866, 199 pp.

Darwin, Emma. *A Century of Family Letters, 1792–1896.* Edited by Henrietta E. Litchfield. London: Murray, 1915, 2 vols. (By permission of John Murray [Publishers] Ltd.)

Davidson, Randall Thomas, and Benham, William. *Life of Archibald Campbell Tait (Archbishop of Canterbury).* New York: Macmillan, 1891, 2 vols.

De Bunsen, Mme Elizabeth S. (Gurney). *Elizabeth Fry's Journeys on the Continent, 1840–1841.* London: Lane, 1931, 208 pp. (By permission of John Lane, The Bodley Head, Ltd.)

Defoe, Daniel. *Due Preparations for the Plague As Well for Soul as Body.* New York: Jensen, 1907, 279 pp.

456

Bibliography

Defoe, Daniel. *A Journal of the Plague Year.* London: Noble, 1720, 376 pp.

de Riedesel, Madame [Frederica]. *Letters and Memoirs Relating to the War of American Independence, and the Capture of the German Troops at Saratoga.* New York: Carrel, 1827, 323 pp.

Dialogues of St. Gregory, Surnamed the Great. Edited by Edmund G. Gardner. London: Warner, 1911, 283 pp.

Diary and Correspondence of Samuel Pepys, F. R. S. Philadelphia: Lippincott, 1855, 2 vols.

Diary of a Southern Refugee During the War. By a Lady of Virginia, 3rd ed., Richmond, Va.: Randolph, 1889, 327 pp.

Diary of Lady Margaret Hoby. Edited by Dorothy M. Meads. Boston: Houghton Mifflin, 1930, 289 pp. (By permission of Routledge and Kegan Paul, Ltd.)

Dickens, Charles. *The Life and Adventures of Martin Chuzzlewit.* London: Nelson, n. d., 897 pp.

Didascalia Apostolorum. Translated by Margaret Dunlop Gibson. London: Clay, 1903, 113 pp.

Directory Cleveland and Ohio City For the Years 1837–38. Cleveland: Sanford and Lott, 1837, 144 pp.

Dock, Lavinia L., and Stewart, Isabel M. *A Short History of Nursing,* 4th ed., New York: Putnam, 1938, 426 pp.

Documents Relative to the Colonial History of the State of New York. Edited by E. B. O'Callaghan. Albany: Weed, Parsons, 1861, 5 vols.

The Documents of the United States Sanitary Commission. New York: 1866–1871, 2 vols.

Dollier de Casson, François. *A History of Montreal 1640–1672.* Translated by Ralph Flenley. London: Dent, 1928, 384 pp. (By permission of J. M. Dent & Sons, Ltd.)

Drane, Augusta Theodosia. *The History of St. Catherine of Siena and Her Companions.* London: Longmans, 1899, 2 vols.

Dunbar, Virginia M. The Origin and Early Development of Two English Training Schools for Nurses. Unpublished paper. London: Florence Nightingale International Foundation, 1936, 188 pp. (By permission of the author.)

Duncon, John. *The Holy Life and Death of the Lady Letice, Vicountess Falkland,* 3rd ed. London: Rich, Royston, 1653, 192 pp.

Dunne, L. *A Trip to Constantinople . . . and Miss Nightingale at Scutari Hospital.* London: Sheppard, 1862, 208 pp.

Early Travels in Palestine. Edited by Thomas Wright. London: Bohn, 1848, 517 pp.

Ellet, Elizabeth Fries (Lummis). *The Women of the American Revolution.* New York: Scribner, 1848, 2 vols.

Emanuel, Cyprian W. *The Charities of St. Vincent de Paul.* Washington: Catholic University of America, 1923, 357 pp. (By permission of Catholic University of America.)

457

Englebert, Omer. *Saint Francis of Assisi.* Translated by Edward Hutton. London: Longmans, 1950, 352 pp. (By permission of Longmans, Green & Co., Ltd.)

An English Translation of the Sushruta-Samhita. Edited by Kaviraj Kunja Lal Bhistragratna. Calcutta: No. 10 Kashi Ghose' Lane, 1907, 3 vols.

The Fifty Earliest Wills in the Court of Probate, London. Edited by Frederick J. Furnivall. London: Trubner, 1882, 200 pp.

Finley, Ruth. *The Lady of Godey's.* Philadelphia: Lippincott, 1931, 318 pp.

Fliedner, Theodor. *Kurzer Abriss Seines Lebens.* Kaiserswerth, 1866.

Forman, J. G. *The Western Sanitary Commission: A Sketch of Its Organization, History, and Aid Given to Freedmen and Union Refugees, with Incidents of Hospital Life.* St. Louis: 1864, 144 pp.

Forster, John. *The Life of Charles Dickens.* Boston: Estes, 1872, 3 vols.

Franklin, Benjamin. *Some Account of the Pennsylvania Hospital from its First Beginning to the Fifth Month, called May, 1754.* Philadelphia: Office of the Gazette, 1817, 145 pp.

Fuller, Thomas. [1654–1734] *Exanthematologia; or a Rational Account of Eruptive Fevers.* London: Printed for Charles Rivington, 1730, 439 pp.

Fuller, Thomas. [1608–1661] *The Historie of the Holy Warre.* Cambridge: Thomas Buck, 1639, 286 pp.

The Genuine Works of Hippocrates. Translated by Francis Adams. London: Sydenham Society, 1849, 477 pp.

Gerberding, G. H. *Life and Letters of W. A. Passavant, D.D.,* 3rd ed. Greenville, Pa.: Young Lutheran Co., 1906, 615 pp. (By permission of The Beaver Printing Company.)

Godlee, Sir Rickman John. *Life of Lord Lister.* London: Macmillan, 1917, 676 pp. (By permission of The Macmillan Company.)

Goodman, Margaret. *Experiences of an English Sister of Mercy.* London: Smith Elder, 1862, 234 pp.

Gregory, William. *The Historical Collections of a Citizen of London in the Fifteenth Century.* Westminster: Camden Society, 1876, 279 pp.

Haldane, Elizabeth C. H. *Mrs. Gaskell and Her Friends.* London: Hodder, 1930, 318 pp. (By permission of Hodder & Stoughton, Ltd.)

Haldane, Elizabeth S. *The British Nurse in Peace and War.* London: Murray, 1923, 282 pp. (By permission of John Murray [Publishers] Ltd.)

Hall, Basil. *Travels in North America in the Years 1827 and 1828.* Edinburgh: Cadell, 1829, 3 vols.

Hall, Francis. *Travels in Canada and the United States in 1816 and 1817.* London: Longmans, 1819, 421 pp.

Hefele, Charles Joseph. *A History of the Councils of the Church From the Original Documents.* Edinburgh: Clark, 1876–1896, 5 vols.

Heidel, Alexander. *The Babylonian Genesis.* Chicago: University of Chicago Press, 1942, 131 pp. (By permission of the University of Chicago Press.)

Henley, Ernest. *In Hospital; Rhymes and Rhythms.* Portland, Me.: Mosher, 1921, 40 pp.

Bibliography

Higginson, General Sir George, G.C.B. *Seventy-one Years of a Guardsman's Life*. London: Smith Elder, 1916, 408 pp. (By permission of John Murray [Publishers] Ltd.)

Hippocrates. *Decorum*. Translated by W. H. S. Jones. London: Heineman, 1923, 4 vols. (Reprinted by permission of Harvard University Press.)

Historic New York: Half Moon Papers. Edited by Maud Wilder Goodwin and Others. New York: Putnam, 1899, 2 vols.

Hoare, Sir Richard Colt. *Recollections Abroad During the Year 1790*. Bath: Crutwell, 1817, 247 pp.

Hodges, Nathaniel. *Loimologia; or, an Historical Account of the Plague in London in 1665*. London: Bell, 1665, 288 pp.

Holzapfel, Herbert. *The History of the Franciscan Order*. Translated by Antonine Tibesar and Gervasse Brinkman. Teutopolis, Ill.: St. Joseph Seminary, 1948, 608 pp.

Hornby, Lady Emelia Bithynia. *Constantinople During the Crimean War*. London: Bentley, 1863, 500 pp.

Hospital Transports, A Memoir of the Embarkation of the Sick and Wounded from the Peninsula of Virginia in the Summer of 1862. Compiled by Frederick Law Olmsted. Boston: Ticknor and Fields, 1863, 167 pp.

Howard, John. *An Account of the Principal Lazarettos in Europe*. London: Johnson, Dilly and Cadel, 1791, 259 pp.

Howe, Julia Ward. *Reminiscences, 1819–1899*. Boston: Houghton Mifflin, 1900, 465 pp. (By permission of Houghton Mifflin Company.)

Hughes, Muriel Joy. *Women Healers in Medieval Life and Literature*. New York: King's Crown Press, 1943, 181 pp. (By permission of Columbia University Press.)

The Idylls and Epigrams of Theocritus Bion and Moschus. Boston: Bibliophile Society, 1905, 3 vols.

Ives, A. G. L. *British Hospitals*. London: Collins, 1948, 50 pp.

Jackson, Oscar L. *The Colonel's Diary: Journals Kept before and During the Civil War by the Late Colonel Oscar L. Jackson of New Castle, Pennsylvania*. Sharon: 1922, 262 pp.

Jameson, Anna Brownell (Murphy). *Sacred and Legendary Art*. Boston: Houghton Mifflin, 1895, 2 vols.

The Jesuit Relations and Allied Documents. Edited by Reuben Gold Thwaites. Cleveland: Burrows, 1896, 73 vols. in 8.

Journals of the American Congress from 1774 to 1788. Washington: Way and Gideon, 1825, 4 vols.

[Keller, Malvina W.] *History of the St. Luke's Hospital Training School for Nurses*. New York: St. Luke's Hospital, 1938, 340 pp. (By permission of the Alumnae Association of St. Luke's Hospital School of Nursing.)

King, E. J. *The Knights Hospitallers in the Holy Land*. London: Methuen, 1931, 336 pp. (By permission of Methuen & Co., Ltd.)

————.*The Rule Statutes and Customs of the Hospitallers, 1099–1310*. London: Methuen, 1934, 224 pp. (By permission of Methuen & Co., Ltd.)

Kingsley, Charles. *Hypatia*. New York: Weeks, n. d., 475 pp.

Kingsley, Charles. *Poems*. London: Oxford University Press, 1913, 348 pp. (By permission of Oxford University Press.)

Knox, John. *An Historical Journal of the Campaigns in North America*. Edited by Arthur G. Doughty. Toronto: Champlain Society, 1914, 1916, 3 vols. (By permission of the Champlain Society.)

La Rochefoucauld-Liancourt, Duke de. *Travels Through the United States of North America, the country of the Iroquois, and Upper Canada in the Years 1795, 1796, and 1797, with an Authentic Account of Lower Canada*. London: Philips, 1799, 2 vols.

Lees, Florence S. *Handbook for Hospital Sisters*. London: Isbister, 1874, 240 pp.

The Legend of S. Francis by the Three Companions. Translated by E. Gurney Salter. London: Dent, 1905, 136 pp. (By permission of J. M. Dent & Sons Ltd.)

Letters of Abelard and Heloise. Translated by C. K. Scott Moncrieff. New York: Knopf, 1926, 264 pp. (By permission of Alfred A. Knopf, Inc.)

Letters of a Family during the War for the Union, 1861–1865. Printed for private distribution, 1899, 2 vols.

Letters of St. Vincent de Paul. Translated and edited by Joseph Leonard. London: Burns, 1937, 614 pp. (By permission of Burns, Oates & Washburne, Ltd.)

Lettres et Conférences de S. Vincent de Paul (Supplément): Procès-Verbaux des Assemblées et des Conseils; Reglements Divers. Paris: 1888.

Liddon, Henry Parry. *Life of Edward Bouverie Pusey*, 4th ed. London: Longmans, 1894–1897, 4 vols.

The Life and Correspondence of the Late Robert Southey. Edited by Charles Cuthbert Southey. London: Longmans, 1850, 6 vols.

Life and Letters of James Hinton. Edited by Ellice Hopkins. London: Kegan Paul, 1878, 371 pp.

The Life and Letters of Rev. William Pennefather. Edited by Robert Braithwaite. New York: Carter, 1878, 536 pp.

The Life and Works of Charles Kingsley. Edited by His Wife. London: Macmillan, 1901–1903, 19 vols.

Life, Letters and Journals of Louisa May Alcott. Edited by Ednah D. Cheney. Boston: Little, Brown, 1928, 352 pp.

Life of Henry Wadsworth Longfellow with Extracts from his Journals and Correspondence. Edited by Samuel Longfellow. Boston: Houghton Mifflin, 1891, 3 vols.

Life of Pastor Fliedner of Kaiserswerth. Translated by Catherine Winkworth. London: Longmans, 1867, 155 pp.

"The Little Flowers" and the Life of St. Francis with the "Mirror of Perfection." New York: Dutton, 1927, 397 pp. (By permission of E. P. Dutton & Co., Inc., and Everyman's Library.)

Livermore, Mary. *My Story of the War: A Woman's Narrative of Four Years' Personal Experience*. Hartford, Conn.: Worthington, 1889, 200 pp.

Bibliography

Longfellow, Henry Wadsworth. *Evangeline, A Tale of Acadie.* New York: Hurst, n. d., 155 pp.

Longshore, J. S. *The Principles and Practice of Nursing or a Guide to the Inexperienced.* Philadelphia: Merrihew and Thompson, 1842, 238 pp.

Longworth's American Almanack, New-York Register, and City Directory: For the Thirtieth Year of American Independence. New York: Longworth, 1805, 410 pp.

Lonsdale, Margaret. *Sister Dora.* Boston: Roberts, 1887, 290 pp.

Ludlow, James Meeker. *Woman's Work in the Church.* London: Strahan, 1866, 317 pp.

McCann, Sister Mary Agnes. *The History of Mother Seton's Daughters, The Sisters of Charity of Cincinnati, Ohio 1809–1917.* New York: Longmans, 1917, 3 vols.

MacNutt, Francis Augustus. *Letters of Cortes.* New York: Putnam, 1908, 2 vols.

Marriott, J. A. R. *The Life and Times of Lucius Cary Vicount Falkland.* London: Rich, Royston, 1653, 192 pp.

Martineau, Harriet. *Biographical Sketches.* New York: Leypoldt, Holt, 1869, 458 pp.

Matheson, Annie. *Florence Nightingale A Biography.* New York: Nelson, n. d., 374 pp.

Melanges d'Archeologie, 1895.

Memoir of the Rt. Hon. Sir John McNeill, G. C. B., and of His Second Wife, Elizabeth Wilson. London: Murray, 1910, 426 pp. (By permission of John Murray [Publishers] Ltd.)

Memoirs and Letters of Sir James Paget. London: Longmans, 1901, 438 pp. (By permission of Longmans, Green & Co., Ltd.)

Memoirs of the Life of Elizabeth Fry, with extracts from her journal and letters, 2nd ed. Edited by Her Two Daughters. London: Hatchard, 1848, 2 vols.

Memoranda, References, and Documents Relating to the Royal Hospitals of the City of London: Prepared and Printed Under the Directions of the Committee of the Court of Common Council, Appointed in Relation to Said Hospitals. London: Taylor, 1836, 107 pp.

Memorial of Two Sisters: Susanna and Catherine Winkworth. Edited by Margaret J. Shean. London: Longmans, 1908, 341 pp.

The Mirror of Perfection of St. Francis of Assisi. Translated by Sebastian Evans. Long Acre, England: Nutt, 1900, 232 pp.

Montalembert, Count de. *Life of Saint Elizabeth of Hungary Duchess of Thuringia.* Translated by Mary Hackett. New York: Kenedy, 1901, 427 pp. (By permission of P. J. Kenedy & Sons.)

Moore, Norman. *The Past and Present State of St. Bartholomew's Hospital.* London: Pearson, 1918, 2 vols. (By permission of C. Arthur Pearson, Ltd.)

Moorman, John R. H. *The Sources for the Life of St. Francis of Assisi.* Manchester: Manchester University Press, 1940, 176 pp.

More, Sir Thomas. *Utopia.* London: Cambridge University Press, 1890, 259 pp. (By permission of Cambridge University Press.)

Morris, E. W. *A History of the London Hospital.* London: Arnold, 1910, 318 pp. (By permission of Edward Arnold [Publishers] Ltd.)

Morton, Thomas G., and Woodbury, Frank. *The History of the Pennsylvania Hospital, 1751-1895.* Philadelphia: Times Printing House, 1895, 561 pp.

Muratori, Lodivico Antonio. *Antiquitates Italicae Medii Aevi.* Milan: Palatine Society, 1738-42, 6 vols.

Newberry, John Strong. *The United States Sanitary Commission in the Valley of the Mississippi during the War of the Rebellion, 1861-1866.* Cleveland: Fairbanks, Benedict, 1871, 536 pp.

———. *A Visit to Fort Donelson, Tenn, for the Relief of the Wounded of Feb'y 15, 1862: A Letter.* 8 pp.

The New Testament.

Nichols, R. H., and Wray, F. A. *The History of the Foundlings' Hospital.* London: Oxford University Press, 1935, 422 pp. (By permission of Oxford University Press.)

Nicholson, Watson. *The Historical Sources of Defoe's Journal of the Plague Year.* Boston: Stratford, 1919, 182 pp.

Nightingale, Florence. *Army Sanitary Administration and Its Reform Under the Late Lord Herbert.* London: McCorquodale, 1862, 11 pp.

[———]. *The Institution of Kaiserswerth on the Rhine, for the Practical Training of Deaconesses.* London: Printed by the Inmates of the Ragged Colonial Training School, 1851, 32 pp.

[———]. *Notes on Hospitals,* 3rd ed. London: Longmans, 1867, 187 pp.

[———]. *Subsidiary Notes as to the Introduction of Female Nursing into Military Hospitals in Peace and War.* London: Harrison, 1858, 133 pp.

Nolan, William. *An Essay on Humanity: or A View of Abuses in Hospitals with a Plan for Correcting Them.* London: Murray, 1786, 49 pp.

Nutting, M. Adelaide, and Dock, Lavinia L. *A History of Nursing.* New York: Putnam, 1907, 1912, 4 vols.

Official Letters to the Honorable American Congress. Written during the War Between the United Colonies and Great Britain by His Excellency George Washington Commander in Chief of the Continental Forces Now President of the United States. New York: Campbell, 1796, 2 vols.

The Old Testament.

Orderly Book of General George Washington, Commander in Chief of the American Armies, Kept at Valley Forge, 18 May-11 June 1778. New York: Lamson, 1898, 54 pp.

Osborne, Sydney Godolphin. *Scutari and Its Hospitals.* London: Dickinson, 1855, 54 pp.

Packard, Francis R. *History of Medicine in the United States.* New York: Hoeber, 1931, 656 pp. (By permission of Paul B. Hoeber, Inc.)

———. *Life and Times of Ambroise Paré (1510-1590) With a New Translation of His Apology and an Account of His Journeys in Divers Places.* New York: Hoeber, 1921, 297 pp.

Bibliography

————. *Some Account of the Pennsylvania Hospital From its first Rise to the Beginning of the Year 1938.* Philadelphia: Engle Press, 1938, 133 pp.

Palestine Pilgrims Text Society. London: The Society, 11 vols.

    II. *Of the Holy Places Visited by Antoninus Martyr (Circa 530 A.D.).* Translated by Aubrey Stewart, 1884, 44 pp.

    V. *Fetullus. Circa 1130 A.D.* Translated by James Rose Macpherson, 1892, 58 pp.

    Description of the Holy Land by John of Wurzburg c. A.D. 1160–1170. Translated by Aubrey Stewart, 1890, 72 pp.

    Theodorich's Description of the Holy Places (Circa 1172 A.D.). Translation by Aubrey Stewart, 1891, 82 pp.

    XII. *Ludolph von Suchem's Description of the Holy Land and of the way Thither. Written in the Year 1350.* Translated by Aubrey Stewart, 1895, 142 pp.

Palladius. *The Paradise of the Holy Fathers.* Translated by Ernest A. Wallis Budge. New York: Duffield, n. d., 2 vols.

Parsons, Frederick Gymer. *History of St. Thomas's Hospital.* London: Methuen, 1932–36, 3 vols. (By permission of Methuen & Co., Ltd.)

Personal Memoirs of John H. Brinton, Major and Surgeon, U.S.V., 1861–1865. New York: Neale, 1914, 361 pp.

Pincoffs, Peter. *Experiences of a Civilian in Eastern Military Hospitals.* London: Williams and Norgate, 1857, 202 pp.

Plato. *Laws.* Translated by R. G. Bury. London: Heinemann, 1926, 2 vols. (Reprinted by permission of Harvard University Press.)

Platt, Elspeth. *The Story of the Ranyard Mission.* London: Hodder, 1937, 128 pp. (By permission of Hodder & Stoughton, Ltd.)

Pliny's Letters. Translated by William Melmoth. New York: Putnam, 1923, 2 vols.

Plutarch's Lives: Alcibiades. Translated by Bernadotte Perrin. London: Heinemann, 1916–1932. Vol. IV of 10-vol. ed. of *Plutarch's Lives.* (Reprinted by permission of Harvard University Press.)

Plutarch's Lives: Lycurgus. Translated by John Dryden. Boston: Little, Brown, 1895. Vol I of 5-vol. ed. of *Plutarch's Lives,* revised by A. H. Clough.

Pöel, Emma. *Life of Amelia Wilhelmina Sieveking.* Translated by Catherine Winkworth. London: Longmans, 1863, 520 pp.

The Poetical Works of Henry Wadsworth Longfellow. Edinburgh: Nimmo, n. d., 633 pp.

Pope-Hennessy, James. *Monckton Milnes; The Years of Promise, 1809–1851.* London: Constable, 1949, 327 pp.

Pope-Hennessy, Una. *Canon Charles Kingsley, A Biography.* London: Chatto & Windus, 1948, 294 pp.

Porter, Whitworth. *A History of the Knights of Malta or the Order of the Hospital of St. John of Jerusalem.* London: Longmans, 1858, 2 vols.

Potter, Henry Codman. *Sisterhoods and Deaconesses at Home and Abroad.* New York: Dutton, 1873, 358 pp.

Bibliography

Procopius. Translated by H. B. Dewing and Glanville Downey. Cambridge, Mass.: Harvard University Press, 1940, 7 vols. (Reprinted by permission of Harvard University Press.)

Public Records of the Colony of Connecticut from October, 1706, to October, 1716, With the Council Journal from October, 1710, to February, 1717. Transcribed by Charles J. Hoadley. Hartford, Conn.: Case, Lockwood and Brainard, 1870, 612 pp.

Ramsey, Grace. *Thomas Grant, First Bishop of Southwark.* London: Smith Elder, 1874, 491 pp.

Rathbone, Eleanor F. *William Rathbone A Memoir.* New York: Macmillan, 1905, 507 pp. (By permission of St. Martin's Press, Inc.)

Rathbone, William. *Sketch of the History and Progress of District Nursing from Its Commencement in the Year 1859 to the Present Date.* New York: Macmillan, 1890, 132 pp.

Raymond of Capua. *Life of Saint Catherine of Sienna.* Translated by the Ladies of the Sacred Heart. Philadelphia: Cunningham, 1860, 432 pp.

Records of the Moravians in North Carolina 1758–1783. Publications of the North Carolina Historical Commission. Edited by Adelaide Lisetta Fries. Raleigh, N.C.: Edwards and Broughton, 1922, 7 vols. (By courtesy of North Carolina State Department of Archives and History).

Reid, Sir T. Wemyss. *Richard Monckton Milnes, The Life, Letters and Friendships of Richard Monckton Milnes, First Lord Houghton.* New York: Cassell, 1891, 2 vols.

Report of the Committee Appointed on the 29th inst. to Visit the Military General Hospitals In and Around Washington. Washington: 1861. Document No. 23, *The Documents of the United States Sanitary Commission.* New York: 1866–71.

Richards, Linda. *Reminiscences of Linda Richards America's First Trained Nurse.* Boston: Whitcomb and Barrows, 1911, 121 pp.

Rickards, E. C. *Felicia Skene of Oxford A Memoir.* London: Murray, 1902, 387 pp. (By permission of John Murray [Publishers] Ltd.)

Robinson, Deaconess Cecilia. *The Ministry of Deaconesses.* London: Methuen, 1898, 241 pp.

The Rule of St. Benedict. Translated by Cardinal Gasquet. London: Chatto, 1925, 130 pp. (By permission of Chatto & Windus.)

Ryder, Edward. *Elizabeth Fry Life and Labors of the Eminent Philanthropist, Preacher and Prison Reformer.* New York: Walker, 1883, 381 pp.

Sabatier, Paul. *Life of St. Francis of Assisi.* Translated by Louise Seymour Houghton. New York: Scribner, 1921, 448 pp.

St. Basil. *The Letters.* Translated by Roy J. Deferrari. New York: Putnam, 1926, 4 vols.

St. Bonaventura. *Life of St. Francis.* Translated by E. Gurney Salter. San Francisco: Nash, 1931, 187 pp.

Schermerhorn, Elizabeth Wheeler. *On the Trail of the Eight-Pointed Cross.* New York: Putnam, 1940, 421 pp.

Bibliography

Select Historical Documents of the Middle Ages. Translated and edited by Ernest Flagg Henderson. London: Bell, 1896, 477 pp.

Select Letters of St. Jerome. Translated by F. A. Wright. London: Heinemann, 1933, 510 pp.

A Select Library of the Nicene and Post-Nicene Fathers of the Christian Church, 1st ser. New York: Christian Literature Co., 1888, 14 vols.

A Select Library of Nicene and Post-Nicene Fathers of the Christian Church, 2nd ser. New York: Christian Literature Co., 1890–, 14 vols.

Seymer, Lucy Ridgely. *A General History of Nursing*. New York: Macmillan, 1949, 332 pp.

Sheldon, George. *A History of Deerfield, Massachusetts*. Deerfield, 1895, 2 vols.

The Shutting Up of Infected Houses as it is practised in England, Soberly Debated. Anonymous, 1665.

Simcoe, Elizabeth Posthuma (Gwillin). *The Diary of Mrs. John Graves Simcoe*. Toronto: Briggs, 1911, 440 pp. (By permission of Ryerson Press.)

Sisterhoods; Schools for Nurses. London: Benrose, 1866, 37 pp.

Skene, James Henry. *With Lord Stratford in the Crimean War*. London: Bentley, 1883, 352 pp.

Smith, George. *History of Delaware County, Pennsylvania*. Philadelphia: Ashmead, 1862, 581 pp.

South, J. F. *Facts Relating to Hospital Nurses*. London: Richardson, 1857, 33 pp.

South After Gettysburg Letters of Cornelia Hancock from the Army of the Potomac 1863–1865. Edited by Henrietta Stratton Jacquette. Philadelphia: University of Pennsylvania Press, 1937, 173 pp. (By permission of University of Pennsylvania Press.)

Southey, Robert. *Journal of a Tour in the Netherlands in the Autumn of 1815*. London: Heinemann, 1903, 264 pp. (Reprinted by permission of William Heinemann, Ltd., and Harvard University Press.)

———. *Sir Thomas More; or Colloquies on the Progress and Prospects of Society*. London: Murray, 1829, 2 vols.

[Stanley, Mary]. *Hospitals and Sisterhoods*. London: Murray, 1854, 154 pp.

Stanmore, Lord. *Sidney Herbert Lord Herbert of Lea A Memoir*. London: Murray, 1906, 2 vols. (By permission of John Murray [Publishers] Ltd.)

The Statutes at Large: Being a Collection of All the Laws of Virginia, from the First Session of the Legislature, in the Year 1619. Edited by William Waller Hening. Richmond: Cochran, 1819–23, 13 vols.

Stow, John. *Annales, or a Generall Chronicle of England, begun by John Stow, continued and augmented by Edmond Howes*. London: 1615, 998 pp.

———. *A Survay of London*. Edited by Henry Morley. London: Routledge, 1890, 446 pp. Longer edition, 2 vols.

Sussex Archeological Collections. Sussex: 1848–, 91 vols.

465

Bibliography

I. *Extracts from the Journal and Account Book of the Rev. Giles Moore, Rector of Horsted Keynes, Sussex, from the Year 1655 to 1679*. 1848, pp. 65–127.

XX. Rev. Edward Turner. *Ancient Parochial Account Book of Cowden, 1704*. 1868, pp. 91–119.

XXIII. Thomas Ross, Esq. *Hastings Documents, 1601*. 1871, pp. 85–118.

Swisshelm, Jane Grey. *Half a Century*, 2nd ed. Chicago: Swisshelm, 1880, 363 pp.

[Taylor, Fanny M.] *Eastern Hospitals and English Nurses: The Narrative of Twelve Months' Experience in the Hospitals of Koulali and Scutari*, 3rd ed. London: Hurst and Blackett, 1857, 356 pp.

Theodoric of Thuringen. *Vita Sancte Elisabethae*. Amsterdam: 1725, 4 vols.

Thomas of Celano. *The Life of St. Clare*. Translated by Fr. Paschal Robinson. Philadelphia: Dolphin, 1910, 167 pp. (By permission of the Dolphin Press.)

————. *Lives of St. Francis of Assisi*. Translated by A. G. Ferrers Howell. London: Methuen, 1908, 169 pp. (By permission of Methuen & Co., Ltd.)

Thorp, Margaret Farrand. *Charles Kingsley 1819–1875*. Princeton, N.J.: Princeton University Press, 1937, 212 pp.

Tooley, S. A. *The History of Nursing in the British Empire*. London: Bousfield, 1906, 392 pp.

————. *The Life of Florence Nightingale*. London: Bousfield, 1904, 344 pp.

Twining, Louisa. *Workhouses and Pauperism and Women's Work in the Administration of the Poor Law*. London: Methuen, 1898, 271 pp.

"Una and Her Paupers:" Memorials of Agnes Elizabeth Jones. By her Sister. New York: Routledge, 1872, 497 pp.

Vertot, Abbé René Aubert de. *The History of the Knights of Malta*. London: Strahan, 1727, 5 vols.

Villehardouin, Goeffroi and de Joinville. *Memoirs of the Crusades*. Translated by Sir Frank Marzials. London: Dent, 1908, 340 pp. (By permission of E. P. Dutton & Co., Inc., and Everyman's Library.)

Vincent, Thomas. *God's Terrible Voice in the City*. 1667, 262 pp.

Vitruvius. *On Architecture*. Translated by Frank Granger. New York: Putnam, 1931, 2 vols.

Wakefield, Priscilla (Bell). *Excursions in North America*, 2nd ed. London: Darton and Hawry, 1810, 420 pp.

Walt Whitman. Edited by Mark Van Doren. New York: Viking Press, 1945, 698 pp.

Walt Whitman and the Civil War. Edited by Charles I. Glicksberg. Philadelphia: University of Pennsylvania Press, 1933, 201 pp. (By permission of University of Pennsylvania Press.)

Warrington, Joseph. *The Nurse's Guide*. Philadelphia: Thomas, Cowperthwaite, 1839, 131 pp.

Watson, John F. *Annals of Philadelphia, Being a Collection of Memoirs, Anecdotes, & Incidents of the City and Its Inhabitants from the Days of*

466

the Pilgrim Founders. Philadelphia: Hunt, 1830, 740 pp. + 78 on New York City.

Wheeler, Henry. *Deaconesses, Ancient and Modern.* New York: Hunt and Eaton, 1889, 315 pp.

Whitman, Walt. *The Wound Dresser.* Edited by Richard M. Bucke. New York: Bodley Press, 1949, 200 pp.

Wiley, Samuel T. *Cyclopedia of Delaware County, Pennsylvania.* Richmond, Ind.: Gresham Publishing Co., 1894, 500 pp.

William Archbishop of Tyre. *A History of Deeds Done Beyond the Sea.* Translated and annotated by Emily Atwater Babcock and A. C. Krey. New York: Columbia University Press, 1942, 2 vols. (By permission of Columbia University Press.)

Willison, George F. *Saints and Strangers.* New York: Reynal & Hitchcock, 1945, 513 pp.

Woman's Mission: A Series of Congress Papers on the Philanthropic Work of Women. Edited by Baroness Burdett-Coutts. New York: Scribner, 1893, 485 pp.

The Women of the South in War Times. Compiled by Matthew Page Andrews. Baltimore: Norman, 1923, 466 pp. (By permission of Remington Putnam Book Company, Baltimore 1, Md.)

Woodham-Smith, Cecil. *Florence Nightingale.* New York: McGraw-Hill, 1951, 382 pp.

Woolsey, Abby Howland. *A Century of Nursing.* New York: Putnam, 1950, 172 pp.

Woolsey, Jane Stuart. *Hospital Days.* New York: Van Nostrand, 1870, 182 pp.

Worcester, Alfred. *Nurses and Nursing.* Cambridge, Mass.: Harvard University Press, 1927, 173 pp. (Reprinted by permission of Harvard University Press.)

The Workes of that Famous Chirurgion Ambroise Parey. Translated by Thomas Johnson. London: Cotes, 1634, 1175 pp.

Works of John Robinson, Pastor of the Pilgrim Fathers. London: Snow, 1851, 3 vols.

Wormeley, Katharine Prescott. *The Cruel Side of the War, With the Army of the Potomac.* Boston: Roberts, 1898, 210 pp.

Wright, Mrs. D. Giraud (Louise Wigfall). *A Southern Girl in '61.* New York: Doubleday, Page, 1905, 258 pp. (By permission of Doubleday & Company, Inc.)

Xenophon. *Memorabilia and Oeconomicus.* Translated by E. C. Marchant. New York: Putnam, 1923, 532 pp.

Year Book 1941 City of Charleston South Carolina. Charleston, S.C.: City Council, 1942, 256 pp.

Bibliography

NEWSPAPERS AND PERIODICALS

Baltimore Catholic Mirror, Feb. 25, 1862.

Beale, Lionel S. "Nursing the Sick in Hospitals, Private Families, and Among the Poor," *Medical Times and Gazette,* Dec. 6, 1873, pp. 630–632.

"Cabildo Archives, French Period," *Louisiana Historical Quarterly,* Vol. III (1920), pp. 555–556. (By permission of *Louisiana Historical Quarterly.*)

Catholic World, April, 1880, pp. 55–63.

Cobbe, Frances Power. "Workhouse Sketches," *Macmillan's Magazine,* Vol. III (November, 1860–April, 1861), pp. 448–461.

Cruzat, Heloise Hulse. "The Ursulines of Louisiana," *Louisiana Historical Quarterly,* Vol. II, No. 1 (January, 1919), pp. 5–23. (By permission of *Louisiana Historical Quarterly.*)

Disselhoff, D. "The Deaconesses of Kaiserswerth: A Hundred Years' Work," *International Nursing Review,* Vol. IX, Nos. 1–4 (1934), pp. 19–28. (By permission of International Council of Nurses.)

"Editorial," *Medical and Surgical Reporter,* Nov. 8, 1862, p. 160.

"Female Nurses in Military Hospitals," *American Medical Times,* July 18, 1861, pp. 25–26, 30.

[Gooch, Robert]. "Protestant Sisters of Charity," *Blackwood's Edinburgh Magazine,* July–December, 1825, pp. 732–735.

[————]. *London Medical Gazette,* 1827, pp. 55–58.

Hart, Ernest. *Fortnightly Review,* April, 1866.

Howson, J. S. "Deaconesses; or the Official Help of Women in Parochial Work and in Charitable Institutions," *Quarterly Review,* September, 1860, pp. 342–387.

Hume, Edgar Erskine. "El Hospital de Jesus Nazareno de la Ciudad de México, fundado en 1524, es al más antiquo de America y Presta Todavia sus Servicios," *Gaceta Medica de México,* Vol. LVIII, Suppl. No. 4 (August, 1938), p. 10. (By permission of Academia Nacional de Medicina de México.)

————. "Medical Work of the Knights Hospitallers of St. John of Jerusalem," *Bulletin of the Institute of the History of Medicine,* May, June, July, 1938, pp. 399–468, 495–613, 677–819.

"Lady Nurses," *Godey's Lady's Book and Magazine,* Vol. LXXXII (January–June, 1871), pp. 188–189.

"Letter to the Editor of the *London Times,*" *London Times,* Apr. 15, 1857.

London Times, June 1, 1860.

"Miss Nightingale," *Illustrated London News,* Feb. 24, 1855, p. 175.

Nasatir, A. P. "Royal Hospitals in Colonial Spanish America," *Annals of Medical History,* November, 1942, pp. 481–503. (By permission of Paul B. Hoeber, Inc., and *Annals of Medical History.*)

[Nightingale, Florence]. "A Note on Pauperism," *Fraser's Magazine,* March, 1869, pp. 281–290.

Bibliography

————. "The Reform of Sick Nursing and the Late Mrs. Wardroper, The Extinction of Mrs. Gamp," *British Medical Journal*, Dec. 31, 1892, p. 1448.

————. "Sick-Nursing and Health-Nursing," *Woman's Mission: A Series of Congress Papers on the Philanthropic Work of Women*, pp. 184–198.

[————.] "Una and the Lion," *Good Words*, June 1, 1868, pp. 360–366.

"The Nightingale Fund," *The Lancet*, June 22, 1872, pp. 873–874.

"The Nightingale's Song to the Sick Soldier," *Punch*, Vol. XXVII (1854), p. 184.

"The Nurses for the East," *Illustrated London News*, Nov. 4, 1854, pp. 447–448.

O'Connor, Stella. "Charity Hospital of Louisiana at New Orleans: An administrative and Financial History, 1736–1941," *Louisiana Historical Quarterly*, Vol. XXXI (1948), pp. 1–109.

Ogle, John W. "Nurses for the Sick Poor," *Medical Times and Gazette*, Apr. 11, 1874, pp. 395–396.

"On the Early History and Modern Revival of Deaconesses," *Church Quarterly Review*, Vol. xlvii (1899), pp. 302–341.

Pall Mall Gazette, 1866.

"Pay of Female Nurses," *Medical and Surgical Reporter*, Sept. 10, 1864, p. 32.

"Report of the Commissioners on Metropolitan Infirmaries," *The Lancet*, July 1, 15, 29; Aug. 12, 26; Nov. 18, 1865; Nov. 4, 11, 1871, pp. 25–26, 45–49, 66–68, 69, 80, 88, 129, 172.

"Report of Committee on the Training of Nurses," *Transactions of the American Medical Association*, 1869, pp. 161–174. (By permission of the *Journal of the American Medical Association*.)

"Report of the Lancet Sanitary Commission on Night Nursing in the London Hospitals," *The Lancet*, Nov. 4, 1872, pp. 642–680.

Richards, Laura E. "Letters of Florence Nightingale," *Yale Review*, Winter, 1935, pp. 326–347. (By permission of *The Yale Review*, copyright Yale University Press.)

Sarma, P. J. "Hindu Medicine and Its Antiquity," *Annals of Medical History*, May, 1931, pp. 318–324.

"Sick Wards in Workhouses," *Saturday Review*, June 30, 1866, p. 780.

"The Sick in the Workhouse," *Saturday Review*, Mar. 10, 1866, pp. 294–295.

"Sidelights on Louisiana History," *Louisiana Historical Quarterly*, Vol. I, No. 3 (1917–1919), p. 110. (By permission of *Louisiana Historical Quarterly*.)

Sigerist, Henry E. "The Need for an Institute of the History of Medicine in India," *Bulletin of the History of Medicine*, February, 1945, pp. 113–116. (By permission of the *Bulletin of the History of Medicine*.)

"Sisterhoods in England," *Saturday Review*, Aug. 25, 1866, p. 233.

"Text of William Shippen's First Draft of a Plan for the Organization of the Military Hospital During the Revolution," *Annals of Medical History*,

Vol. I, No. 2 (Summer, 1917), pp. 174–176. (By permission of Paul B. Hoeber, Inc., and the *Annals of Medical History*.)

"Two Noble Women," *Harper's Weekly,* June 6, 1857, p. 353.

Weigall, Rachel. "An Elizabethan Lady," *Quarterly Review,* July, 1911, pp. 119–138. (By permission of John Murray [Publishers] Ltd.)

[Whitman, Walt]. *New York Leader,* Mar. 15, 22, 29; Apr. 12, 19; May 3, 17, 1862.

[———]. *New York Times,* Feb. 26, 1863; Dec. 11, 1864.

"Who is Mrs. Nightingale?" *London Times,* Oct. 30, 1854.

Index

An asterisk (*) preceding an item in the index refers to a numbered reading in the text. The number of the reading is given in *italics*.

Index

Index

475